SUDDEN DEATH: MEDICINE AND RELIGION IN EIGHTEENTH-CENTURY ROME

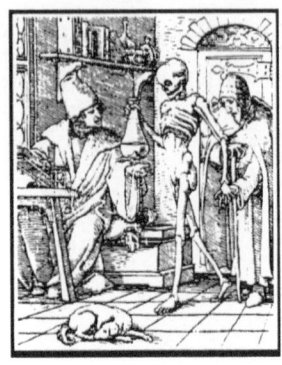

The History of Medicine in Context

Series Editors: Andrew Cunningham and Ole Peter Grell

Department of History and Philosophy of Science
University of Cambridge

Department of History
Open University

Sudden Death: Medicine and Religion in Eighteenth-Century Rome

MARIA PIA DONATO

C.N.R.S. Institut d'Histoire Moderne et Contemporaine, Paris, France and University of Cagliari, Italy

Translated by Valentina Mazzei

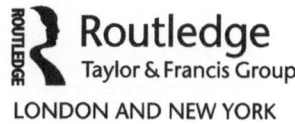

Routledge
Taylor & Francis Group

LONDON AND NEW YORK

First published in paperback 2024

First published 2010 by Ashgate Publishing

Published 2016
by Routledge
4 Park Square, Milton Park, Abingdon, Oxon OX14 4RN

and by Routledge
605 Third Avenue, New York, NY 10158

Routledge is an imprint of the Taylor & Francis Group, an informa business

British Library Cataloguing in Publication Data
A catalogue record for this book is available from the British Library

The Library of Congress has cataloged the printed edition as follows:
Donato, Maria Pia.
  [Morti improvvise. English]
  Sudden death : medicine and religion in eighteenth-century Rome / by Maria Pia Donato.
    pages cm. – (The history of medicine in context)
  Revised translation of: Morti improvvise / Maria Pia Donato. Roma : Carocci, c2010.
  Includes bibliographical references and index.
  ISBN 978-1-4724-1873-9 (hardcover)
  1. Sudden death–History–18th century. 2.
  Death–Religious aspects–Catholic Church–History of doctrines–18th century. 3.
  Medicine–Religious aspects–History–18th century. 4. Medicine–Italy–Rome–
  History–18th century. 5. Lancisi, Giovanni Maria, 1654-1720. De subitaneis mortibus. I. Title.
  RB150.S84D6613 2014
  618.92'026–dc23
                                                                    2014012045

  ISBN: 978-1-4724-1873-9 (hbk)
  ISBN: 978-1-03-292590-5 (pbk)
  ISBN: 978-1-315-61127-3 (ebk)

DOI: 10.4324/9781315611273

Contents

Acknowledgements

I have contracted many debts of gratitude in the course of research for this book, which I am now glad to pay back. First of all, I thank Massimo Bucciantini, who gave me the idea for this volume during a joint seminar in early modern history and history of science at the University of Cagliari in 2007. I also would like to thank Michele Camerota, the best scholar, colleague and friend I have had the pleasure to work with at the University of Cagliari.

Alessandro Pastore, Biagio Salvemini, Marcello Verga and Maria Antonietta Visceglia read the final draft and gave me valuable suggestions, for which I am grateful. I am indebted to the many scholars and friends who offered advice and help: Federico Barbierato and Erminia Irace first of all, Elisa Andretta, David Armando, Elena Brambilla, Marina Caffiero, Giovanna Capitelli, Massimo Cattaneo, Sandra Cavallo, Harold J. Cook, Filippo de Vivo, Guido Giglioni, Ottavia Niccoli, Marilyn Nicoud, Domenico Rocciolo. My gratitude also goes to Bradford Bouley, Jill Kraye, Robert Sayre and Tessa Storey for their invaluable help with the English translation.

I would like to thank, in addition, colleagues and friends at the Warburg Institute and the former Wellcome Trust Centre for the History of Medicine at UCL in London for assisting me with their knowledge and kindness over the years, especially Anita Pollard and Natalie Clarke. The Wellcome Library for the History and Understanding of Medicine proved an invaluable resource, and I am grateful to the Library staff. I would also like to thank the Organisers Committee of the History of Pre-modern Medicine seminars at the Wellcome Library for inviting me to discuss my research in March 2014. The research for this book has benefited from the support of several institutions – the University of Cagliari, the University of Milan, École française de Rome – which all deserve a mention. I am, moreover, grateful to Andrew Cunningham and Ole P. Grell for agreeing to publish the English translation in the 'History of Medicine in Context' series, which they edit, to Emily Yates, of Ashgate, who supervised the publication, and to Tricia Craggs and Lindsey Brake for their help with the copy-editing. Finally, as always, I wish to thank my family and, especially, Luc Berlivet, if only for the happy days we spent in the libraries of London, Paris and Rome and for all the cups of coffee (a great cephalic, as Lancisi and Baglivi would have said) he made me.

Abbreviations and Translator's Notes

ACDF	Archive of the Congregation for the Doctrine of the Faith, Vatican City
ASR	Archivio di Stato, Rome
ASV	Archivio Segreto Vaticano
ASVR	Archivio Storico del Vicariato, Rome
BLR	Biblioteca Lancisiana, Rome
BNF	Bibliothèque Nationale de France, Paris
BNR	Biblioteca Nazionale Vittorio Emanuele II, Rome
DBI	*Dizionario biografico degli italiani*, Rome, 1961–
Diario di Clemente XI	Ms ASV, Archivio Borghese I 578, *Diario del pontificato di Clemente XI*
SM	G.M. Lancisi, *De subitaneis mortibus*, Rome, 1707
Valesio	F. Valesio, *Diario di Roma*, ed. G. Scano, Milan 1977–79
VL	Vatican Library

Translations are the translator's unless stated otherwise.

Quotations from Lancisi's *De subitaneis mortibus* refer to the first Roman edition of 1707 by Buagni. A modern English translation of the book is also available, namely *Translation of De subitaneis mortibus (On Sudden Death)*, trans. P.D. White and A.V. Boursy, New York, 1971.

Introduction

In 1705 and 1706, an 'epidemic' of sudden deaths terrorised the city of Rome. Romans were already exhausted by war, economic difficulties and natural calamities. People of all ages and social conditions died without any apparent cause or recognisable symptoms, so unexpectedly as to have no time to make their last repentance, thus endangering their spiritual salvation. Fear spread like wild fire. While doctors puzzled over the nature of the ailment, Pope Clement XI ordered the civic health authorities to launch a public investigation and perform autopsies on the dead. The medical inquiry lasted from January to March 1706 and was the first of its kind to be performed in a European city. Furthermore, it resulted, the following year, in the publication of the important treatise *De subitaneis mortibus* (*On sudden death*) by the papal physician Giovanni Maria Lancisi, one of the earliest modern scientific investigations into death.

With the 1706 investigation and Lancisi's book, death became a political instrument enabling physicians to establish their authority and serving a variety of other purposes: confronting health emergencies, developing scientific knowledge, and understanding and containing illness and mortality. This new approach to death separates modern medicine from the Hippocratic and Galenic tradition. Moreover, the events that occurred in Rome marked a change in the attitude of physicians towards the dying. In an attempt to cope with something as terrifying as unexpected death, medical practitioners adopted an interventionist stance, the outcome of which, in the long term, was the birth of emergency medicine. Although real progress in resuscitation techniques did not occur until the nineteenth century, the change of attitude dates back a century earlier to the sudden death 'epidemics' in papal Rome.

Investigating sudden death as a medical, legal and religious issue, this book shows how medicine broke free from the Hippocratic tradition, which regarded death as the obvious limit of the physician's capacity, and how death became a proper object of scientific discourse and action, paving the way for the development of methods of control over the following three centuries.

Today, the material and symbolic management of death is no longer confined to religion. In modern industrial societies, death is mainly entrusted to medicine from the outset, so that it can be delayed by means of treatments (including transplants and cardio-pulmonary resuscitation (CPR)) and health and demographic surveillance systems, so that its progress can be made painless and dignified, and so that afterwards it can be defined, ascertained and explained, especially when it occurs in suspicious circumstances. It is true that in recent times many aspects of the modern medicalisation of death have been questioned in Western countries in light of a variety of political, ethical and religious issues. A revision of the definition and treatment of death is being demanded from a religious or philosophical perspective, though with contrasting arguments and diverging, even opposing, aims. The power and knowledge of medicine over death has been challenged by those who demand that individuals should be empowered with respect to the end of their lives or, conversely, by those who wish to subject them to the laws of the state or the Church.

Sudden death, perceived for hundreds of years as the ultimate threat to body and soul, encapsulates the contradictions of the modern medicalisation of dying. In theory, it comes close to the widespread wish for a quick, painless demise.[1] But things are very different in reality. Sudden deaths – whether from work-related accidents, road accidents, brain or cardiovascular incidents, or unexpectedly swift complications of known pathological conditions – are nowadays completely medicalised, sometimes against the will of the (often unconscious) sufferer, and emergency medical interventions expose the dying to the risk of having to survive artificially with the aid of machines. In everyday practice, sudden death is overloaded with extremely sensitive ethical and deontological issues. Emergency resuscitation (in itself a problematic procedure, which is sometimes performed on those who have explicitly expressed a desire not to undergo it) cannot always restore the superior cerebral activity needed for social interaction and other autonomous vital functions in the patient. What is the status of someone in this position? Are they dead or alive? When can organs be donated? It is well known that in the late 1960s, in connection with organ transplantation, the definition and diagnosis of death shifted from a traditional cardiovascular to a cerebral criterion. A brain-based criterion, however, has also proven elusive.[2] In other

---

[1]   S. Timmermans, *Sudden Death and the Myth of CPR*, Philadelphia, 1999. The modern vision of sudden death as preferable to a long agony in hospital is discussed in P. Ariès, *Western Attitudes Toward Death: From the Middle Ages to the Present*, trans. P.M. Ranum, Baltimore and London, 1974. However, B.G. Glaser and A.L. Strauss, *Time for Dying*, Chicago, 1968, demonstrates that both doctors and nurses react negatively to the unexpected death of patients in hospitals.

[2]   The cerebral criterion, soon after its definition by the Harvard Committee in 1968, drawing on medical research on brain localisation and specialisation, was – and still is – the object of heated debate and conflicting judicial decisions based on the distinction between the encephalic trunk, the brain and the cortex. See, among a vast and growing literature, D. Lamb, *Death, Brain Death, and Ethics*, London, 1985; R.M. Zaner, ed., *Death: Beyond Whole-Brain Criteria*, Dordrecht, 1988; S.J. Youngner, R.M. Arnold and R. Schapiro, eds, *The Definition of Death: Contemporary Controversies*, Baltimore and London, 1999; F.P. de Ceglia, ed., *Storia della definizione di morte*, Milan, 2014. For awareness of the persisting perplexities concerning the definition of death and the 'grey area' between life and death, see

words, new concerns about dying with dignity have not replaced older fears of being abandoned while still alive.[3] Moreover, though in most cases CPR fails to achieve its declared aim of bringing the victim of a sudden crisis back to life, medicine draws tremendous social and cultural legitimation from the myth of resuscitation, which it is not eager to renounce.

With contemporary medicine constantly pushing the limits of death towards technological criteria,[4] and in a society accustomed to the medical management of death (and ready to criticise medicine when it fails to do so), sudden death seems tragically unnatural. It is, at the least, ambiguous. And indeed, the authority of medical-legal experts is still closely connected to unexpected death. In modern Western society, 20 per cent of deaths every year occur without warning, out of their 'natural' time and place. All these deaths need to be explained and made acceptable.[5] Today, as in the past, forensic medicine serves this purpose. Among other things, it preserves the value of morbid anatomy by resorting to autopsy, a practice that historically marked the beginnings of the modern science of the body, though it is now largely replaced by contemporary methods of clinical investigation and medical imaging.[6]

It needs to be emphasised that the 'taming of death' by means of medicine, as examined in this book, does not encompass the dramatically successful cures which, starting from the late eighteenth century, progressively and exponentially reduced mortality in the Western world. Death began to be controlled before the onset of these new healing methods; the shift was mainly ideological and epistemic in nature, though it profoundly affected the social and professional authority of physicians. It consisted, above all, in the investigation of normal and pathological processes starting from corpses (no longer used exclusively to study the structure of healthy human bodies, as in Renaissance anatomy),[7] and laid claim to areas and topics of knowledge and action that were once the preserve of

---

G. Agamben, *Homo Sacer: Sovereign Power and Bare Life*, trans. D. Heller-Roazen, Stanford, 1998, largely inspired by Foucault; from a Christian stance, see J.P. Bishop, *The Anticipatory Corpse: Medicine, Power, and the Care of the Dying*, Notre Dame, IN, 2011.

3   M.S. Pernik, 'Brain Death in a Cultural Context: The Reconstruction of Death, 1967–1981', in *The Definition of Death*, ed. Youngner et al., pp. 3–33; J. Bourke, *Fear: A Cultural History*, London, 2005.

4   W.R. Albury, 'Ideas of Life and Death', in *Companion Encyclopedia of the History of Medicine*, ed. W.F. Bynum and R. Porter, London, 1993, vol. 1, pp. 249–80.

5   S. Timmermans, *Postmortem: How Medical Examiners Explain Suspicious Deaths*, Chicago, 2006.

6   L.S. King and M.C. Meehan, 'A History of Autopsy', *American Journal of Pathology*, 73, 1973, pp. 514–44.

7   Initially, normal anatomy was regarded as a branch of *medicina theorica* and natural history, a 'useless' (that is, devoid of strictly practical aims) form of knowledge, full of moral and religious implications; see R.K. French, *Dissection and Vivisection in the European*

religious and political authorities. According to Michel Foucault, the epistemic inclusion of death in eighteenth-century medical experience allowed medicine to take the first hesitant steps away from the ancient Hippocratic-Galenic tradition, which had viewed death as the obvious and insurmountable limit of the relationship of *pietas* between doctor and patient; it enabled physicians to develop a new scientific discourse and affirm their power/knowledge over life.[8]

Several different circumstances were necessary for the first steps in that direction to be taken, and this is precisely what happened in Lancisi's Rome. In the first place, there was the dreadful nature of the sudden deaths and the widespread alarm they caused among both the populace and the social elite. Second, there was Roman medicine's long-standing excellence in normal and pathological anatomy and the vitality of local scientific institutions (often disregarded by history of science).[9] Rome was thus able to draw on the intellectual resources offered by mechanical philosophy and Galilean science to develop a new understanding of life and death, as is evident in Lancisi's treatise *On Sudden Death*. Finally, there were special political and religious circumstances: on the one hand, the distinctive features of the papal monarchy and the specific notion of 'good rule' (*buon governo*) within the ecclesiastical government of the Papal States,[10] as well as the popes' patronage of science; on the other hand, the events that took place during the pontificate of Clement XI. His ambitious international policies, including intervention in the War of the Spanish Succession, produced great economic and political difficulties for the Papal States and for the Apostolic See, leading to the failure of his reform programme. The evolution of Catholic theology and of religious sensibilities at the end of the seventeenth century, together with the prevalence of rigorism, are also essential for understanding both the fear aroused by sudden death and the attitude of the Church authorities, who were not willing to make allowances for a supernatural interpretation of the events and therefore favoured a different solution to the health crisis.[11]

Renaissance, Aldershot, 1999; A.R. Mandressi, *Le regard de l'anatomiste: dissections et invention du corps en Occident*, Paris, 2003.

   [8]   M. Foucault, *The Birth of the Clinic: An Archaeology of Medical Perception*, trans. A.M. Sheridan Smith, London, 1973 (originally published in 1963).

   [9]   For innovative recent studies on science in early modern Rome, see A. Romano, 'La science moderne, ses enjeux, ses pratiques et ses résultats en contexte catholique: réflexions romaines', in *Rome et la science moderne: entre Renaissance et Lumières*, ed. A. Romano, Rome, 2008, pp. 3–44. See also M.P. Donato and J. Kraye, eds, *Conflicting Duties: Science, Medicine and Religion in Rome 1550–1750*, London, 2009.

   [10]   P. Prodi, *The Papal Prince. One Body and Two Souls: The Papal Monarchy in Early Modern Europe*, trans. S. Haskins, Cambridge, 1987.

   [11]   G. Signorotto, *Inquisitori e mistici nel Seicento italiano: l'eresia di Santa Pelagia*, Bologna, 1989; E. Brambilla, *Corpi invasi e viaggi dell'anima: santità, possessione, esorcismo*

It is significant that the events narrated in this book occurred in early eighteenth-century papal Rome, the centre of a troubled Catholicism in search of reform. Acting neither in contradiction to nor in competition with religion, medicine dealt with death at the specific request of ecclesiastical authorities. The Church established the limits of the medical investigation and also the hierarchy of values, which might be reassessed but not subverted. It was in these precise historical circumstances that doctors were permitted to venture into the territory of death under the aegis of religious authority. The consequences, however, were far-reaching, and later in the eighteenth century, in the age of Enlightenment and reform, medicine would begin to challenge religion and gradually take over its supreme position with regard to death.

The aim of this book is to explore an early episode in the long (and uneven) history of how physicians gained control over death. The 1706 investigation into the causes of the spate of sudden deaths that terrorised Rome, together with Lancisi's treatise *On Sudden Death*, laid the first conceptual, ideological and technical foundations of the medicalisation of death that we still experience in our times.

Notwithstanding the resonance of this topic with today's public debates, the differences between the past and the present cannot – and must not – be played down. How can the present situation be compared to the early eighteenth century, with its collegiate organisation of medicine, limited medicalisation of society, subordination of science to religion, restricted scope of medical intervention and eclectic medical culture, which, while aspiring to establish a new science of the body, had not yet emerged from the shadow of the ancients? Unlike specialists of different disciplines who have retraced past events in order to shed light on the most burning contemporary issues,[12] the historian studies past events in themselves, exploring change regardless of the direction it eventually took.

Also, although this book is about death, it is not directly derived, in terms of method, from the work of those historians of mentality who in the 1970s made death into a full-fledged historical topic (Philippe Ariès, Michel Vovelle and others). At that time, many of the human sciences began to engage with this topic, thrilled by the changes in the social organisation of death and the new medical-technical opportunities to manipulate it (the first heart transplant was

---

dalla teologia barocca alla medicina illuminista, Rome, 2010.

[12]   See, for instance, C.A. Defanti, *Soglie: medicina e fine della vita*, Turin, 2007. Defanti is an Italian neurologist and an expert in intensive care, who was involved in the tragic and hotly debated case of Eluana Englaro, a young woman who remained in a permanent vegetative state for 17 years before her family could obtain the legal right to suspend artificial nutrition and hydration in 2009; see also D. Steila, *Vita/morte*, Bologna, 2009. For a criticism of presentism in the use of history in medico-ethical debates, see Pernik, 'Brain Death in a Cultural Context'.

performed in 1967);[13] today thanatology is still a major area of research.[14] The focus of this book is different. Admittedly, one of the issues it treats is how, at the beginning of the eighteenth century, a city perceived sudden death and reacted to its threats, how fear was socially constructed and how solutions were devised by resorting to different belief systems (medicine and religion). Nevertheless, my main topic is the role of medicine in society, and I focus on a particular time and place – Rome under Clement XI – in order to understand how different levels of reality and various figures interacted with each other and to offer a reconstruction of the circumstances, the motives and the resources that brought about scientific and cultural innovation.

As is well known, the revisionism that cultural history, along with the history of science, has undergone for several decades now demands that ideas, including scientific ones, should be firmly connected to the social context in which they were first expressed. This book sets out to explore a creative process and to put it into its historical context. My 'externalist' focus on a precise time and place does not, however, exclude a finely-grained 'internalist' analysis of scientific and medical works. Far from it. My aim is not only to identify the intellectual, social and political conditions that gave rise to these writings – including those held in little esteem by the history of medicine and science – but also to evaluate them against the background of broader long-term cultural phenomena such as Galenism, Galilean science and Counter-Reformation Catholicism.

Specific contexts produce specific types of knowledge and styles of thought.[15] Indeed, I am convinced that only an 'ecological' approach to a precise historical

---

[13]   Sociology got there before history, with classic works such as E. Morin, *L'homme et la mort dans l'histoire*, Paris, 1951; G. Gorer, *The Pornography of Death* (1955), now in G. Gorer, *Death, Grief and Mourning*, Garden City, NY, 1965, pp. 192–9; J. Mitford, *The American Way of Death*, New York, 1963. In the 1970s, the experts from various disciplines who became interested in death shared the more or less explicit assumption that modern Western society had removed death from public life and thus made it 'obscene', and that criticism of such concealment was therefore necessary; see J.-D. Urbain, 'Morte', in *Enciclopedia*, vol. 9, Turin, 1980, pp. 519–55. My own research starts from a different premise, inspired by the work of Foucault: in modern society, regardless of the individual experience of dying, death has been made the object of science, from which we derive ways of knowing, institutions and policies. See also L. Prior, *The Social Organisation of Death: Medical Discourse and Social Practices in Belfast*, Basingstoke and London, 1989.

[14]   M. Sozzi, *Reinventare la morte: introduzione alla tanatologia*, Rome and Bari, 2009; for a critical overview of recent studies in the Catholic context, see A. Prosperi, 'Il volto della Gorgone: studi e ricerche sul senso della morte e sulla disciplina delle sepolture tra Medioevo ed età moderna', and M.A. Visceglia, 'Conclusione', in *La morte e i suoi riti in Italia tra medioevo e prima età moderna*, ed. F. Salvestrini, G.M. Varanini and A. Zangarini, Florence, 2007, pp. 3–29 and 483–96.

[15]   L. Fleck, *Genesis and Development of a Scientific Fact*, ed. T.J. Trenn and R.K. Merton, trans. F. Bradley and T.J. Trenn, Chicago, 1981. Furthermore, by focusing on the interactions

context can explain two essential points of the story narrated in this book: the particular period in which it took place and the religious origin of the changing attitude towards the end of life. There is a broad consensus among historians that the eighteenth century witnessed a profound alteration in the collective stance on life, health and death, and that the middle of the century saw the birth of a new scientific discourse on death, along with a political and philanthropic willingness to have a positive impact on people's lives. Secularisation and the rejection of fatalism are commonly regarded as the main features of the changing attitude towards death, in general,[16] and sudden death, in particular, which ceased to be regarded as divine punishment and *mala mors*. In this study, I argue that the shift of the physicians' approach to death occurred earlier than is generally thought and that the facts surrounding the spate of sudden deaths in eighteenth-century Rome represented the initial break with tradition. This was the first time that the obligation of physicians to intervene at the end of life had been formulated, altering the attitude that had guided them for thousands of years in treating dying patients. Interestingly, though, the roots of this change are to be found in religion as much as in medicine. The new stance is connected to a shift in Catholic theology and piety and the rise of rigorism in the late seventeenth and early eighteenth centuries; these factors partially explain why the 'revolution of death' began in papal Rome.

In what follows I shall investigate sudden death as a public health issue, as a scientific question and as a moral and theological problem. The book is divided into three parts, which correspond to distinct perspectives: that of the town, of medical learning and of the Roman Catholic Church. Each of these entails focusing on specific sources and on periodisation, and, over the course of the book, the reader will be taken from Rome under Clement XI to Enlightenment Europe.

Part I deals with the reactions to sudden deaths in Rome in the winter of 1705 and 1706. Chapter 1 narrates the first attempts to explain the causes of the sudden deaths. The initial response from the civil and ecclesiastical authorities was to resort to religion and to attribute the tragic events to divine wrath. This allowed them not only to control fear, but also to impose social discipline on Roman society and consolidate their hold on religious life and customs. Meanwhile, a lively medical debate arose as to the causes of these incidents and the best remedies. The pope ordered his personal physician, Giovanni Maria Lancisi, and the civic medical authorities to perform a series of dissections in the university anatomical theatre in order to discover the 'true causes' of

---

between a context, a scientific community and a style of thought, in the wake of Fleck, it is possible to avoid a cumulative and linear history of science: styles of thought are, in fact, unstable because the conceptual elements change when placed in different configurations.

[16] D. Hervieu-Léger, 'Mourir en modernité', in *Qu'est-ce que mourir*, ed. J.-C. Ameisen, D. Hervieu-Léger and E. Hirsch, Paris, 2003, pp. 87–105.

the deadly events. Autopsies enabled the *protomedicus* (First Physician) and the papal physician to rule out any significant risks to the population and to restore public confidence. The crisis, consequently, became a success both for the pope and for the medical officials. Chapter 2 delves into the intellectual and institutional circumstances behind the use of this modern research tool and examines those who were involved in it. Chapter 3 traces the follow-ups to the 1706 investigation and shows how afterwards the College of Physicians in Rome and the medical profession as a whole took a more active role in public life. The successful management of that emergency resulted in the integration of health and medical issues in the policies of the early eighteenth-century papacy. This process was helped by the positive reassessment of the authority of physicians, building on the empirical foundations provided by autopsies; in the health emergencies that followed, pathological anatomy – that is, the anatomy of diseased organs and tissues – became an essential argument for giving a larger and wider scope to medicine.

The second part of the book is devoted to the history of medicine as a science. Chapter 4 examines how sudden death and death, in general, were interpreted in both ancient and early modern Galenic medicine and how Lancisi revised the entire issue in light of the mechanical physiology of his day in the treatise *On Sudden Death*. One of the main features of Lancisi's work is the importance assigned to pathological anatomy as a method for investigating death and understanding life. Chapter 5 analyses the epistemic foundations and practical consequences of Lancisi's method of observing lesions detected on the dissecting table in order to get back to the pathological process that produced them and also, to some extent, to guide diagnosis. In the scholarly literature, this method is usually associated with G.B. Morgagni's *De sedibus et causis morborum per anatomen indagatis* (*On the seats and causes of diseases as investigated by anatomy*, 1761) and the School of Paris in Revolutionary France. I argue that the customary view that the systematic employment of human dissection for pathology dates to the late eighteenth century should be revised. However, the distinctiveness of early eighteenth-century medical culture should not be seen solely from a theological perspective. A close analysis of Lancisi's treatise reveals the specific features of the early anatomo-pathological method, while the works of his contemporaries show that, in the same period and within the same professional community, different notions of illness and different uses of corpses coexisted.

Part III deals with the ethical and religious implications of sudden death. Where is the line that separates life and death located? What should the physician do when confronting death? What roles are played by medicine and by religion in dealing with those who are dying? Chapter 6 presents a comparison between medical and religious literature on the physician's responsibilities towards the dying. Traditionally, despite differences on several key points, medical and ecclesiastical authors had generally agreed that physicians should not attempt to treat the dying. This attitude began to change, however, at the beginning of the eighteenth century; here, too, the events in Rome and Lancisi's book marked a turning point. In order to explain why this change occurred in papal Rome, Chapter 7 delves into contemporary theological debates, showing how the rigorist emphasis in the moral theology of the Catholic Church during the second half of the seventeenth century increased popular fears concerning the salvation of an individual who died suddenly, which paved the way for a new and more active role for medicine. The crisis of Baroque piety thus led to two apparently conflicting phenomena: on the one hand, it strengthened the fear surrounding sudden death; on the other hand, it empowered contemporary natural philosophy to deal with it. In this way, a new alliance of science and faith was forged, in which religion was defended from the sceptics and libertines and cleansed of the taint of undisciplined devotion. This did not, however, preclude the need for a religious response to the fears associated with sudden death. As demonstrated in Chapter 8, the papacy responded by setting in motion the canonisation of Andrea Avellino, a cleric of the Theatine congregation. A personification of the heroic virtues for which the Church stood, Avellino had died of apoplexy, and the miracles he was credited with also made him the ideal protector of devout Catholics terrified by the prospect of sudden death.

The three parts of the book work together to portray how an early modern society coped with the most frightening of events and how the boundaries between medicine and religion were redrawn, when death ceased to be regarded as beyond the realm of scientific investigation.

PART I
Sudden Death and the Physician's Role in Society

Chapter 1

Fears

Prologue: A Mysterious Chain of 'Accidents'

On Thursday 17 December 1705, the learned antiquarian Francesco Valesio noted in his diary the strange case of a 'certain greengrocer in Piazza Navona who was stricken by apoplexy while walking out of a tavern and fell immediately dead'.[1]

Similar cases had been reported since the previous spring.[2] Then, over the summer and the autumn, there had been reports of 'sudden deaths and apoplectic accidents and most serious ailments'.[3] The first isolated episodes took an alarming turn when, on 9 January 1706, two more victims of sudden death where discovered, an innkeeper and a greengrocer near the Chiesa dell'Anima, and only three days later 'a poor woman who died unexpectedly in her bed was found in the S. Urbano alley'.[4] The following week another chronicler noted that 'many people died of apoplexy'.[5]

Sudden death was dreaded by any Christian. It was considered as shameful and despicable as violent death.[6] An invocation to ward it off could be found in any prayer book, and litanies to the saints pleaded for protection *a subitanea et improvisa morte*.[7] Especially daunting since it threatened the salvation of the soul, sudden death was also dangerous for the corpse, as it might be withheld from consecrated land, as happened to an unfortunate prostitute who died 'after

---

[1]   Valesio, vol. 3, p. 513.

[2]   Ibid., vol. 3, p. 335, on the death of a bookkeeper 'struck by an apoplectic accident'; p. 375, on the death of a fiscal of the Senatorial tribunal; p. 414, on two other inexplicable deaths. News on similar accidents had already been reported in *Diario di Clemente XI*, November 1703, fols 181v–182r.

[3]   *Diario di Clemente XI*, fol. 215, 7 October 1705, reports the case of a 'curialist [who] died of an apoplectic accident while he was presenting a case'. Valesio, vol. 3, p. 388, 16 May 1705, notes that 'a certain greengrocer died suddenly while he was drinking merrily at the Leoncino inn, and a woman in Monti passed to the other life in a similar way; and many have been struck with apoplectic accidents this week'.

[4]   Valesio, vol. 3, p. 535.

[5]   *Diario di Clemente XI*, fol. 223.

[6]   P. Ariès, *The Hour of Our Death*, trans. H. Weaver, London, 1981, pp. 12–13.

[7]   *Rituale Romanum Pauli V P.M. iussu editum*, Rome, 1615, p. 70.

dining merrily ... and since she passed away without repenting, her corpse was buried outside the city walls'.[8]

The chain of deaths continued incessantly. Valesio noted in his diary 18 cases in the period from January to March 1706: a poor woman 'walking out of the Traspontina Church' and a 'wretched, crippled beggar', and then peasants, craftsmen, 'Messina the Jesuit priest', servants and prelates. The death of the young footman of the Marquis Spada, who passed away 'sitting by the fire in the home of a prostitute',[9] seemed to embody the *exempla* that for centuries had admonished Christians to avoid all opportunities for sin where the end might catch them by surprise: dances, games and houses of ill repute. Fear quickly spread throughout Rome. What was happening? The horrific spectacle of the contorted bodies in the city streets turned these events into a public calamity. The demise of a servant of Cardinal Sacripanti who, 'while serving his master at the door of the carriage on his return to St. Peter's ... fell suddenly dead, to the utter dismay of the cardinal who ordered that the carriage be stopped immediately and assistance given to bring him back to life, all in vain', caused enough sensation to be reported in the *avvisi* dispatched to all parts of Italy from the papal city.[10]

People had been living in fear for years. The seventeenth century had ended in a difficult and uncertain situation for the temporal and spiritual power of the papacy, beset by famine, adverse weather conditions and poverty, against a backdrop of war and pestilence. With the new century, a succession of calamities struck with such violence and was accompanied by signs so sinister as to herald even more desolation.

The War of the Spanish Succession threatened the territorial integrity of the Papal States. The politics of neutrality of the Apostolic See – 'a dangerous resolution for a weak party', as the famous scholar and annalist Ludovico Antonio

---

[8]   Valesio, vol. 3, p. 566. As stated in the *Rituale romanum*, jews, infidels, heretics, schismatics, the excommunicated and manifest sinners (including those who committed suicide, although it was difficult to ascertain their fault, especially for persons drowned in rivers) were excluded from consecrated burial. On the burial area outside the city walls at Porta Flaminia, also called Muro Malo, see A. Menniti Ippolito, 'Il "vecchio recinto" del Testaccio: agli inizi della sepoltura degli acattolici in Roma', in *The Protestant Cemetery in Rome: The 'Parte Antica'*, ed. A. Menniti Ippolito and P. Vian, Rome, 1989, pp. 15–90. On the threat of sudden death to convert prostitutes, see T. Storey, *Carnal Commerce in Counter-Reformation Rome*, Cambridge, 2008, pp. 47–50.

[9]   Valesio, vol. 3, pp. 542–3, 549.

[10]   Ms BNR, Vittorio Emanuele 790, fol. 115, 23 January 1706: 'several apoplectic accidents causing the sudden death of several persons befell on Sunday, among whom the footman to Cardinal Sacripanti while he was attending to the carriage of His Eminence, who stepped out of the carriage to help him, but too late since he was dead'. Further accounts of apoplectic accidents in Rome are reported in the *Gazzetta di Bologna*, 9 March and 12 April 1706.

Muratori would say – immediately revealed its weakness. Rome, the centre of diplomacy of the Catholic world, turned into the theatre of an unprecedented struggle. Fights, scuffles and brawls involving the opposing factions were frequent, and the fabricated news of an attempt to kidnap the pope's nephew made the situation so tense as to appear out of control.[11] An actual uprising broke out in September 1701, provoked by the intrigues of Cavalier della Macchia, whereby 'the city looked as if it would rebel altogether, with rising cries and suspicions as it became filled with armed people, nor did anybody know whether they sided with Philip V or with the Emperor'.[12] There was no way of recovering peace. The following year an observer reckoned that 'if diligence is not applied, there is the danger that some Sicilian vespers may break out'.[13]

The uncertain fortunes of the war, exacerbated by the House of Savoy abandoning the French side and allying with the Imperialists, took a turn for the worse. After the incursion of the imperial troops in Ferrara in 1701, many episodes of border violation between the French and the Austrian armies ensued. In 1704, the Ficarolo diplomatic incident – when the French occupied the locale previously freed by their adversaries in the name of papal neutrality – made enemies of the imperial troops stationed along the Po River, who then proceeded to a new invasion of Ferrara in 1705.[14] Meanwhile, as a result of the widespread destruction and shortages caused by the warring armies, feeding Rome required an enormous effort on the part of the congregations of the Annona and the Grascia, all to the detriment of the impoverished provinces.[15]

Nature's destructive force compounded with troubles created by man. Since the close of the seventeenth century, the weather had showed no sign of relenting. In March 1702 'a whirlwind and a sudden hailstorm did great damage' causing the death of some workers, and it was immediately followed by reports from Naples and Benevento announcing the eruption of Vesuvius (some

---

[11]   L. Muratori, *Annali d'Italia*, vol. 12, Rome, 1744, p. 4; S. Tabacchi, 'L'impossibile neutralità: il papato, Roma e lo Stato della Chiesa durante la guerra di successione spagnola', *Cheiron*, 39–40, 2003, pp. 223–43.

[12]   *Diario di Clemente XI*, fols 57v–70v, quotation fol. 60r.

[13]   G.V. Gravina, *Carteggio politico (1690–1712)*, ed. A. Sarubbi, Naples, 1971, p. 217.

[14]   L. von Pastor, *History of the Popes from the Close of the Middle Ages*, trans. E. Graf, vol. 33, London, 1957, pp. 24–41.

[15]   On the Annona, which supplied grains to the capital and controlled the price of bread, see J. Revel, 'Le grain de Rome et la crise de l'Annone dans la seconde moitié du XVIIIe siècle', *Mélanges de l'École Française de Rome: Moyen Âge, Temps modernes*, 84, 1972, pp. 201–81; M. Martinat, *Le 'juste marché': le système annonaire romain aux XVIe et XVIIe siècles*, Paris, 1994; D. Strangio, *Crisi alimentari e politica annonaria a Roma nel Settecento*, Rome, 1999. The congregation of the Grascia regulated the commerce of meat and all related products; see H. Gross, *Rome in the Age of Enlightenment: The Post-Tridentine Syndrome and the Ancien Regime*, Cambridge, 1990, ch. 7.

tremors were felt in Rome too), 'upon which calamity such strong winds, heavy rainstorms and hailstorms followed that the whole earth may be engulfed'.[16] Due to the heavy rain, the Tiber first burst its banks and dragged away a number of unfortunate bystanders, then overflowed at the end of December and 'rotten, putrefied corpses [were seen] floating in the Tiber, which caused great fear'.[17]

Worse was yet to come. In January 1703 Rome was hit by an earthquake, the most unexpected and swiftest of catastrophes, reaping death and destruction in a matter of moments. Tremors were so strong that 'the bells pealed by themselves... [and] the population was struck with horror, Rome was turned into a maelstrom of shrieks and wails ... and everybody threw themselves at the feet of the confessors to pour out their sins'.[18] Many slept in the open for days, and although there was a limited amount of damage, shrieks and prayers 'made this calamity appear greater than it really was'.[19] At the beginning of February, a more violent earth tremor added to the general fear. Several localities on the Appennines were razed to the ground, hundreds of victims were counted in Norcia, Cascia and Aquila, 'nor can the havoc and fright that was in Rome be expressed ... because over April, May and June more tremors were felt, and everyone was constantly alarmed, fearing the worst'.[20] The seismic activity continued into the month of October. Then, an incredibly violent hailstorm caused the death of several animals, as one chronicler claimed.[21] Nature raged with unabated fury.[22]

An endless stream of alarming events and omens heralding further disasters exacerbated fear and instilled the suspicion that some divine or diabolical plan was at work. Not long before the earthquake, for instance, a worker was swallowed by a chasm near the Aurelian walls and 'most horrifyingly, the body was never

---

[16]   *Diario di Clemente XI*, fol. 102v, 13 March 1702; *Distinta relazione dell'orribile, e spaventoso terremoto, accaduto alli 14 del presente mese di marzo nella città di Benevento*, Rome, 1702.

[17]   *Diario di Clemente XI*, fol. 148v; B. Abbati, *Epitome metheorologica de' tremoti, con la cronologia di tutti quelli che sono occorsi in Roma dalla creatione del mondo ... Con la relatione non solo di questi, ma dell'inondatione del Tebro ancora*, Rome, 1703.

[18]   *Diario di Clemente XI*, fol. 153.

[19]   Ibid., fol. 155; Muratori, *Annali*, p. 14.

[20]   Muratori, *Annali*, p. 15; P. De Carolis, *Relazione generale delle rovine e mortalità cagionate dalle scosse del terremoto de 14 gennaro e 2 febbraro 1703 in Norcia, Cascia e loro contadi*, Rome, 1703; *Relazione de' danni fatti dall'innondazioni, e terremoto nella città dell'Aquila, ed in altri luoghi circonvicini*, Rome, 1703; *Veridica, e distinta relazione, overo diario de' danni fatti dal terremoto dalli 14. Gennaro, sino alli 2. di Febraro 1703*, Rome, 1703.

[21]   *Diario di Clemente XI*, fol. 181r.

[22]   On the 'great storm' of 1703 in Britain, see I. Golinski, *British Weather and the Climate of Enlightenment*, Chicago, 2007, pp. 41–52.

found'.[23] Pope Clement XI's inspection of the flooded Tiber was enough to spark the rumour that 'as soon as he raised his hands, the water began to lower, a truly admirable and prodigious act that can be deemed a miracle of the pontifical authority'.[24] Sinister planetary conjunctions led astrologists to predict ill-fated times. In 1703 the whole of Rome was 'upset by the prediction which was found in a certain book by a self-proclaimed astrologist called Albigini from Florence, a mighty fortunate man in his delusions, as it has been said that he has been always right this year'.[25] The price of the book went up from 25 *baiocchi* to 4 *giuli*, 'from which we can gather the ingenuity of the Florentines, who know how to extract great gain from such trifles', commented Valesio cuttingly.[26] A year later, all it took was a fire, and immediately 'it was said that this was a manifest and clear sign of future calamities'.[27] Everyday life was beset by disconcerting scenes heightening tension, as happened in February 1703, when a hot-headed youth ('who was punished', a chronicler points out) hit himself repeatedly with a stone in front of the Chiesa Nuova 'saying that at the seventh hour the earthquake would strike again, something that alarmed people greatly when the news spread around Rome'.[28] In fact, as another witness reports, 'in the furthest areas of the city, altering the facts as is customary in idle talk, it was claimed that an infant had spoken'.[29] The cardinal vicar suspended all night processions and had the streets patrolled by guards in order to calm people's minds.

The most anguishing episode occurred during the earthquake in February 1703. The renowned physician and lecturer at the university of Rome Giorgio Baglivi relates it in a report – *De terremoto romano* – that he wrote in the style of Hippocrates. The earthquake had already put everybody out of their minds when

> before midday, it was rumoured that fateful destruction loomed over everyone and that the ancient city was to end in ruins. In the middle of the night that same day, some infamous and iniquitous men dared to roam the neighbourhoods and districts and knock on almost all the doors of the houses where the inhabitants, still frightened, had only just retired, awakening them from sleep; people, terrified by the sudden commotion, and at that time fearing the worst, could hear the voices of those men running hither and thither and rejoicing in the public fears.

---

[23]   *Diario di Clemente XI*, fol. 150r.

[24]   Ibid., fol. 149v.

[25]   Gravina, *Carteggio politico*, p. 262. The tract alluded to is *Trattato astrologico di quanto influiscono le stelle dal cielo a pro, e danno delle cose inferiori per tutto l'anno 1703*, Florence, [1702].

[26]   Valesio, vol. 2, p. 526.

[27]   *Diario di Clemente XI*, fol. 199v, 13 November 1704.

[28]   Ibid, fol. 162v.

[29]   Valesio, vol. 2, p. 526.

> Word was that the Supreme Pontiff had predicted that at the tenth hour of the night the whole city would perish, that it would be the last day for all inhabitants, and that a papal decree ordered everybody to leave their homes at once and seek to save themselves. The Romans, terrified by these unexpected rumours, uncertain and unaware of what they should do, at first began to shake, and then, stunned and pale with fear, fled to the public places and open spaces. The common people, more inclined to credulity, fled first ... [women] in tears besought God, and pulling their children from their breasts ... incessantly lifted them towards the heavens ... All prayed ... that innocent children and the humble be spared the wrath they deserved for their sins.[30]

The Governor of Rome, Ranuccio Pallavicini, sent soldiers and policemen to surround the houses and convince the inhabitants that the rumours had been spread 'through the intentions of thieves'. However, the culprits were never identified, 'though searched for with the utmost diligence'. According to Baglivi, who was indeed quite sceptical, 'not only the populace but also many sensible people believe that such disturbance was not man's but the devil's work', not least because similar events happened simultaneously in more than one place.[31] The anonymous author of a *Journal of the Pontificate of Clement XI* (*Giornale del pontificato di Clemente XI*) judged the facts to be 'the work of the Devil', because

> At the same moment in time, there was a knock at the door of all the houses in this city ... and what caused more amazement was that the same happened at the houses in the nearby villages ... and most remarkably nothing went missing from any of the houses left open by their inhabitants, which shows that it was not (as many believed) the thieves' doing, all the more so as all efforts to track down the accomplices were in vain.[32]

An unofficial report on the incident refrained from passing judgement on its origin, refusing to judge whether it was caused by criminal intent 'as it is probable, or ... by execrable impiety' or even by 'a truly diabolical art'. It did not make any

---

[30]   G. Baglivi, *Opere complete medico-pratiche ed anatomiche*, Florence, 1842, pp. 596–677, quotation at pp. 619–20. On Baglivi, see the entry by M. Crespi in DBI, vol. 5, 1963; *Alle origini della biologia medica: Giorgio Baglivi tra le due sponde dell'Adriatico*, special issue of *Medicina nei secoli*, 12, 2000.

[31]   Baglivi, *Opere*, p. 621. According to Valesio, vol. 2, pp. 507–8, 'nor did fear take hold solely of persons of low status, but princes and princesses alike fled with little or no clothes on them', and 'the nuns, whose doors were knocked upon, could scarcely be contained [in their convents]'. During the penitential ceremonies in St Peter's the next day, some 'beat themselves with iron chains, others flogged themselves until they bled, some had chains to their feet, others carried the heaviest of crosses'.

[32]   *Diario di Clemente XI*, fol. 160v.

mystery, however, of how the 'fright and the commotion was most arduous to describe'.[33] In truth, the memory of this episode remained alive for decades.[34]

After a few months of relative calm, during which public works for the modernisation of the city were launched (for example the Port of Ripetta, the Clementino granary), yet another earthquake was felt at the beginning of 1705. The news of Emperor Leopold's death 'had great resonance in the city of Rome ... as everyone believed that things would get more and more complicated and confused'.[35] The papal court's ephemeral hopes for peace were shattered by the news of the imperial election of Joseph I, who refused to sign the customary act of submission to the pope and withdrew his ambassador from Rome. Meanwhile, relations with the Spanish monarch Philip V, whom the pope had not yet formally recognised, deteriorated.[36] On 26 July 1705, having reconquered Brabant and part of Flanders, Eugene of Savoy entered Milan and assumed control over Northern Italy, launching multiple raids into the Papal States and reclaiming several imperial fiefs. The nuncio Giovanni Antonio Davia, already banned from court, was expelled from Vienna. Nor were these the only troubles for the Apostolic See: Johann Wilhelm, Count Palatine of the Rhine, expanded religious freedom in his states to the detriment of Catholics; the struggle for the Polish throne escalated; the *Vineam Domini* bull enacted in 1705 against the Jansenists raised resentment against the curia in the French parliaments and clergy, while Catholics in the Orient suffered new persecutions.[37] An era had ended and no new stability was in sight; everything was in turmoil. Then, the mysterious sudden deaths began.

Natural Disasters, Human Sins, Divine Aid

To cope with the disaster, Clement XI immediately mobilised the weapons of piety. Already on 4 January 1703 he had granted special indulgences to all those who begged 'God's help for the present need of the Church'[38] and had led the recitation of litanies in person. He then went in procession to the Lateran

---

[33] L.A. Chracas, *Racconto istorico de' terremoti sentiti in Roma e in parte dello Stato ecclesiastico e in altri luoghi la sera de' 14 di gennaio, e la mattina de' 2 di febbraio del anno 1703*, Rome, 1704, pp. 108–9.

[34] D. Gagliardi, *Dell'infermo istruito*, vol. 2, Rome, 1720, pp. 128–9.

[35] *Diario di Clemente XI*, fols 208v–209r.

[36] H. Kamen, *The War of Succession in Spain 1700–15*, Bloomington, IN, 1969, pp. 387–90.

[37] S. Reboulet, *Histoire de Clément XI Pape*, Avignon, 1752, p. 174; Pastor, *History of the Popes*, pp. 102–3, 184–218, 365–85.

[38] *Clementis Undecimi pont. max. Bullarium*, Rome, 1723, pp. 24–5, 4 January 1703.

basilica and climbed the Holy Steps on his knees 'weeping bitterly'.[39] The echo of his devotion reverberated throughout Catholic Europe at war.[40] The following month, after the destruction brought about by the earthquake, the pope returned to the Holy Steps, 'which he climbed on his knees and with his head bared', and summoned a penitential procession to which 'all qualities of persons convened in Rome, knights, princesses and high-born ladies together with the commoners'.[41] 'Taking advantage of the terror of earthquakes', the pope also introduced popular missions in Rome. According to the Venetian Ambassador Giovanni Morosini, the tenor of the preachings, delivered day and night in the oratories of the confraternities, was so gloomy as to strike the final blow to the spirit of the anguished Romans.[42] Many deplored the doings of the missionaries, 'who mostly preach ... heaping all the evils of the situation on the most idiotic flock, not bothering about the lack of education of the spiritual ministers to which so little attention is paid, in the confessionals as much as on the pulpits'.[43]

Clement XI proclaimed another extraordinary jubilee for 1704. For two years in a row, 'having learned from experience that the sound of bells ... is very effectual for inciting the people to implore divine succour in the present great needs', he had the bells rung at the time at which the earthquake had struck in February 1703.[44] The secular and the regular clergy, nuns and confraternities, vied with each other in performing good deeds, which were all diligently recorded in a propagandistic booklet published on the first anniversary of the earthquake.[45] A special congregation of prelates and nobles was appointed with the task of finding a way to thank God for his protection against greater harm, and they proposed the suspension of the carnival for five years and that all citizens wear

---

[39]   *Diario di Clemente XI*, fol. 156v; Chracas, *Racconto istorico*, p. 5.

[40]   G. Quenet, *Les tremblements de terre aux XVIIe et XVIIIe siècles: la naissance d'un risque*, Seyssel, 2005, pp. 214–21.

[41]   I am quoting respectively from Chracas, *Racconto istorico*, p. 60, and *Diario di Clemente XI*, fol. 161v.

[42]   C. Morandi, ed., *Relazioni di ambasciatori sabaudi, genovesi e veneti durante il periodo della grande alleanza e della successione di Spagna 1693–1713*, Bologna, 1935, p. 193; J. Coste, 'Missioni nell'agro romano nella primavera del 1703', *Ricerche per la storia religiosa di Roma*, 2, 1978, pp. 165–223. On night missions, see O. Niccoli, 'Riti notturni: le processioni fra Cinquecento e Seicento', in *La notte: ordine, sicurezza e disciplinamento in età moderna*, ed. M. Sbriccoli, Florence, 1991, pp. 80–93.

[43]   Gravina, *Carteggio politico*, p. 233.

[44]   Ms ASVR, Segreteria, Registro degli editti del Vicario 1606–1709, 5 February 1703, repeated on 14 April and 25 May.

[45]   S. Grassi Fiorentino, 'Nella sera della domenica. Il terremoto del 1703 in Umbria: trauma e reintegrazione', *Quaderni storici*, 55, 1984, pp. 137–54.

mourning clothes for a year. Clement XI merely prohibited all entertainment for one year.[46] Later, however, he resolved to suspend the carnival of 1705 too.

Weapons of piety were wielded again when, in 1706, more cases of sudden death plunged Rome into terror again. Once more, the pope banned the carnival, and the city governor prohibited all pastimes and even spiritual performances; hence, 'since there was no entertainment in town', Romans could only gather in Piazza Navona 'to hear the charlatans'.[47] On the anniversary of the earthquake the pope led the procession to Santa Maria in Trastevere, followed by a huge crowd 'remindful of the awful dread'.[48] After the earthquake, the cardinal vicar prescribed the litanies to beg for protection from sudden death (*a subitanea et improvisa morte*);[49] three years later, in March 1706, he published a special liturgy *ad postulandam gratiam bene moriendi*. This special service was extended to the whole Church by Clement XI 'so that at the present time, when so many cases of sudden death are occurring both in the city and elsewhere, we may ask God for the grace of a good and pious death'.[50] At the end of May that same year, the pontiff led another imposing procession to the hospital of Santo Spirito in Sassia, singing the litanies of the saints.[51] The religious fervour was so great that it inevitably gave rise to satire by

> those discontented with the present government, consisting in a hapless tercet, which, falsely exaggerating the little attention given to public affairs, concluded that 'we only attend to some great Oration' alluding equivocally both to the prayers imposed for the indulgences and to his holiness' brother's name [Orazio].[52]

The sudden deaths did not stop. Between April and September 1706, Valesio noted several in his diary.[53] The succession of accidents 'frightened the city, [for they were] an admonishment to live well in God, as many who were striken by this ailment were left crippled or unconscious'.[54] Moreover, on 3 November 1706 another 'long but not so vigorous' earthquake caused further dismay (the

---

[46] Valesio, vol. 2, p. 524.

[47] Valesio, vol. 3, p. 557. The governor's edict was dated 16 January 1706. On charlatans and their performance art, see D. Gentilcore, *Medical Charlatanism in Early Modern Italy*, Oxford, 2006.

[48] *Gazzetta di Bologna*, 16 February 1706.

[49] Ms ASVR, Segreteria, Registro degli editti del Vicario 1606–1708, 5 February 1703.

[50] *Missa ad postulandam gratiam bene moriendi*, Rome, 1706. The Apostolic approval of 27 March 1706 is registered on the copy now held at the British Library, shelfmark 1896.d.7.(34). This decision is mentioned in Reboulet, *Histoire de Clément XI*, p. 173.

[51] Ms BNR, Vittorio Emanuele 790, fol. 151v, 29 May 1706.

[52] Valesio, vol. 3, p. 298, 13 January 1705.

[53] Valesio, vol. 3, especially pp. 637 and 680.

[54] *Diario di Clemente XI*, fol. 235v, 27 August 1706.

city of Sulmona was seriously damaged),[55] while the enemy armies approached the capital threateningly. 'Ubique mors, ubique luctus, ubique desolatio' ('everywhere death, everywhere sorrow, everywhere desolation'): on 2 December 1706 the pope proclaimed yet another universal jubilee to pray for peace and for all other *praesentibus Catholicae Ecclesiae necessitatibus*. During a vehement prayer in the consistory, he even invited the cardinals to set an example by adopting better conduct.[56] Again, the following year, carnival festivities were forbidden along with all other 'carousals', and some unrepentant Romans were thrown in jail for failing to comply with the prohibitions.[57]

At that time, many continued to view natural disasters, especially earthquakes, as God's punishment: 'these horrible effects of secondary causes are scourges, and voices of the Most High, which chastise and bring back onto the path of virtue men lost on the street of vice'.[58] More precisely, despite an increasing disenchantment emerging in scientific writings, no one denied that catastrophes could have supernatural origins, whether it be direct, as divine punishment, or only indirect, that is, as a sign to be interpreted within the design of Providence.[59]

By common consent, diseases might be either a form of heavenly punishment or the deed of the devil and 'demonic persons' too. Such explanations were used, for instance, during the plague of 1656–57.[60] Similar beliefs were widespread in the Roman Church and curia. For years the moral abuses of clergy and laity, the

---

[55]   Quoted from the *Gazzetta di Bologna*, 17 November 1706; *Distinta relazione del danno cagionato dal tremuoto succeduto a di 3. di novembre 1706*, Naples, 1706.

[56]   *Bullarium*, pp. 54–6; *Clementis XI Pont. Max. opera omnia*, vol. 1, Frankfurt, 1729, pp. 23–4.

[57]   *Diario di Clemente XI*, fols 290v–291r.

[58]   V. Teloni, *De terremoti, loro cagioni, effetti, e malori, che producono*, Viterbo, 1703, p. 17; De Carolis, *Relazione generale delle rovine*, p. 15; Abbati, *Epitome metheorologica de' tremoti*.

[59]   A. Placanica, *Segni dei tempi: il modello apocalittico nella tradizione occidentale*, Venice, 1990; F. Deconinck-Brossard, 'Acts of God, Acts of Men: Providence in Seventeenth- and Eighteenth-Century England and France', in *Signs, Wonders, Miracles: Representations of Divine Power in the Life of the Church*, ed. K. Cooper and J. Gregory, Woodbridge, 2005, pp. 356–75; A.-M. Mercier-Faivre and C. Thomas, eds, *L'invention de la catastrophe au XVIIIe siècle: du châtiment divin au désastre naturel*, Geneva, 2008, and for England A. Walsham, *Providence in Early Modern England*, Oxford, 1999.

[60]   P. Correa, *Tractatus de natura, causis, et curatione pestis*, Rome, 1657; A. Kircher, *Scrutinium physico-medicum contagiosae luis, quae pestis dicitur*, Rome, 1658, pp. 66–7; C. Valesio, *Aphorismi Prognostici Hippocratis in febribus acutis commentariis illustratis*, Rome, 1659, on disease in general p. 68, on plague p. 919. On 'manufactured' plague, see P. Preto, *Epidemia, paura e politica nell'Italia moderna*, Rome and Bari, 1987; on the prevailing of naturalism in accounting for epidemics, see P. Slack, *The Impact of Plague in Tudor and Stuart England*, London, 1985.

vices of monks and the immodesty of women had been publicly denounced. The harshest critics believed immorality to be the cause of all persecutions suffered by the Catholic Church. In 1703 the ecclesiastical authorities solemnly proclaimed that the earthquake was nothing less than the manifestation of 'the wrath of God, justly indignant for our sins'; it was therefore imperative to give up 'trafficking, games, licentious revelries and other worldly vanities', since 'divine wrath, justly caused by such profanations, sends public scourges in the form of war, floods, earthquakes, plagues and the like'.[61] A general ban on prostitution was put forward. Zealots at court tried to insinuate in the pope's mind that unless adequate measures were taken, the plague would cross the borders of the Ecclesiastical state, ruining the country and his personal reputation.[62] What if the sudden deaths too were scourges inflicted by divine wrath, or at least signs of God's will?

Preachers and theologians taught that sudden death was the punishment inflicted by God on heathen, obstinate sinners. The Bible narrated many events of this kind, such as the deaths of Ananias and Sapphira (Acts of the Apostles 5.1–11). Ananias' death had been translated into images countless times. One fresco by Pomarancio, for instance, loomed in the Roman basilica of St Mary of the Angels.[63] Apoplexy or fulmination – or being seized by apoplexy as if struck by lightning (this was the Greek etymology of the word apoplexy) – was the punishment meted out to usurers, fornicators, dancers and blasphemers.[64] Comets were sometimes associated with sudden death and could be interpreted both as

---

[61]   *Lettera circolare* of cardinal Carpegna, Rome, 1703.

[62]   Ms ASV, Fondo Albani vol. 1, fols 173–5; vol. 2, fols 61–7; vol. 3, fol. 138, where an anonymous religious person wrote: 'I have heard much murmur not so much from respectable persons but from those who are not held to be sanctimonious, or hypocrites, that in Rome it will not only be allowed to stage commercial comedies but also to organise Carnival masquerades, whereas in all other confining states … all of these things have been forbidden, if only to show respect towards God's disdain, which manifests itself with the scourge of plague as far as the borders of Italy … if truly His Holiness were of this disposition, and our sins then attracted this fearful scourge over Rome or another part of the state, who could ever absolve Your Beatitude from universal blame from the Catholics and the heretics alike.'

[63]   Other well-known representations of this subject are by Masaccio in the Brancacci chapel in S. Maria del Carmine in Florence, and by Raffaello, now in the Victoria & Albert Museum, London. In the seventeenth century, the death of Ananias was especially popular in the Low Countries, as it alluded to the avarice of tradesmen; see A. Pigler, *Barockthemen: Eine Auswahl von Verzeichnissen zur Ikonographie del 17. und 18. Jahrhunderts*, vol. 1, Budapest, 1956, pp. 380–81.

[64]   J. Berlioz, 'La foudre au Moyen Âge: l'apport des exempla homilétiques', in *Les catastrophes naturelles dans l'Europe médiévale et moderne*, ed. B. Bennassar, Toulouse, 1996, pp. 165–74.

a sign and as a cause.[65] If one is to believe the testimony of an anonymous curial officer, the 'fearful cases of sudden death and apoplectic accidents' in Rome were perceived by the people precisely as 'punishment'.[66] In January 1706, proclaiming the indulgences, the Cardinal Vicar Gaspare Carpegna attributed these 'accidents' to the sins of the people and lamented 'how brief was the correction of our conduct, and now, alas, we see that the wrath of God continues because of our obstination in sin, and justly threatens us with ever more serious disasters'. In the following months, he called on all citizens to practise spiritual exercises in order 'to appease the wrath of God' and to avoid 'those scourges of new calamities, which at present impend upon us, willed by His most just indignation'.[67]

In the Papal States similar considerations pertained to religious as well as to civil government. Indeed, calamities offered ecclesiastical authorities an opportunity to tighten their grip on society, at a time when the Spanish hegemony in Italy was waning and new lifestyles were emerging. At the end of the seventeenth century, the neo-Tridentine popes had revived social discipline in order to restore the sacred and exemplary character of Rome through a vigorous combination of charity and repression.[68] The same politics was now reinvigorated. Pope Albani was elected in 1700 with the support of the faction of the *Zelanti* cardinals (and the eventual acceptance of France) in the hope that he would address the serious problems of the Church and the state and the imminent threat of the dynastic crisis in Spain.[69] He soon gave proof of his willingness to continue his predecessors' effort to reform all 'abuses' and correct the lack of accuracy in worship, poor devotional zeal and the excessive freedom

---

[65]   Ms Venice, Archivio di Stato, Inquisitori di Stato, b. 704, *avviso* from Rome, 3 May 1681: 'Monsignor Artus died all of a sudden ... and others have also died of apoplexy this week, from which it appears that the evil forebodings of the comet have begun to occur, the effects of which were already said to begin in the month of May'. I am grateful to Federico Barbierato for this reference.

[66]   *Diario di Clemente XI*, fols 181v–182r.

[67]   Edicts of 11 January, 16 February and 23 April 1706.

[68]   M. Fatica, 'La reclusione dei poveri a Roma durante il pontificato di Innocenzo XII (1692–1700)', *Ricerche per la storia religiosa di Roma*, 3, 1979, pp. 133–79; M. Turrini, 'La riforma del clero secolare durante il pontificato di Innocenzo XII', in *Riforme, religione e politica durante il pontificato di Innocenzo XII 1691–1700*, ed. B. Pellegrino, Lecce, 1994, pp. 249–74.

[69]   On Pope Albani, see S. Andretta, 'Clemente XI', in DBI, vol. 26, 1982. On the factions in the College of Cardinals, see G. Signorotto, 'The *squadrone volante*: "Independent" Cardinals and European Politics in the Second Half of the Seventeenth Century', in *Court and Politics in Papal Rome*, ed. G. Signorotto and M.A. Visceglia, Cambridge, 2002, pp. 177–211; S. Tabacchi, 'Cardinali zelanti e fazioni cardinalizie tra fine Seicento e inizio Settecento', in *La Corte di Roma tra Cinque e Seicento: 'teatro' della politica europea*, ed. G. Signorotto and M.A. Visceglia, Rome, 1998, pp. 139–66.

of clergy and laity.[70] The alarming situation caused by the war, natural disasters and other tragic events paved the way to implementing salutary remedies. By express command of the pope, preaching was directed 'against luxury and domestic vanities' (the spectacular if ephemeral effect was the falling into disuse 'of bonnets with those great tufts and ribbons that were in fashion'),[71] and all were admonished 'to refrain from gallant conversations, the very greatest cause of evil'.[72] The pontiff warned young prelates that 'those who want to advance [in their career] must desist from all improper, idle conversation unworthy of the ecclesiastical status'.[73] The compulsory lessons of Christian doctrine were extended to children. A prison for urchins was established within the Hospice of San Michele, an imposing workhouse and dormitory for the poor equally dispensing care and coercion, founded at the end of the seventeenth century. Exemplary corporal punishment was inflicted on prostitutes, concubines and self-proclaimed witches. Moral surveillance was occasionally so ruthless as to arouse popular resentment. Valesio reports in his diary an episode in 1705. The pope was 'as per his custom on the balcony of his room with his crystal spy-glass' when he saw a man protect a woman from rain with his cloak and had them both arrested. The poor man was accused of adultery, and the pope 'uncustomarily, not only demanded that he be sentenced to 10 years in jail, but that he be publicly whipped'; the same punishment was inflicted on the woman, but the people disapproved the severity of this sentence 'for a crime not fully proven'.[74] The same diarist noted that, during the gloomy carnival of 1705, over two hundred people were arrested on charges of 'debauchery and revelry'.[75]

A special Congregation for Ecclesiastical Discipline first established in 1696 was reactivated to assist the ordinary congregations of cardinals. Rome witnessed long forgotten scenes of monastic discipline imposed forcibly, when the obligation of common life was imposed on the nuns of the Concezione near the Arco dei Pantani.[76] Zealots denounced carousing in the convents and all

---

[70]   F. Bianchini, 'Risposta ... alla Santità di ... Clemente papa XI sul principio del suo glorioso pontificato', in his *Opuscula varia*, Rome, 1753, vol. 2, pp. 252–309.

[71]   Valesio, vol. 2, p. 490.

[72]   Ibid., p. 499; ms ASVR, Segreteria, Registro degli editti del Vicario 1606–1708, 17 January 1703. According to Chracas, *Relazione*, pp. 14–15, the pope told the preachers that 'the pestiferous sources of our crimes' were the 'scarce reverence to churches, diminished observance and celebration of holy days, abominable neglect on the part of the fathers in the education of their children ... licence in conversation which has been too great for some time, and finally the immodesty of women in luxury and lascivious attire'.

[73]   Morandi, *Relazioni di ambasciatori*, p. 193.

[74]   Valesio, vol. 3, pp. 316–17 and passim; *Diario di Clemente XI*, fol. 138r–v and fol. 23v.

[75]   Valesio, vol. 3, p. 321.

[76]   Ibid., vol. 3, p. 574. Being under the supervision of a cardinal, rather than the male order's superiors, the nuns of the Consolazione had always claimed a privileged status; see

sorts of excesses in celebrating the monacation of novices.[77] The Cardinal Vicar Carpegna (who had been in charge since 1671 and embodied the continuity between the austere pontificates of the late seventeenth century and the new century) seized the opportunity to extend his jurisdiction over the regular clergy, notwithstanding the limitations imposed on his powers by the reform of tribunals in 1692.[78] At his behest, a flurry of edicts was issued to ban entertainment, to regulate the behaviour of clergy and laity, to force everyone to abide by the obligations of his or her status.[79] Some measures acted as simple reminders of the canonic dictates in force, while others were unprecedented, like the prohibition on women studying music with male teachers. Wigs, a highly fashionable accessory, had already been prohibited for the clergy in 1681, 1691 and 1699, and the ban was reaffirmed in 1703. In 1705 a priest was imprisoned for missing the academies of casuistry, the attendance of which was mandatory for confessors. The rector of the charitable hospice for indigent priests in Borgo, 'who had been entertained in the home of two beautiful young women',[80] met the same fate. In December 1706 a long, detailed edict was emanated *About the life and honesty of ecclesiastics and especially about dress and clerical tonsure* (*Circa la vita ed onestà degl'ecclesiastici e specialmente circa l'abito e tonsura clericale*). The vicar's henchmen roamed the city, partly to control political conversations and partly to moralise public customs, so much so that there were a few incidents, the worst of which involved two young artists, *pensionnaires* at the French Academy.[81]

In such tragic times death could certainly not be neglected. In 1704 the cardinal vicar forbade the removal of any objects from cemeteries, in order to preserve the martyrs' sacred relics (the custodian of the relics, Marco Antonio

---

S. Andretta, *La venerabile superbia: ortodossia e trasgressione nella vita di suor Francesca Farnese (1593–1651)*, Turin, 1994, pp. 180–88.

[77] Ms ASV, Fondo Albani, vols 2–5; *Della giurisdittione e prerogative del Vicario di Roma: opera del canonico Antonio Cuggiò segretario del tribunale di sua Eminenza*, ed. D. Rocciolo, Rome, 2004, pp. 61, 294–302.

[78] D. Rocciolo, 'Introduzione', ibid., pp. 15–24. On the vicar's and other tribunals in Rome, see I. Fosi, *Papal Justice: Subjects and Courts in the Papal State, 1500–1750*, trans. T.V. Cohen, Washington, DC, 2011. On late seventeenth-century episcopalism, see C. Donati, 'La Chiesa di Roma tra antico regime e riforme settecentesche (1675–1766)', in *Storia d'Italia, Annali 9, La Chiesa e il potere politico dal Medioevo all'età contemporanea*, ed. G. Chittolini and G. Miccoli, Turin, 1986, pp. 721–66.

[79] Ms ASVR, Segreteria, Registro degli editti del Vicario 1606–1708; Segreteria, Raccolta di editti e altre materie 1700–1720, b. 9. On women fashion and the moderation of luxury, see ms ASV, Fondo Albani, vols 1, 3 and 4.

[80] Valesio, vol. 3, pp. 318, 307.

[81] *Correspondance des directeurs de l'Académie de France à Rome avec les surintendants des bâtiments*, ed. A. de Montaiglon, vol. 3, Paris, 1889, pp. 158–70.

Boldetti, undertook a systematic study of them).[82] Cardinal Carpegna then turned his attention to funeral rites. He forbade that corpses be laid out on the ground, specifying that they were always to be placed 'on the bier'. He commanded that deceased priests be laid out in their holy garments. In 1706, in the midst of the sudden death crisis, he felt compelled to further stress the rules of the Roman Catholic ritual concerning the transportation of corpses, prohibiting the use of 'coaches and carriages'.[83] In 1707 Carpegna had the customary funeral ordinances reprinted in a volume, together with all new edicts and decrees on the matter, intended for parish curates. The following year, he sternly admonished all members of the clergy and confraternities yet again not to exact more than what was due for funerals. Alas, greed in the presence of death was indeed a problem that had beset the Church for centuries.[84]

Doctors in Action against the 'Epidemic'

The anxieties of the people of Rome could be alleviated with prayers and processions, encouraging them to draw spiritual profit from the events. Up to a certain point, fear could be used as an instrument to impose social discipline. Nevertheless, one question remained: why so many sudden deaths? God's inscrutable will might be their final cause, as devout Catholics assumed, yet it was still necessary to ascertain the material and natural causes. What was killing so many helpless citizens?

Initially, isolated cases 'were attributed to the instability of the season, now cold North winds, now burning Sirocco having blown'.[85] Fingers were then pointed against chocolate, a tasty habit of the Romans. Some suspected that 'the great frequency [of apoplexy] in our time stems perhaps from abuse of

---

[82]   M.A. Boldetti, *Osservazioni sopra i cimiteri de' santi martiri, ed antichi cristiani di Roma*, Rome, 1720. On the conservation of relics, see [Cuggiò], *Della giurisdittione e prerogative del Vicario*, pp. 112–18.

[83]   The first edict is recorded with the date 4 February 1706 in ms ASVR, Segreteria, Registro degli editti del Vicario 1606–1708; the others are in *Bullarium*, pp. 310–12, 317.

[84]   *Statuta antiqua de Officio camerarij cleri Romani, et iuribus funeralibus ecclesiarum, præsertim parochialium Almae Vrbis, una cum additionibus, seu declarationibus novissime ... Adiecta taxatione emolumentorum funeralium ad communem intelligentiam vulgari sermone impressa: cum appendice diversorum edictorum, decretorum, et decisionum ad eadem statuta pertinentium*, Rome, 1707; *Bullarium*, p. 321. See also V. Harding, *The Dead and the Living in Paris and London*, Cambridge, 2002; I. Ait, 'I costi della morte: uno specchio della società cittadina medievale', in *La morte e i suoi riti in Italia tra medioevo e prima età moderna*, ed. F. Salvestrini, G.M. Varanini and A. Zangarini, Florence, 2007, pp. 275–321.

[85]   Valesio, vol. 3, p. 388.

chocolate, which greatly fattens the blood'.[86] Coffee, a more recently introduced drink that was advertised as an excellent 'cephalic',[87] was next in the dock, soon joined by the indictment of the quality of tobacco and the abuse of liquors. There were fears that some kind of contagion might be spreading. The city of Rome, still haunted by memories of the plague of 1656, had been spared from the contagion from Dalmatia in 1684 and again from the plague from Apulia in 1690–91, but pestilences crept up to its borders.[88] In the general confusion, people blamed 'at one moment, the rotten quality of the tobacco, at another the fetid exhalations from past earthquakes, then again the abuse of chocolate, and finally an unknown virus in the atmosphere'.[89]

Fear was general. So many people were dying all of a sudden. Nothing of the sort had ever been witnessed before. Somehow or other, early modern cities had learned to react to the plague by implementing a more or less sophisticated quarantine at the first signs of this depressingly familiar disease. However, they were still uncertain as to how to identify and address other dangers to public health. News of 'new apoplectic accidents ... in people of all ages, young and old' spread in a flash.[90] Rome had no mortality records other than the parish records compiled for religious purposes, and rumours circulated unchecked. Any unusual occurrence sufficed to make 'Death transform his scythe into a horrid trumpet and fill the whole city with a frightful whisper', a situation that urgently necessitated 'the supervision of those who govern and the assistance of those who attend to the care of the bodies'.[91]

It was the duty and the prerogative of university-trained physicians to lavish their learning and counsel. Ever since ancient times, a doctor had principally

---

[86] Baglivi, *De praxi medica*, in *Opere*, pp. 124–5. In contrast, he considered coffee excellent in that 'it cures headache after lunch'. Consumption of chocolate had become rather widespread in the mid-seventeenth century during times of fasting, despite some opposition on the part of canonists and moralists.

[87] *Virtù del Kafe bevanda introdotta nuovaente nell'Italia con alcune osservazioni per conservar la sanità nella vecchiaia*, Rome, 1671; *Dichiaratione delle virtù della bevanda del caffè*, Rome, 1683. In 1642, the College of Physicians banned the publicising of coffee mentioning the diseases it purportedly healed. In 1676 the same prohibition was extended to tobacco, chocolate, coffee and liqueurs.

[88] A. Corradi, *Annali delle epidemie occorse in Italia dalla prime memorie fino al 1850*, vol. 2, Bologna, 1973 (anastatic of the 1865–94 edition); M.P. Donato, 'La peste dopo la peste: economia di un discorso romano (1656–1720)', *Roma moderna e contemporanea*, 14, 2006, pp. 159–74.

[89] SM, 'Occasio scribendi', unpaginated.

[90] *Diario di Clemente XI*, fol. 235v, 27 August 1706.

[91] A.N. Bernabei, *Dissertazione delle morti improvvise*, Rome, 1708, p. 4. On the recording of deaths, see C.M. Cipolla, 'I libri dei morti', and C. Sbrana, 'Le registrazioni di morte a Roma', in *Le fonti della demografia storica in Italia*, vol. 2, Rome, 1972, pp. 851–66 and 869–74.

been expected to name and explain diseases, prior to actually treating them.[92] Indeed, since the very first foundation of universities, learned medicine had differentiated itself from the 'mechanical' branches of the healing art precisely for taking on the task of supplying explanations *per causas* and the prestige of the *auctoritates*. These were the foundations upon which rested both the tripartite hierarchy of physicians, surgeons and apothecaries, and the mutually beneficial relationship between medical doctors and political power, especially in organisms as fragile and dangerous as cities. The privileges enjoyed by doctors as members of the upper classes in the social hierarchy of *ancien régime* society entailed several obligations, among which was dispensing free treatment to the poor and responding to requests from the authorities.[93] The fact that at the beginning of the eighteenth century Galenism was openly questioned did not relieve doctors of their duty to deal out explanations and recommendations. It simply made their task more difficult.

According to a dominant hypothesis of the time, sudden deaths were a direct outcome of earthquakes. The author of the manuscript journal of Clement XI noted that 'this ailment began to occur more frequently after the earthquake'.[94] The *avvisi* reporting the death 'by apoplectic accident' of Monsignor Rota and of Marquis Muti, on 27 March 1706, relate that physicians reckoned that 'this malign influence proceeds from the earthquakes of the past few years, and they believe it alters air and produces such bad quality'.[95] The idea that earthquakes corrupt air was a very ancient one and yet continually updated.[96] In his *De terremoto romano*, Baglivi wrote that during the earthquake of 1703, 'many, hit by apoplexy, died all of a sudden', and that because of the wars, floods and

---

[92] D. Gourevitch, *Le triangle hippocratique dans le monde gréco-romain: le malade, sa maladie et son médecin*, Rome, 1984, pp. 255–88; N.G. Siraisi, *Medieval and Early Renaissance Medicine: An Introduction to Knowledge and Practice*, Chicago, 1990; R.K. French, *Medicine before Science: The Business of Medicine from the Middle Ages to the Enlightenment*, Cambridge, 2003. On the fear of unknown disease, see D. Gentilcore, 'The Fear of Disease and the Disease of Fear', in *Fear in Early Modern Society*, ed. W.G. Naphy and P. Roberts, Manchester, 1997, pp. 184–208.

[93] R. Palmer, 'Physicians and the State in Post-Medieval Italy', in *The Town and State Physician in Europe from the Middle Ages to the Enlightenment*, ed. A.W. Russell, Wolfenbüttel, 1981, pp. 47–61.

[94] *Diario di Clemente XI*, fol. 223, 18 January 1706.

[95] Ms BNR, Vittorio Emanuele 790, fol. 133. Monsignor Rota's apoplexy was reported · in the *Gazzetta di Bologna* of 12 April 1706 too.

[96] J. Henderson, 'The Black Death in Florence: Medical and Communal Reactions', in *Death in Towns: Urban Responses to the Dying and the Dead 100–1600*, ed. S.R. Bassett, Leicester, 1992, pp. 136–50.

earthquakes, apoplexy 'has become familiar in the last 10 years'.[97] The toxic exhalations could be released from the cracks in the earth or from the corpses of the victims, and such an explanation was deemed valid both within the framework of Aristotelianism (air was corrupted qualitatively and 'essentially') and within the corpuscular paradigm of the moderns, which had gained momentum in the late seventeenth century.

Indeed, several physicians set out to explain the sudden deaths occurring in Rome. A number of tracts were published between 1706 and 1709: one *Lettera informativa intorno le cause delle morti improvise* (*Letter of information concerning the causes of sudden deaths*) by Angelo Evangelista, *Romanorum lachrymae subitaneis mortibus effusae exsiccantur* (*Dr da Sylva eases the tears the Romans shed because of the sudden deaths*) by Manoel da Sylva Pereyra, a *Dissertazioni delle morti improvvise* (*A Dissertation on sudden deaths*) by Antonio Nicola Bernabei, and a *Trattato dell'apoplessia* (*Treatise on apoplexy*) by Domenico Mistichelli.[98] This list should be completed with the Protomedicus and his officials' manuscript reports and the treatise *De subitaneis mortibus* by the papal physician Giovanni M. Lancisi, which will be discussed in the next chapter.

The sheer number of opinions expressed over the course of those dramatic months is a measure of the widespread apprehension caused by sudden death. But it is also true that it was the physicians' intervention that eventually transformed isolated accidents into a public affair affecting an entire community. In fact, in the towns of early modern Europe, threats to public health offered physicians an opportunity to gain greater visibility than at any other time. An outbreak of plague and of any other contagion and 'errant illness' sparked public debates on the nature, causes and appropriate treatment for each. A sanitary crisis provided a chance for the medical profession to reaffirm its usefulness to society, and for a single physician an opportunity to stand out. Any practitioner was entitled to express his thoughts. Unanimity was not required as long as compliance with the accepted scientific canons and respect for the established professional hierarchy were ensured.[99] In other words, not only was the *consilium* a moral imperative for the doctor, it was also a social necessity.

---

[97]   Baglivi, *Opere*, pp. 611, 608 and 762–3, where he relates Marcello Malpighi's autopsy and explains the autopsy findings imputing ailments to the 'noxious effluvia still excited by many earthquakes ... [which] may be fomites for this epidemic apoplexy'.

[98]   All published in Rome, in 1706, 1706, 1708 and 1709 respectively.

[99]   K. Park, *Doctors and Medicine in Early Renaissance Florence*, Princeton, 1985; D. Harley, 'Honour and Property: The Structure of Professional Disputes in Eighteenth-Century English Medicine', in *The Medical Enlightenment of the Eighteenth Century*, ed. A. Cunningham and R.K. French, Cambridge, 1990, pp. 138–53; M. Pelling, 'Public and Private Dilemmas: The College of Physicians in Early Modern London', in *Medicine, Health and the Public Sphere in Britain, 1600–2000*, ed. S. Sturdy, London, 2002, pp. 27–42.

Obviously, this necessity was all the stronger the more the medical market was thriving. And when it came to the number of medics, no city could rival Rome. At the beginning of the eighteenth century, the papal city (where a population of approximately 132,000 lived) boasted an exceptional ratio of doctors per inhabitants.[100] If one added the medical trainees in service in hospitals, major and minor surgeons, phlebotomists, midwives, pharmacists, empirics and charlatans, Rome was a veritable medical Mecca. And yet, it continued to attract newcomers.[101] Despite the competition, there was a good chance of securing a stable position and this was a perfect reason to settle in Rome. The city boasted a dense network of health institutions. Hospitals were the concrete expression of the popes' charity as well as an instrument of spiritual and temporal government. The five major hospitals –Santo Spirito, San Giacomo of the Incurables, San Salvatore near the Lateran, Consolazione and Fatebenefratelli on the Tiberina Island – had a large staff of doctors and surgeons. The importance of these institutions was so great that the appointed primary physicians and head surgeons enjoyed a leading position in the professional community and in Roman society. Further medical staff were employed more or less permanently in the madhouse of Santa Maria della Pietà and in the hostels run by the foreign communities (the so-called Nations) and confraternities.[102] Health care for the poor, placed under the control of the

---

[100] C.M. Cipolla, *Public Health and the Medical Profession in the Renaissance*, Cambridge, 1976, p. 82, estimates the number of physicians per 10,000 inhabitants as follows: Florence 1630: 4.1; Palermo 1575: 2.7; Milan 1591: 3.7; Bologna 1630: 6.8; Rome 1656: 11.6; Rome 1675: 12.6; Antwerp 1585: 2.2; Lyon 1620: 2.2; Paris 1626: 2.1; Amsterdam 1641: 3.7. In Rome, 160 university-trained physicians were enrolled in the official list of authorised medical practitioners in 1703 in a population of 134,528; see Gross, *Rome in the Age of Enlightenment*, table 1. For comparison with London, see M. Pelling and C. Webster, 'Medical Practitioners', in *Health, Medicine and Mortality in the Sixteenth Century*, ed. C. Webster, Cambridge, 1979, pp. 165–235. On France, see L. Brockliss and C. Jones, *The Medical World of Early Modern France*, Oxford, 1997, pp. 198–208. On the minor branches of the healing arts in Rome, see A. Calabrini, M. Marta and S. Ricci, *I barbieri di Roma: collegio dei barbieri e parrucchieri di Roma, cinque secoli e mezzo di attività*, vol. 1, *1443–1870*, Rome, 1985; A. Kolega, 'Speziali, spagirici, droghieri e ciarlatani: l'offerta terapeutica a Roma tra Seicento e Settecento', *Roma moderna e contemporanea*, 4, 1998, pp. 311–48; Gentilcore, *Medical Charlatanism*.

[101] Among authorised physicians, those who had gained their doctorate at La Sapienza in Rome numbered 82 per cent in 1703, 72 per cent in 1709 and 78 per cent in 1715; however, only 40.5 per cent in 1703 and 43 per cent in 1715 were born in Rome (my calculations are based on A.L. Bonella, 'La professione medica a Roma tra Sei e Settecento', *Roma moderna e contemporanea*, 4, 1998, pp. 349–66).

[102] For an overview of hospitals and charitable institutions, see C.B. Piazza, *Eusevologio romano, ovvero delle opere pie di Roma*, Rome, 1698; M. Piccialuti, *La carità come metodo di governo: istituzioni caritative a Roma dal pontificato di Innocenzo XII a quello di Benedetto*

Office of Papal Charities, should also be mentioned. Moreover, every convent, every noble household and *familia* of cardinals had its own physician. The aristocratic overpopulation, the relatively old age of the political elite and the many job opportunities made the pope's city a real magnet for ambitious young licentiates and experienced practitioners alike.

The background of the experts who wrote about the mysterious 'epidemic' of sudden deaths reflects the complexity of the medical scene in Rome: three private practitioners, da Sylva, Bernabei and Evangelista; a hospital doctor, Mistichelli; and the pope's archiater, Giovanni Maria Lancisi. Like many physicians practising in Rome, Mistichelli and Bernabei came from the Marche (they were respectively from Fermo and Cossignano and had both graduated from the University of Fermo), while Evangelista was from Zagarolo near Rome and had studied in the capital, and da Sylva had gained his doctorate in Coimbra. A couple of them had already sought celebrity through the printing press.[103]

Rome's supranational character, as the 'theatre of the World' where people from all nations and countries met, meant that excellent career opportunities were open to foreigners. Medical practice was regulated by a chartered body of 12 to 14 members, the Roman College of Physicians, but unlike those of many other Italian towns, the Roman college remained accessible to non-natives.[104] Sponsored by the pope and cardinals, a number of famous foreigners had also

---

XIV, Turin, 1994. On the mental asylum, see L. Roscioni, *Il governo della follia: ospedali, medici e pazzi nell'età moderna*, Milan, 2003.

[103] A. Evangelista, *De aquae usu, et abusu in febribus dissertatio problematica*, Rome, 1703. Mistichelli's observations on a monstrous foetus and on the hearing nerve were published in *Lettres de G. Desnoues ... et de mr. Guglielmini ... sur différentes nouvelles découvertes*, Rome, 1706, pp. 173–88 and 205–11.

[104] As dictated by the 1531 statutes, admission to the College was reserved to Roman *cives*, but in reality these only made up between 23 and 30 per cent of the overall College members, according to the data I have drawn from the *Nomina et cognomina DD. Collegii Romani Medicorum*, appended to the *Statuta collegii DD. almæ Vrbis medicorum ex antiquis romanorum pontificum bullis congesta, et hactenus per Sedem Apostolicam recognita, et innouata*, Rome, 1676. In 1676 the new statute confirmed the status quo, requesting only that colleagues be domiciled in Rome. For medical chartered colleges and their 'wide' or 'closed' configuration, see C. Webster, 'Thomas Linacre and the Foundation of the College of Physicians', in *Essays on the Life and Work of Thomas Linacre c.1460–1524*, ed. F. Maddison, M. Pelling and C. Webster, Oxford, 1977, pp. 198–264; E. Brambilla, 'La medicina del Settecento: dal monopolio dogmatico alla professione scientifica', in *Storia d'Italia*, *Annali 7, Malattia e medicina*, ed. F. Della Peruta, Turin, 1984, pp. 5–147, and her *Genealogie del sapere: università, professioni giuridiche e nobiltà togata in Italia (XIII-XVII secolo)*, Milan, 2005; A. Pastore, *Le regole dei corpi: medicina e disciplina nell'Italia moderna*, Bologna, 2006, pp. 125–54. Several towns of the Papal States had their own college, such as Bologna, on which, see G. Pomata, *Contracting a Cure: Patients, Healers and the Law in Early Modern Bologna*, Baltimore and London, 1998.

taught at the University of Rome, La Sapienza. As the historiographer of La Sapienza Pantaleone Balsarini put it in the mid-eighteenth century, 'in Rome it is highly profitable to apply oneself to the study of medicine, which allows great advancement', and

> Most of them [the physicians] have carriages, lead splendid lives, though they are nearly all offspring of poor men ... Generally, it is more profitable to devote oneself to medicine than to law, if only because doctors get to be acquainted with popes, cardinals, princes and princesses.[105]

Acquaintances were in fact always necessary. For physicians as much as for prelates, members of the curia and artists, success and advancements depended on their ability to gain entry into the complex, multi-centric system of patronage in that maze of institutions and courts that governed early modern Rome.[106] Hence, it was imperative to take advantage of any opportunity to increase one's visibility. The history of medicine in Rome is unsurprisingly interspersed with controversies sparked by a wide range of topics – Tiber waters, public baths, the use of vitriol – that could be turned into public issues, often with an antiquarian overtone in order to please the cultivated ears of princes, cardinals or even the pope.[107] To a certain extent, the sudden deaths during Clement XI's papacy at the beginning of the eighteenth century fall within this scheme. The problem was there. Anyone could see it looking at the wretched cadavers of those who passed away unexpectedly on the public streets without any material or spiritual assistance. Physicians could certainly not evade the obligation nor miss an opportunity to give their answer.

---

[105] Ms Rome, Biblioteca Alessandrina 60, P. Balsarini, *Memorie della Sapienza*, fol. 237.

[106] On patronage and careers in Rome, see, in a vast body of scholarship, W. Reinhard, *Freunde und Kreaturen: 'Verflechtung' als Konzept zur Erforschung historischer Führungsgruppen Römische Oligarchie um 1600*, Munich, 1979; R. Ago, *Carriere e clientele nella Roma barocca*, Rome and Bari, 1990; W. Reinhard, 'Papal Power and Family Strategy in the Sixteenth and Seventeenth Centuries', in *Princes, Patronage and the Nobility: The Court at the Beginning of the Modern Age, 1450–1650*, ed. R.G. Asch and A.M Birke, Oxford, 1991, pp. 329–56; M.A. Visceglia, 'Burocrazia, mobilità sociale e patronage alla corte di Roma tra Cinque e Seicento: alcuni aspetti del recente dibattito storiografico e prospettive di ricerca', *Roma moderna e contemporanea*, 3, 1995, pp. 11–55.

[107] N.G. Siraisi, *History, Medicine, and the Traditions of Renaissance Learning*, Ann Arbor, 2007; A. Clericuzio, 'Chemical Medicines in Rome: Pietro Castelli and the Vitriol Debate (1616–1626)', in *Conflicting Duties: Science, Medicine and Religion in Rome 1550–1750*, ed. M.P. Donato and J. Kraye, London, 2009, pp. 281–302.

A New Plague? The First Tentative Answers from Medicine

Did all the deaths depend on the same cause? Was it just apoplexy or syncope, which could be traced back to the nosology of the ancients, or a new phenomenon? Why were widely different categories of people equally affected? Was the ailment endemic or epidemic, and maybe even contagious? Could anything be done to prevent death? And what was sudden death, after all?

Let us deal for now with da Sylva and Evangelista, whose short tracts were the first to be issued from the printing presses, in 1706. Their on-the-spot texts reveal how an eclectic early eighteenth-century medicine, still firmly rooted in Galenism, dealt with an unusual event. Their approach implies playing down the issue of death in itself, viewed as an inescapable fact and an accepted actuality of the doctor–patient relationship, while shifting the focus onto the ordinary categories of medical practice.

Faithful to Hippocrates and Galen, in his *Romanorum lachrymae subitaneis mortibus effusae exsiccantur*, da Sylva omits to define or discuss sudden death. As for the incidents in Rome, he defends the usefulness of the classical notion of epidemics as a widespread ailment, a 'common malady' which strikes people of different sex, conditions and dispositions. In spite of their differences, he claims, all the people that had been seized experienced 'difficulty in breathing, anxiety of heart, oppression and anguish, a hazy dizziness'. Consequently, they all suffered from the same epidemic disease, which is by definition a disease caused by universal causes. And what cause could be more universal than air? Da Sylva is adamant in his verdict: it is an epidemic disease that 'originates from air'.[108] More precisely, he agrees with the most widespread current hypothesis, and considers it to be corruption of air caused by terrestrial exhalations due to the earthquakes. These 'vitriolic, arsenical and nitrous' exhalations, which ordinarily only cause light fevers and are dispelled by the sun, disperse in higher, lethal quantities during earthquakes. A cursory recollection of historical writings from Livy onwards confirms the correspondence between earthquakes and epidemics.

Why then were terrestrial exhalations harmful if the same chemical elements are found in healthy bodies? How could the latency time between the earthquakes and the outbreak of the disease be explained? These were age-old questions indeed. Da Sylva evokes an unspecified 'efficient fermentative agent' whose 'harmful arsenical and vitriolic quality' disposes the blood to stagnation and 'through coagulation it hinders circulation and thus, life'.[109] Despite his respect for tradition, da Sylva draws on a modern theory that had already proven very popular in medical practice across Europe – that is, the circulatory

---

[108]   M. da Sylva, *Romanorum lachrymae subitaneis mortibus effusae exsiccantur*, Rome, 1706, pp. 9–10.

[109]   Ibid., pp. 14 and 16.

physiopathology sketched by Frans de la Boë Sylvius and Thomas Willis. According to their teachings, fever and other ailments were an effect of an imbalance in the natural movements of the blood, and mainly of a lack or excess in the fermentative movement, brought about by an imbalance of chemical components.[110] The Portuguese physician stresses how blood stagnation resulting from chemical imbalance poses a greater danger than the simple slowing down of the blood circulation caused by a 'plain' plethora (superabundance). Only an expert physician can distinguish between the two ailments: if blood stagnation focuses on the heart, the patient experiences *praefocatio* (choking), brings his hand to his chest, sweats and has an intermittent pulse, whereas a plethora focusing on the brain would make the patient feel headache, ringing in the ears, vertigo and aphasia. In order to help the 'afflicted nature', da Sylva recommends a series of medicines capable of 'dissolving' stagnation and reactivating circulation.[111] He also endorses phlebotomy as the most effective remedy. He reports stories of successful treatments, and does not omit to tell the tragic story of a monk who died because an 'empirical and foolhardy' surgeon neglected to carry out the prescribed bloodletting. Readers are thus warned of the dangers they might encounter unless they follow doctor's orders.

Contrary to da Sylva, in his *Lettera informativa* Angelo Evangelista is against the idea of an epidemic raging in Rome. Although he does not question the canonical definition of epidemic as 'common disease', he underscores that the symptoms experienced by the dying were varied: 'some, losing consciousness, collapsed to the ground bleeding from their mouths ... others were struck while lying in bed ... others, slumbrous and delirious, were seized by strong convulsions'.[112] Evangelista does not contest the authority of the ancients but he prefers a more modern vocabulary full of chemical and mechanical metaphors. He uses the classical (and outdated) explanation of apoplexy as a result of 'slow, sometimes putrid, rancid phlegm overflowing in the brain, holding and blocking the flow of vital spirits',[113] but he specifies that it is caused by 'bad mixtures in the

---

[110] W.F. Bynum and V. Nutton, eds, *Theories of Fever from Antiquity to the Enlightenment*, London, 1981; A.G. Debus, *Chemistry and Medical Debate: van Helmont to Boerhaave*, Canton, MA, 2001; A. Clericuzio, 'La chimica della vita: fermenti e fermentazione nella iatrochimica del Seicento', *Medicina nei secoli*, 15, 2003, pp. 227–46. To oversimplify their medical theories, Sylvius maintained that acids dissolved the blood whereas Willis believed they generally coagulated it.

[111] Da Sylva, *Romanorum lachrymae*, p. 35.

[112] A. Evangelista, *Lettera informativa intorno le cause delle morti improvise*, Rome, 1706, unpaginated.

[113] According to traditional physiology, vital spirits carried by the blood from the heart are transformed into animal spirits within the brain ventricles. These animal spirits produce sense and motion in the nerves; apoplexy occurs when the ventricles are obstructed by morbid matter. This account of apoplexy was undermined, more than by the simple discovery of the

blood, from which some sparks, similar to burning acid, passed into the nerves'; depending on the 'greater or lesser resistance which they found, they produced a diversity of symptoms of varying severity, and in greater or lesser time either killed or maimed'.

In fact, according to Evangelista, none of the recent deaths could be deemed to be unexpected. The unfortunate patients of his who died swiftly (he names several) were already suffering 'from other ailments, which were hidden initially', and especially 'slow fevers, but of a bad sort'. Indeed all is lost when the 'feverish ferment ... no longer fitting in the vessels, almost tyrannically occupies principal parts like the chest and the head'. As he explains, the noxious ferment is a 'very strong ferment or juice of an alien and perverse nature', which is produced mostly from food, according to the true teachings of Hippocrates and 'the new Hippocrates' Thomas Sydenham. Besides, Evangelista also praises Harvey, Charleton and Willis. Among the causes of the fatal ailment he also points to blood 'filled with nitro-sulphur, usually called elastic, from which the vessels become thicker too and sometime they lacerate'; unfit to achieve proper circulation, stagnant blood becomes acidic and corrodes the distressed vessels.

Da Sylva and Evangelista do not share the same views on treatment, either. Actually, there were few physicians who did agree on a remedy against the danger of unexpected death efficacious enough to reassure the distressed people of Rome. The usefulness of phlebotomy, for instance – for decades a controversial topic – was still a matter for heated debate. While da Sylva and Bernabei recommended this practice, Evangelista regarded bloodletting as 'always very dangerous', whereas Mistichelli warned against those 'blood-thirsty doctors who cannot undertake care of the sick without a lancet in the hand of the surgeon'.[114] Obviously, all of them insisted on the necessary caution in prescribing remedies. After all, prudence was the cornerstone of the canonical *methodus medendi*. As Bernabei put it, 'medicines are like excellent, precious and varied fabrics ... for clothes, but one wants a well trained tailor who may make a well fitting and suitable dress'.[115]

Hence, two physicians like da Sylva and Evangelista do not agree on the identification of the causes and the interpretation of the signs of sudden death, or on the treatments to prevent it. Their attitudes are also discordant. The Portuguese doctor is committed to the defence of the ancients, whereas the Italian Evangelista displays a more progressive, conciliatory stance. They are both testimonies to

---

circulation of the blood, by seventeenth-century research on the brain, which moved the main functions from the ventricle to the cortex and the deep cerebral structures. See Chapter 4 for more details on this topic.

[114]   D. Mistichelli, *Trattato dell'apoplessia*, Rome, 1709, p. 119. On bloodletting, see I.W. Müller, *Blutengeltherapie im 17. und 18. Jahrhundert*, Wolfenbüttel, 1985. Helmontians were especially opposed to bloodletting, and Evangelista does in fact refer to van Helmont.

[115]   A. Bernabei, *Dissertazione delle morti improvvise*, Rome, 1708, p. 43.

that plural, eclectic medicine that had replaced Galenism without abandoning it altogether. In truth, at the beginning of the eighteenth century, new and diverging theories contradicting or complementing the enduring tenets of humoral medicine had but increased the pluralism characterising early modern medicine.[116]

Nonetheless, da Sylva and Evangelista have much in common. In the first place, they resort to circulatory physiology and fermentation theory as the key to explain the sudden deaths of 1705 and 1706. Although circulatory physiology had been at the core of medical thinking for over half a century, it still provided a valuable resource for practical medicine insofar as it enabled a new stance on pathology.[117] The old notion of humoral plethora, for instance, could be adjusted into a more modern version to suit the discovery of blood circulation and the theory of fermentation. Second, the two physicians agree on the role of noxious exhalations and 'bad air', although the former advocates a qualitative chemical notion of corrupt air, while the latter favours a kind of corpuscularianism postulating the joint action of corpuscles and particles. As regards style of exposition, their discursive techniques and style of reasoning are also similar. Their demonstrations proceed from definitions (of diseases in general) to particulars (the sick patients), and from these to the identification of universal causes that encompass them all.[118] Their desire to provide exhaustive explanations – inherent in the social role of university-trained physicians – keeps both authors within the tradition of scholastic medicine. Although they briefly allude to autopsies performed on the corpses – something that we shall discuss later – they base the validity of their method on their own practice. Successful (or failed) *curationes* provide *a posteriori* evidence on diagnosis and treatment.

Another feature that da Sylva and Evangelista have in common is that instead of discussing death – what sudden and unexpected death is, and whether it is possible to foresee and prevent it – their analysis focuses on disease, putting more emphasis on prevention than on treatment. Accordingly, they agree on one point: nobody is safe unless they adopt a moderate and orderly lifestyle, the 'right and regulated life' recommended by the doctor. Both are adamant that the preservation of good health, and of life itself, consists mainly in controlling the six non-naturals. After all, warns da Sylva, 'gluttony kills more than the sword'.[119]

---

[116] Brambilla, 'La medicina del Settecento'.

[117] R.G. Frank, *Harvey and the Oxford Physiologists: A Study of Scientific Ideas*, Berkeley, 1980.

[118] I. Maclean, *Logic, Signs and Nature in the Renaissance: The Case of Learned Medicine*, Cambridge, 2002.

[119] Da Sylva, *Romanorum lachrymae*, p. 25. The so-called non-naturals (that is, elements that are not physical components of the body but have an effect upon it) were food and drink, air, motions and stillness, evacuation and retention, sleep and wakefulness, and the motion of the soul. They were the core of *regimina sanitatis*, on which see H. Mikkeli, *Hygiene in the Early Modern Medical Tradition*, Helsinki, 1999; M. Nicoud, *Les régimes de*

Such a preventative and behavioural approach to health can be found in all the authors writing on the subject of sudden death, regardless of their theories. Antonio Bernabei, for instance, identifies the main cause of sudden death in acids from food and corrupt air (equally caused by earthquakes, planetary influence and the exhalations of corpses). He suggests several preventative measures in order to remove 'from the bodies the bad dispositions they may have and remove those humours that can bring a man to the edge of the precipice': live in the mountains, dispel fumes in the air, make use of tobacco which can stir 'the dormant spirits in the brain', drink coffee, tea or chocolate, wines and sorbets, and, last but not least, 'live happily', since fear is the enemy of health.[120] According to Domenico Mistichelli, 'the dietary treatment' consists in 'not abusing the six non-natural things' while the 'preventive treatment'

> amounts to a certain way of life consisting on the one hand of a perfect diet, and on the other of the use of appropriate remedies ... whence one will live the days of one's life free from that prolonged death that is fear of sudden death.[121]

The 'moral' and individual approach to illness, one of the most enduring teachings of the ancients, was shared by experts and laypersons alike in dealing with sickness.[122] From this particular point of view, physicians speak a language that transcends theoretical differences and is accessible to all. Among other things, such an approach to health and illness helped explain why a certain illness affects some and spares others, an agonising question in the face of epidemics, especially when evidence of contagion was lacking as in the case of the sudden deaths in Rome. The reason for discrepancy is to be found in individual dispositions (in Evangelista's words 'the greater or lesser resistance found') and in the person's way of living.[123] Traditional medical authority was grounded precisely in this approach. Indeed, the university-educated physician related to his patient as an adviser, providing guidance for an overall action in order to restore good health, rather than a particular medicine for a specific disease. Knowledge (of the nature and causes of a disease), judgement (on each individual case) and advice (on how to preserve and restore health) were the fundamental means of conveying medical professional

---

santé au Moyen Âge: naissance et diffusion d'une écriture médicale (XIIIe–XVe siècle), Rome, 2007. For everyday practice of regimens, see S. Cavallo and T. Storey, *Healthy Living in Late Renaissance Italy*, Oxford, 2013.

[120]   Bernabei, *Dissertazione delle morti improvvise*, pp. 42, 45 and 84.

[121]   Mistichelli, *Trattato dell'apoplessia*, pp. 159 and 162–3.

[122]   R. Jütte, 'The Social Construction of Illness in the Early Modern Period', in *The Social Construction of Illness*, ed. J. Lachmund and G. Stollberg, Stuttgart, 1992, pp. 23–38.

[123]   A. Pastore, 'La morte e la peste: note sulla trattatistica medica della prima età moderna', in *Il medico di fronte alla morte (secoli XVI–XXI)*, ed. G. Cosmacini and G. Vigarello, Turin, 2008, pp. 33–51.

ideology.[124] They were also what set apart doctors of philosophy and medicine from charlatans. Not surprisingly, none of the Roman physicians mentioned above fails to expose the malpractice of unlicensed rivals, who intoxicate their gullible patients with aggressive, unspecific remedies made up 'of mercury, antimony, powders from Sicily, alabaster, steel, magnesia, and a thousand others of similar nature, which anybody is able to sell, even if they are not physicians'.[125]

Thus, while addressing a problem that they themselves made somehow collective, da Sylva and Evangelista interpret the issue of sudden death from the stance of individuals and as a matter of personal responsibility. Respectful of the Hippocratic-Galenic tradition which, despite theoretical updates, continues to be the basis of their conception of health and disease, their discussion leaves out the issue of death as such (which remains the insurmountable limit of the doctor–patient relationship). According to this traditional approach, physicians play a pastoral role similar in many ways to that of clergymen. After all, the temperance and sobriety that they recommend are in line with the moderate conduct expected of all good Christians. Incidentally, a greater authority was granted to medical opinion if it coincided with religious precepts[126] – did not the clergy preach fasting and abstinence as the only way to escape divine wrath and an unfortunate demise?

In conclusion, physicians in Rome did respond promptly to the general alarm caused by the 'epidemic' of unexpected deaths. As doctors of philosophy and medicine, they were required to provide guidance through their explanations of the causes of the frightful accidents and their advice on the way to prevent them – a task which they did not fail to fulfil, though they could not really impose rules of conduct as religious authorities could aspire to do, at least in papal Rome.[127] The question, however, is not so much whether physicians were

---

[124] H.J. Cook, 'Good Advice and Little Medicine: The Professional Authority of Early Modern English Physicians', *Journal of British Studies*, 33, 1994, pp. 1–31.

[125] Bernabei, *Dissertazione delle morti improvvise*, p. 7.

[126] A. Wear, *Knowledge and Practice in English Medicine, 1550–1680*, Cambridge, 2000, pp. 178–84.

[127] Plague outbreaks provided an opportunity to experiment with new instruments of social control and elaborate dystopias of authoritarian societies, as underscored by C. Jones, 'Plague and its Metaphors in Early Modern France', *Representations*, 53, 1996, pp. 97–127; Pastore, *Le regole dei corpi*, pp. 37–62. It should be noted anyway that a discrepancy persisted between the prudent and individualist medical approach to disease, including plague, and the urgency of political responses to it; see M. Dinges, 'Pest und Staat: von der Institutionengeschichte zur sozialen Konstruktion?', in *Neue Wege in der Seuchengeschichte*, ed. M. Dinges and T. Schlich, Stuttgart, 1995, pp. 71–103; M. Nicoud, 'I medici e l'ufficio della sanità a Milano nel Quattrocento', in *Le epidemie nei secoli XIV–XVII*, ed. A. Leone and G. Sangermano, Salerno, 2007, pp. 93–111. Segregation and containment of people suffering from the French pox, practised at the end of the fifteenth century, was soon discontinued,

willing to assume their traditional role in society, but if this was still consistent with the demands of society and political power; whether in fact the authority of the experts should not be re-established on the basis of new types of evidence and proof, by directly confronting death and the corpse.

and hospitals for 'incurables' lost their connotation of institutions of confinement; see J. Arrizabalaga, J. Henderson and R. French, *The Great Pox: The French Disease in Renaissance Europe*, New Haven, CT, 1997.

Chapter 2

The Medico-legal Enquiry on Sudden Death, or: The Truth of the Body and the Public Role of Physicians

An Anatomo-pathological Investigation 'at the Pope's Command'

All biographers of Clement XI invariably mention the calamities and 'unusual mortality' that Pope Albani had to brave. Armed with the weapons of faith he faced 'any dangerous, frightful and strange event that might ever occur ... in the twenty years during which he steered the apostolic vessel amid unceasing storms'.[1]

In truth, spiritual weapons were not the only resource the pope employed to halt the horror of sudden deaths. A prince as well as a pastor and a bishop, Clement had to attend to his temporal duties equipped with something more than just 'indulgences'. Hence, in order to restore calm and public confidence, he resorted to science. Very soon, at the beginning of 1706, he ordered the *protomedicus* (the state's Lead Physician who supervised and attended to all 'things pertaining to medicine')[2] and the papal secret *archiater* (the pope's first physician) to conduct an investigation.

It was the first time that science had been called upon to confront a sanitary crises other than the plague or similar pestilential fevers. Doctors were asked to give an expert opinion on the rising number of suspicious deaths; more precisely, their assignment was to 'investigate in depth the true causes of the rampant deaths by way of dissection of those who had died suddenly'.[3] The pope commanded that some corpses – exclusively men of modest condition – be publicly dissected in the anatomical theatre at Sapienza University, which was normally reserved for the anatomy lessons performed on the bodies of executed criminals. The Governor of Rome, Ranuccio Pallavicini, put men and means at

---

[1] *Vite degli arcadi illustri*, vol. 4, Rome, 1727, p. 12; S. Reboulet, *Histoire de Clément XI Pape*, Avignon, 1752, p. 173; P.-F. de Lafitau, *La vie de Clément XI souverain pontife*, Padua, 1752, pp. 169–71.

[2] The definition is taken from the ms *Discorso dell'inconvenienti che nascono nella medicina* by the Roman Protomedicus Lorenzo Garzonio (1619), ms ASR, Università di Roma, b. 61, fol. 776.

[3] Quoted from the dedicatory epistle and the *Occasio scribendi* in SM, page unnumbered.

the service of the appointed physicians to facilitate their work. A sensible and vigorous prelate, Pallavicini had already shown his ability by settling the quarrels and riots between the French and the Imperial factions that had upset Rome in connection with the War of the Spanish Succession. He had also acted promptly and energetically against the hoodlums who had terrorised Romans during the 1703 earthquake. Promoted to cardinal in May 1706, he would regrettably end his career on 30 June 1712 by falling victim to apoplexy himself.

The first autopsy was performed on the victim that had caused the most sensation, Cardinal Sacripanti's footman. On 18 January 1706 his corpse was examined in the anatomical theatre of the *studium* in the presence of the highest political and medical authorities and before an audience of doctors, surgeons and medical students. Michelangelo Paoli and Gaspare Reali, physicians of the apostolic palaces, and the doctor surgeon in charge of the city's prisons also attended. Incisions were carried out by the university official *sector*, Domenico Simoncelli.[4]

Of course, it was not the first time that corpses had been cut open in public. Albeit still infrequent, the dissection of corpses for didactic, legal or medical purposes was a widespread practice in the foremost European cities and universities.[5] Rome had been one of the main centres of the 'anatomical Renaissance' of the sixteenth century,[6] and dissections had been carried out in the university theatre since 1512.[7] It had then been the adoptive hometown of a group of celebrated anatomists, including Bartolomeo Eustachi, Juan Valverde de Amusco, Realdo Colombo and Arcangelo Piccolomini, who had profited from the pope's aspiration to promote the *studium urbis* and established anatomy as an academic discipline.[8] We shall leave aside for the moment discussion of

---

[4]   Ms BLR, Lancisi 300, fol. 264. Simoncelli had carried out research on the auditory nerve and the pineal gland; see *Lettres de G. Desnoues ... et de mr. Guglielmini ... sur différentes nouvelles découvertes*, Rome, 1706, pp. 205–11. On the division of tasks during dissections, see A. Carlino, *The Book of the Body: Anatomical Ritual and Renaissance Learning*, trans. J. Tedeschi and A.C. Tedeschi, Chicago, 1999.

[5]   R. French, *Dissection and Vivisection in the European Renaissance*, Aldershot, 1999; R. Mandressi, *Le regard de l'anatomiste: dissections et invention du corps en Occident*, Paris, 2003.

[6]   N.G. Siraisi, 'Life Sciences and Medicine in the Renaissance World', in *Rome Reborn: The Vatican Library and Renaissance Culture*, ed. A. Grafton, Washington, DC, 1993, pp. 169–98. Prohibition of the practice of dissection by the Church has been disproved by historians and a growing number of studies have reappraised the role played by the Church in its development. See, for instance, A. Paravicini Bagliani, *Medicina e scienze della natura alla corte dei papi nel Duecento*, Spoleto, 1991, pp. 269–79.

[7]   Carlino, *Book of the Body*, pp. 85–92.

[8]   A. Cunningham, *The Anatomical Renaissance: The Resurrection of the Anatomical Projects of the Ancients*, Aldershot, 1997.

dissections in hospitals, which also underwent great development in the second half of the seventeenth century.

It was also not the first time that doctors had been asked to examine corpses as experts and for legal purposes. Such practice went as far back as the thirteenth century and was particularly developed in countries under Roman Law,[9] and obviously in Rome, which was the seat of important tribunals with supranational jurisdiction, such as the Sacra Rota. Autopsies constituted a form of expert proof that was validated by both doctrine and practice. It was precisely a papal protomedicus, Paolo Zacchia, who codified it most authoritatively in his lengthy and successful *Quaestiones medico-legales*.[10] In truth, criminal justice was possibly the only field in Rome where doctors – together with the surgeons employed by the city governor – had exclusive jurisdiction upon death. It was their duty to inspect corpses that presented lesions or wounds and were found in suspicious circumstances. Otherwise, bodies were normally released to the deceased's family, parochial church or confraternity.

Occasionally, dissections of bodies were also performed in other contexts, always conferring scientific and professional distinction to physicians in their role as experts.[11] After the Council of Trent, canonisation procedures required doctors to carry out necropsies on the bodies of the candidates for sainthood. In Counter-Reformation Rome, several 'holy anatomies' had been performed, like that of Filippo Neri, founder of the Oratorians, in 1595.[12] As regards popes, whether or not they were considered for canonisation, their corpses were incised before the administration of funeral rites so as to exclude any suspicion of

---

[9] The first documented forensic autopsy was carried out in Bologna in 1302, according to A. Simili, 'The Beginning of Forensic Medicine in Bologna', in *International Symposium on Society, Medicine and Law*, ed. H. Karplus, Amsterdam, 1973, pp. 91–100. The medical expert witness role assumed increasing importance in parallel with the stabilisation of modern legal systems, and so did autopsy. See C. Crawford, 'Legalizing Medicine: Early Modern Legal Systems and the Growth of Medico-legal Knowledge', in *Legal Medicine in History*, ed. M. Clark and C. Crawford, Cambridge, 1994, pp. 89–116; A. Pastore, *Il medico in tribunale: la perizia medica nella procedura penale d'antico regime (secoli XVI–XVIII)*, Bellinzona, 1998.

[10] Published between 1621 and 1661, and on which see A. Pastore and G. Rossi, eds, *Paolo Zacchia: alle origini della medicina legale, 1584–1659*, Milan, 2008.

[11] A. Carlino, 'Il cadavere esibito: le poste in gioco dello spettacolo anatomico della medicina rinascimentale', *Micrologus*, 7, 1999, pp. 405–19.

[12] On 'holy autopsies', see K. Park, *Secrets of Women: Gender, Generation, and the Origins of Human Dissection*, New York, 2006, pp. 39–76, 161–80; E. Andretta, 'Anatomie du Vénérable dans la Rome de la Contre-réforme: les autopsies d'Ignace de Loyola et de Philippe Neri', in *Conflicting Duties: Science, Medicine and Religion in Rome 1550–1750*, ed. M.P. Donato and J. Kraye, London, 2009, pp. 255–80; B.A. Bouley, 'Contested Cases: Medical Evidence, Popular Opinion, and the Miraculous Body', in *Médecine et religion: collaborations, compétitions, conflits (XIIe–XXe siècles)*, ed. M.P. Donato et al., Rome, 2013, pp. 139–62.

homicide or simply to ascertain the cause of death, especially if they had passed on swiftly and unexpectedly. One such case, and possibly the first one, seems to have been that of Alexander V, who died suddenly in Bologna in 1410.[13] Subsequently, eight popes were subjected to post-mortem examination in the course of the sixteenth century, and almost all popes underwent the same procedure in the following century.[14] Autopsies were soon extended to cardinals and members of the aristocracy, as reliance on this practice to provide dependable empirical evidence of specific diseases increased.[15] By the end of the seventeenth century the practice had become customary, and autopsies of illustrious men and noble women were carried out in the domestic environment and made public through printed or manuscript reports. Last but not least, authorities could at times call for autopsies at the first signs of contagious disease in order to evaluate the situation and officially proclaim a state of emergency. When the plague struck Rome in 1656, for instance, two autopsies were immediately performed before quarantine was organised.[16]

Sudden death was *ipso facto* considered suspicious in all of the medico-legal literature. Only a medical expert could ascertain whether death was caused by poisoning or trauma or, conversely, by natural causes.[17] After all, murderers might very well be at work in that gloomy winter of 1706. All of Rome remembered the affair of the infamous 'venomous women' who, in 1657, taking advantage of the plague outbreak, had peddled 'pitchers of distilled water mixed with arsenic and quicksilver, with which many women had killed their husbands and other relatives'.[18] Their victims died 'without knowledge or understanding of their own ailment and ... though they were dead, they looked as if they were alive and

---

[13]   It is mentioned by the renowned surgeon Pietro d'Argelata, *Cirurgia*, Venice, 1497. On papal funeral rituals, see A. Paravicini Bagliani, *The Pope's Body*, trans. D.S. Peterson, Chicago, 2000, pp. 99–143; M.A. Visceglia, *Morte e elezione del papa: norme, riti e conflitti*, Rome, 2013. On medical expert witness reports on royal bodies, see G. Ricci, *Il principe e la morte: corpo, cuore, effigie nel Rinascimento*, Bologna, 1998, pp. 61–75.

[14]   R. Palmer, 'Medicine at the Papal Court in the Sixteenth Century', in *Medicine at the Courts of Europe, 1500–1837*, ed. V. Nutton, London, 1990, pp. 49–78.

[15]   N.G. Siraisi, 'Segni evidenti, teoria e testimonianza nelle narrazioni di autopsie del Rinascimento', *Quaderni Storici*, 36, 2001, pp. 719–44.

[16]   P. Savio, 'Ricerche sulla peste di Roma degli anni 1656–1657', *Archivio della Società romana di storia patria*, 95, 1972, pp. 113–42, esp. pp. 139–40.

[17]   E.H Ackerknecht, 'Early History of Legal Medicine', in *Legacies in Law and Medicine*, ed. C.R. Burns, New York, 1977, pp. 249–71, underlines the cautious position of F. Fideli's *De relationibus medicorum libri quatuor*, Palermo, 1602, especially pp. 345–9. See also *Il methodus testificandi di G.B. Codronchi*, ed. C. Puccini et al., Bologna, 1987, p. 27. A case of sudden death attributed to poison after post-mortem examination had revealed coagulated blood in J. Schenck, *Observationes medicarum rariores libri VII*, Lyon, 1644, p. 265.

[18]   G. Gigli, *Diario Romano (1608–1670)*, ed. G. Ricciotti, Rome, 1958, p. 486.

asleep', which aroused fears that a 'new kind of contagion' might be spreading.[19] Sixteenth- and seventeenth-century medical literature offers several examples of autopsies carried out in the presence of health officials on the victims of sudden death without apparent cause.[20] In 1651 suspect occurrences of abrupt death in Rome led doctors to perform a number of autopsies; a few years later, during the papacy of Alexander VII, 'many corpses of persons who died all of a sudden were opened by Giovanni Trullo, papal surgeon, who observed the rupture of blood vessels in the chest or in the head'.[21] However, Trullo's investigation had not the pomp, nor the procedures of the one disposed half a century later by Clement XI.

The sole fact that in 1706 the dissections were performed at the express command of the pope made the investigation into the mysterious deaths tremendously significant. The involvement of the highest medical figures in Rome further contributed to its prominence. Francesco Valesio recorded the momentous event in his diary on Monday, 18 January:

> Today, at La Sapienza, the protomedicus oversaw the opening of the corpse of Cardinal Sacripante's footman, who had died suddenly the day before; and in his brain they found oozed blood, which is deemed to have caused his death.[22]

On 3 February, Valesio recorded the autopsies of a labourer and a footman whose corpses were opened 'by pontifical order' once again in the presence of the protomedicus. The following month it was a barber's turn to be dissected.

In what constituted an unprecedented occurrence, a total of seven autopsies were performed in rapid succession at the university anatomical theatre in order to dispel any doubt. A report was compiled on behalf of the protomedicus by the College of Physicians' First Counsellor, Giacomo Sinibaldi, while Alessandro Pascoli, lecturer of anatomy and surgery at La Sapienza and ordinarily in charge of university anatomies, took pains to circulate relevant information.[23] The

---

[19] I quote from V. Paglia, *La morte confortata: riti della paura e mentalità religiosa a Roma nell'età moderna*, Rome, 1982, p. 128. On criminality during sanitary crisis, see A. Pastore, *Crimine e giustizia in tempo di peste nell'Europa moderna*, Rome and Bari, 1991, esp. pp. 187–204.

[20] D. Terilli, *De causis mortis repentinae tractatio in qua etiam disputatur quid sit mors et vita in genere et quae mortis causae communes, singula vero quae de causis mortis repentinae enarrantur*, Venice, 1615, pp. 2, 60.

[21] Reported by D. Panaroli, *Iatrologismorum, seu medicinalium observationum Pentecostae quinque*, 2nd edn, Rome, 1652, pp. 128–31, and in SM, p. 122.

[22] Valesio, vol. 3, p. 540.

[23] Sinibaldi, born in Rome, the son of a prominent physician, was professor of *materia medica* and later of theoretical and practical medicine at Sapienza University. In 1681, he compared Willis' and Sylvius's theories of fevers in a tract entitled *Dell'abuso dei vescicatori*, which was one of the first systematic discussions of the fermentative and circulation doctrines

wide dissemination of the results of the autopsies can be gathered from the fact that Valesio (the son of a medical doctor, but not one himself) was able to note down a concise record of them in his diary: in February the investigative medical committee 'found hydrops in the chest of the labourer and oozed blood in the heart of the footman', while the barber was deemed the victim of an 'aneurysm in the heart'.[24] News of the conclusions from the official investigation can be found in a variety of sources, including non-medical ones.[25]

And the results were decidedly positive. Indeed, post-mortems allowed the protomedicus to issue a reassuring verdict. There was no contagion, nor could there be any talk of a true epidemic. Every case proved to be the outcome of a different pathological condition, for the most part caused by defects in the composition and the circulation of the blood, in line with the then fashionable theories of blood fermentation and coagulation. The authorities stated that, just as everyone believed, earthquakes might also have contributed releasing noxious exhalations in the air. All things considered, Romans could be reassured. No mysterious pestilence plagued the city, and the repeated occurrences of sudden death were fully explicable by the experts on the evidence of post-mortem examinations.

The papal physician Giovanni Maria Lancisi, appointed by the pope to supervise the investigation, came to the same conclusions. In the dedicatory epistle of his theoretical and practical treatise *De subitaneis mortibus* (*On Sudden Death*), initially circulated in manuscript and printed in 1707, Lancisi praised Pope Clement XI because

> When the terror of sudden death had been rampant in the city for months, nothing, except imploring divine aid, came to your mind before the idea that, once the causes had been discovered, the evil would be extirpated.[26]

Lancisi reiterated as often as he could that the investigation had been carried out at the express command of the pope, every time emphasising the importance of necropsy in the solution to the mystery of the sudden deaths. The autopsies at La Sapienza were recounted in detail in the second book of the treatise. According to Lancisi, the diversity of lesions that were found in each of the examined corpses

---

in Rome. On Pascoli, see L. Guerrini, *Il grande affare della sapienza umana: scienza e filosofia nell'opera di Alessandro Pascoli (1669–1757)*, Florence, 2000, and Pascoli's own *Opere scelte*, ed. C. Vinti, M. Bastianelli and A. Allegra, Perugia, 2007.

[24]   Valesio, vol. 3, pp. 549, 570.

[25]   References to the protomedicus' report can be found in A. Evangelista, *Lettera informativa intorno le cause delle morti improvise*, Rome, 1706, and M. da Sylva, *Romanorum lachrymae subitaneis mortibus effusae exsiccantur*, Rome, 1706, pp. 9–10, 31. Unfortunately this document seems not to have survived, and its content can only be indirectly surmised.

[26]   SM, dedicatory epistle, unnumbered page.

constituted the most significant result yielded by dissection. Such lesions were situated mostly in the heart, in the large blood vessels and in the brain meninges of the deceased, and therefore clearly pointed to pre-existing conditions:

> Not a few were taken away with the indication of a blood vessel in the chest or in the abdomen already weakened by a varix or aneurysm which suddenly ruptured. Many died because of severe apoplexy caused by the blood intercepted and effused in the brain. Finally, others died because of severe, persistent spasms or paralysis in the *praecordia*, or due to an obstruction in the passages of the heart or large blood vessels.[27]

Consequently, post-mortem evidence showed that each death could be ascribed to specific, individual causes and was merely the tragic outcome of pre-existing conditions. There was no epidemic illness or pestilence to be afraid of, as 'in great part, the deaths were not of people in good health, but ... [of people] whose health had been for some time overtly or covertly weakened'.[28] Lancisi expatiated upon death and the circumstances by which it might be considered unexpected. This was indeed a rare occurrence, according to the papal physician, and one that is invariably preceded by a phase of pathological condition upon which, however brief, doctors might be able to act before the final crisis. Five cases were then expounded in greater detail in the book: a 'syncopal apoplexy'; a syncope due to enlargement, prolapse and aneurysm of the heart; a cerebral congestion; an apoplexy following convulsions of the meninges and of the heart; and an aneurysm in the pulmonary artery with sudden rupture of the vena cava.

As for Rome, Lancisi observed that the unusual mortality resulting from unexpected accidents counterbalanced the decreased incidence of other seasonal affections. Drawing on Hippocrates, particularly on the Hippocratic treatise *On Airs, Waters and Places* in which the negative effects of seasonal changes were expounded, he argued that climate had most certainly precipitated the crisis. The abrupt shifts between warm and cold periods and the southern winds had arguably increased the normal dispersion of the volatile components of corporeal fluids, causing irregularities in their composition and movement. These in turn damaged the solid parts of the body, as revealed by dissection in examining the corpses of people seized by sudden death. The archiater also underlined the role of food and lamented the dangers to which the poorest of the population were exposed. The poor could in fact easily fall victim to rotten food and to improper medication by charlatans. Therefore, stricter control on all branches of the healing art, always recommendable, was now urgent, together with other sanitary and charitable measures to improve the general welfare of the citizens of

---

[27] SM, pp. 113–14.
[28] SM, p. 114.

Rome. In line with several colleagues who had already intervened in this debate, however, Lancisi also recommended a sober lifestyle and moderate regimen as the best preventative measure against sudden death. And he did not refrain from putting forward a curative strategy, presenting a number of medicinal remedies which had been tested successfully during the most acute phase of the supposed 'epidemic', so that

> If ever conditions should arise similar to those of last year, doctors might find protective measures founded on the present investigation, so that ... fragile persons can be wholly protected from the danger of death or at the least gain time ... to atone for their sins and recommend themselves to God.[29]

Hence, the protomedicus and the papal physician were able to produce two reassuring verdicts in the light of the *sensata cognitio* of dissections, and through the trustworthy testimony of a legitimate group of learned experts. With the support of the pope (who had granted access to the bodies), medical officials could successfully and authoritatively base their explanations and reassurances on the empirical evidence of post-mortems. 'The Holy Father's command to unearth the hidden truth with the anatomist's knife', to use Lancisi's words,[30] put an end to speculation and fear. True, cases of unexpected death continued – no less than eight were recorded by Valesio from April to October 1706[31] – but they were divested of the frightful, obscure aura they initially had. Although the debate among medical practitioners did not give any sign of relenting after the official investigation was closed, none could but take the autopsies into account and relinquish any talk of mysterious facts or supernatural causes whatsoever.

In short, it was a great success for all the parties involved in the investigation. In the mid-seventeenth century, Pope Alexander VII's decisive action in tackling the tragic outbreak of the plague had shown how a health crisis could engender consensus; 50 years later, Pope Albani resorted to the same strategy in facing an unprecedented threat that was promptly accounted for by his doctors. Fear gave way to celebration as Clement XI was saluted as a charitable and enlightened prince. In the immediate wake of the investigation, so as to further enhance the medical establishment's authority and give additional proof of the pope's concern, the protomedicus seized the opportunity to order a general inspection of all tobacco sellers. Since noxious exhalations had not been ruled out as a possible factor in the spate of mortality, measures were adopted to improve the salubrity of the city: trees were planted in the streets and in the squares 'for the benefit of all, since the heat of the sun, particularly in summer, is usually noxious

---

[29] SM, p. 126.
[30] SM, p. 113.
[31] *Diario di Clemente XI*, fol. 235v; *Gazzetta di Bologna*, 21 September 1706.

to health'; the small lake Marta was drained; new rules for the collection of waste were enacted and thorough cleaning of houses and cellars was carried out 'under the watch of his Holiness, our Lord, who with paternal charity and zeal tends to the health and safety of his subjects'.[32]

The Reasons for Success: the Protomedicate, the Roman College of Physicians and the Governance of Medicine

As has already been discussed, corpses had been dissected well before 1706. However, in that year, autopsies were performed for both medical and legal purposes on an unusually high number of bodies, and in the context of a wide-ranging, official and widely publicised investigation ordered by the pope. It was also the first time that the anatomo-pathological method had been applied not to individuals but to confront a public health issue. Furthermore, it was employed not to ascertain the existence of a familiar disease (like the plague) but to investigate the causes of death and the nature of unknown illness. According to some historians of medicine, this was indeed the 'first epidemiological investigation on a non-transmissible condition' carried out using a method that was later to become established, albeit by slow, uneven progression.[33] Why, might one ask, did such remarkable innovation originate in Rome? Up until then, nothing particularly differentiated the pontifical capital from other early modern cities in which the dissection of corpses was practised, a lively medical community operated and generic forms of health surveillance were in place. So why Rome?

Presumably, the critical political situation at the beginning of the eighteenth century gave impetus to Clement XI's determination to act decisively and thus give a clear signal of the government's vigilance. Was it not the pope's habit to watch over the city with his crystal spy-glass leaning over his balcony? War on the borders, public disorder in the streets, crimes still unpunished (such as the prank of the fabricated order to the citizens to vacate their homes during the earthquake), all contributed to an explosive situation that any untoward event might ignite. It was common knowledge that criminal gangs often took advantage of sanitary emergencies to commit their crimes, and only three

---

[32]   Edicts of the Presidente delle strade (Supervisor of the streets) Nicolò del Giudice of 17 February 1706; the Treasurer Lorenzo Corsini, 30 April 1706; the Presidente delle strade Fabrizio Augustini, 21 January 1707 and 14 April 1707.

[33]   J.O. Leibowitz, *The History of Coronary Heart Disease*, Berkeley, CA, 1970, p. 75. The Roman medical investigation is discussed in C.A Wunderlich, *Handbuch der Pathologie und Therapie*, 2nd edn, vol. 1, Stuttgart, 1852, p. 53; H. Haeser, *Lehrbuch der Geschichte der Medicin und der epidemischen Krankheiten*, 3rd edn, vol. 2, Jena, 1881, pp. 600–602, 630; M.D. Altschule, *Essays on the Rise and Decline of Bedside Medicine*, Bangor, PA, 1988, p. 64.

years had passed since the fear of plague-spreaders had come back to the city.[34] Accordingly, post-mortem examinations were conducted in the presence of the prison surgeon (who was officially in charge of writing up police reports in cases of murder or other criminal offences) and of the judges and notary of the governor's tribunal to serve a dual purpose: underlining the official nature of the procedure and sending an explicit warning to potential scoundrels. At any rate, in September 1706 the freshly appointed Governor Francesco Caffarelli issued new stringent measures against loafers and layabouts.

Generally, in his administration of temporal as well as of spiritual affairs, Giovan Francesco Albani strove to advance the reforms implemented over the previous decades. These reforms were common to most European monarchies of the time and aimed at promoting absolutism without upsetting the overall balance of powers of corporatism on which rested *ancien régime* society. In the case in point, the measures taken in Rome highlighted the authoritarian traits of the ecclesiastical monarchy in line with a traditional concept of 'good rule' (*buon governo*); the pope, however, was now no longer seen as the mere guarantor of good governance but as an active agent, and enabled as such to alter social relations.[35] In other words, Pope Albani favoured a strong government under the direct authority of the sovereign pontiff that was liable to regain credit both within the state and beyond. The vigorous management of the sudden death crisis was arguably an instance of such policy.

However, the political motives underlying the 1706 events cannot completely account for the response to the crisis. After all, it was the first time that doctors were called upon to confront a threat to public safety. Unlike other cities in Italy, Rome did not have a permanent health board overseeing public health nor a health and demographic surveillance system. A special congregation composed

---

[34]   P. Preto, *Epidemia, paura e politica nell'Italia moderna*, Rome and Bari, 1987, pp. 100–102.

[35]   P. Prodi, *The Papal Prince. One Body and Two Souls: The Papal Monarchy in Early Modern Europe*, trans. S. Haskins, Cambridge, 1987, pp. 33–6, regards the end of the seventeenth century as a period of decline for the papal monarchy. Conversely, M. Rosa, 'Aspetti del pontificato di Innocenzo XII', in *Riforme, religione e politica durante il pontificato di Innocenzo XII 1691–1700*, ed. B. Pellegrino, Lecce, 1994, pp. 9–22, underscores the concentration of power brought about by late seventeenth-century reforms and the influence of French absolutism. S. Andretta, 'Clemente XI', in DBI, vol. 26, 1982, pp. 302–20, insists on the disproportion between the scale of Pope Albani's ambitions and the actual outcomes of his politics. See also V. Reinhardt, *Überleben in der frühneuzeitlichen Stadt: Annona und Getreideversorgung in Rom 1563–1797*, Tübingen, 1991, pp. 147–474; S. Tabacchi, 'Le riforme giudiziarie nella Roma di fine Seicento', *Roma moderna e contemporanea*, 5, 1997, pp. 155–76; S. Tabacchi, *Il Buon Governo: le finanze locali nello Stato della Chiesa (secoli XVI–XVIII)*, Rome, 2007, pp. 338–74. On the general periodisation of Italian history, see M. Verga, 'Tra Sei e Settecento: un'età delle preriforme?', *Storica*, 1, 1995, pp. 89–122.

exclusively of prelates was established only in the event of plague outbreaks, resorting to physicians only as consultants, at best. Ordinary administrative bodies such as the congregation of the Sacra Consulta had some generic competence in the salubrity of rural areas.[36] Of course, in Rome, as much as elsewhere, there were corporative structures such as the College of Physicians and the Protomedicate charged by the central power with the supervision of all healing practices, whose role in promoting innovation should not be overlooked.

Strictly speaking, the College regulated doctorates, licences and patents, and arbitrated contention among practitioners, whereas it was the protomedicus' duty to 'deal with, govern, order and regulate the affairs pertaining to the College and punish whosoever exercises the medical or chemical art without a licence'.[37] More specifically, he conducted an annual visit to the apothecaries and supervised medical practice in Rome and its surroundings and in a large part of the Papal States. Since in *ancien régime* society policing the corporative organisation was conceived as the first and best way to defend public health, both institutions acquired remarkable power in the course of the sixteenth century. Their strength was further fostered by the consolidation of the papal monarchy.[38] Flexible policies, the presence of strong and respected personalities

---

[36] According to F.A. Zaccaria, *Lo Stato presente o sia la relazione della Corte di Roma già pubblicata dal cav. Lunadoro ... ritoccata, accresciuta, ed illustrata*, vol. 2, Rome, 1774, p. 118, the Consulta had 'supreme criminal and civil jurisdiction ... it hears the petitions of the people against governors, rectors and other state officials, rectifies unjust taxation imposed on subjects; hears vassals' complaints against feudal lords ... watches over the salubrity of the provinces, and dispenses the orders that are necessary to keep away contagious diseases that might strike, and disposes all of the provisions needed to ensure the tranquillity of the state'. On early modern health boards, see C.M. Cipolla, *Public Health and the Medical Profession in the Renaissance*, Cambridge, 1976; C.M. Cipolla, *Miasmas and Disease: Public Health and the Environment in the Pre-Industrial Age*, trans. E. Potter, New Haven and London, 1992. More particularly on Venice, where a very active health board operated, see N.E. Vanzan Marchini, *I mali e i rimedi della Serenissima*, Vicenza, 1995.

[37] I quote from article XIV of the 1531 College *Statuta*, on which see F. Garofalo, *Quattro secoli di vita del Protomedicato e del Collegio dei medici di Roma: regesti dei documenti dal 1471 al 1870*, Rome, 1950. For a more general overview, see D. Gentilcore, "All that pertains to medicine": Protomedici and Protomedicati in Early Modern Italy', *Medical History*, 38, 1994, pp. 121–42; D. Gentilcore, *Healers and Healing in Early Modern Italy*, Manchester, 1998; A. Pastore, *Le regole dei corpi: medicina e disciplina nell'Italia moderna*, Bologna, 2006, pp. 125–54. The difference between the consulting prerogatives of Protomedicates and the executive capacities of health boards is underlined by G. Pomata, *Contracting a Cure: Patients, Healers, and the Law in Early Modern Bologna*, Baltimore and London, 1998, p. 13.

[38] L.A. Braconi, 'Materiali d'archivio per la storia del Collegio medico romano nel Seicento e nel Settecento', *Annali di storia delle università italiane*, 4, 2000, pp. 27–38; E. Andretta, *Roma medica. Anatomie d'un système médical: Rome, XVIe siècle*, Rome, 2012.

with close connections to the papal court and tighter relations with the curia than with the (less powerful) municipal administration enabled the College and the Protomedicate to manage the complex but flourishing health marketplace of the capital successfully and even extend their ambitions to the provincial market.[39] And although the seventeenth century marked a period of relative difficulty for both institutions, characterised by social and intellectual disruptions and culminating in the plague of 1656,[40] nonetheless the College and the protomedicus successfully regained trust of the people and authority in the last decades of the century.

The revival of the two institutions encompassed three main strands: increased control over medical education and practice, intervention in matters of public health and intellectual renovation. A long phase of reorganisation was indeed launched aiming at centralisation and rationalisation. Its main outcomes included the revision of all licences for the minor healing arts (1671), the institution of a register (*matricola*) of physicians approved for practice after a period of apprenticeship (1673), the reform of the College's statutes (1676), new agreements with the corporation of apothecaries and, most importantly, the creation of a 'permanent magistrature' within the College, consisting of four doctors elected for life who would take on the role of protomedicus in turn. Despite sporadic failings, the corporate system was sensibly strengthened and its sphere of influence significantly expanded.[41] At the same time, the public face of the two chief medical institutions was boosted by activities such as chemical analysis of mineral waters[42] and the gathering of demographic records 'for the

---

[39]   On municipal government in early modern Rome in relation to papal government, see L. Nussdorfer, *Civic Politics in the Rome of Urban VIII*, Princeton, 1992.

[40]   M.P. Donato, 'La peste dopo la peste: economia di un discorso romano (1656–1720)', *Roma moderna e contemporanea*, 14, 2006, pp. 159–74.

[41]   A. Kolega, 'Speziali, spagirici, droghieri e ciarlatani: l'offerta terapeutica a Roma tra Seicento e Settecento', *Roma moderna e contemporanea*, 4, 1998, pp. 311–48; M.P. Donato, 'La medicina a Roma tra Sei e Settecento: una proposta di interpretazione', *Roma moderna e contemporanea*, 13, 2005, pp. 99–114. For actions to infringe the customary *ius doctorandi* of institutions other than the College of Physicians, in the framework of Clement XI's attempt to revive the Roman *studium* and limit the autonomy of local political bodies in the Papal States, see ms ASR, Università di Roma, b. 4 and 16, and M.R. Di Simone, *La "Sapienza" romana nel Settecento: organizzazione universitaria e insegnamento del diritto*, Rome, 1980. After the suppression of his criminal jurisdiction brought about by the overall reform of Roman tribunals (1692), in 1699 the protomedicus obtained from the Consulta the right to be assisted by armed men while carrying out inspection of apothecaries: ms ASR, Università di Roma, b. 58, fasc. 61.

[42]   During the pontificate of Innocent XI, for instance, physicians tested the chemical composition and quality of the *Acqua acetosa* water because of a number of presumed unexpected deaths 'following its consumption'; see ms ASR, Università di Roma, b. 58, fasc. 51. Experiments and chemical analysis of other mineral waters are reported, for example,

many observations that may be done surrounding the quality of air and other affairs concerning public health'.[43] Meanwhile, the intellectual make up of the College also changed as a result of the admission of younger colleagues whose education had taken place in the years from 1660 to 1680, a time of rapid theoretical and ideological renewal for medicine. Opening up to novel scientific ideas, Roman corporative authorities thus came to represent a wider spectrum of the positions and tenets that coexisted in the medical world, thus rebutting criticism and blunting discontent.[44]

In other words, although at the beginning of the eighteenth century collegiate regulatory bodies and the hierarchic organisation of medical practice were often the focus of criticism and conflict in many parts of Europe, the papal Protomedicate and Roman College of Physicians were dynamic and relatively powerful institutions. They had resisted the erosion of the dogmatic monopoly of learned medicine by modernising regulations, extending their jurisdiction and opening up to innovative ideas. Each had also renewed its ties of alliance with the pontifical monarchy, at that time also actively seeking to extend its power. It is no accident that, between October 1705 and January 1706, the pope, 'applying his paternal piety to the long and healthy preservation of his subjects', restored the autonomous civil and criminal jurisdiction of the College.[45]

---

in C. Fontana, *All'Eminentissimi ... Cardinali della Sacra Congregatione dell'Acque. Esposto*, Rome, 1694; C. Meyer, *Nuovi ritrovamenti dati in luce per eccitare l'ingegno de' virtuosi*, Rome, 1689; F. Bianchini, *Opuscula varia*, Rome, 1753, vol. 1, pp. 35–50; P.A. Giulianelli, *Essame delle acque di Civita Vecchia, e di Trevi*, Rome, 1701. On the controls on tobacco manufactures, see ms ASR, Università di Roma, b. 58, fasc. 56.

[43] In all likelihood, physicians inspired the cardinal vicar's decision to list, from 1702 onwards, births and deaths in the *stati delle anime*, the parish registers, as stated in ms ASVR, *Istruzzione circa il modo di comporre lo stato delle anime nella città di Roma ... secondo il calcolo che si fa ogn'anno per ordine del'E.mo Sig.re Cardinale Vicario, 1600–1710*. I am grateful to Massimo Cattaneo for bringing this document to my attention.

[44] Donato, 'La medicina a Roma'. The College established connections with scientific institutions abroad and participated in research on the chemical composition of the blood initiated by R. Vieussens and inspired by Boyle's work (ms London, Royal Society Archives, Class. Papers XIV (i) 53 and RBC 8, fols 177–9, later published in *Philosophical Transactions*, 22, 1700–1701, pp. 599–610, and in Lancisi, *Opera*, vol. 2, Geneva, 1718, pp. 257–67). On the strained relations within the corporate medical organisation at the end of the seventeenth century, see E. Brambilla, 'La medicina del Settecento: dal monopolio dogmatico alla professione scientifica', in *Storia d'Italia, Annali 7, Malattia e medicina*, ed. F. Della Peruta, Turin, 1984, pp. 5–147, esp. pp. 33–9. A similar evolution of the London College of Physicians is analysed by T.M. Brown, 'The College of Physicians and the Acceptance of Iatromechanism in England, 1665–1695', *Bulletin of the History of Medicine*, 44, 1970, pp. 12–30.

[45] The quotation is from an edict issued by the Cardinal Chamberlain on 6 October 1705, now in ASR, Università di Roma, b. 58, fasc. 58.

It can therefore be argued that the College's recent evolution contributed to inducing the Roman medical establishment to promote, rather than hinder, an innovation that potentially increased its authority in the shadow of the monarch. In concordance with their ambitions, Roman medical magistrates undertook the task of uncovering the causes of sudden death through 'repeated dissections' with the full awareness that the medical inquest – ordered by the pope in the midst of what was universally perceived as a great danger to the population – would strengthen their prestige and possibly extend their prerogatives over the life and death of the citizens.

The Quest for Evidence

I have argued that the success of the 1706 investigation resulted from the underlying general political and administrative orientations of the papal monarchy at the turn of the seventeenth and eighteenth centuries, as well as from the institutional evolution of the two main health authorities in the capital city. Admittedly, these trends were common to other European states at the time, and occasionally encompassed health issues in the framework of mercantilist or early cameralist policies.[46] However, the pope's authority over the temporal as well as the spiritual, and the pronounced paternalism connected to the double nature of the papal monarchy made Rome unique and a particularly favourable context for innovation.

A further decisive element, and in a way peculiar to the case in point, was the cultural context of early eighteenth-century Rome. One of the major protagonists of the events discussed, the papal physician Giovan Maria Lancisi, offers us a revealing clue in this respect. In the dedicatory epistle prefacing his treatise *De subitaneis mortibus*, Lancisi extolled Clement XI as a generous protector of learning, and invited him to make of Rome an 'Attic Academy' of all modern sciences. Lancisi thus placed the Sapienza medical inquest (and his own treatise, of course) under the aegis of the pope as part of Albani's project for the political and cultural revival of Rome.

---

[46]   R.A. Dorwart, 'The Royal College of Medicine and Public Health in Brandenburg-Prussia, 1685–1740', *Medical History*, 2, 1958, pp. 13–23, H.J. Cook, *The Decline of the Old Medical Regime in Stuart London*, Ithaca and London, 1986 and A. Lunel, *La maison médicale du Roi: XVIe–XVIIIe siècles. Le pouvoir royal et les professions de santé (médecins, chirurgiens, apothicaires)*, Seyssel, 2008, point at a similar institutional dynamic in other contexts and analyse how the monarchy used the corporative structure of the capital city in an attempt to extend its control over the healing professions in the whole state, although the major eighteenth-century intellectual, social and political transformations eventually collapsed corporatism, as shown, among others, by L. Brockliss and C. Jones, *The Medical World of Early Modern France*, Oxford, 1997.

Ever since his election in 1700, Clement XI – who had been educated in the refinements of modern French culture – followed an ambitious, sophisticated agenda, combining the widespread post-Westphalia expectations of Church reform and the transformation of the European mind.[47] It represented the 'last flare of curialism, but at the same time a project of reform and a yearning for Christian universalism'.[48] The arts and letters, the sciences, the splendours ancient and modern were meant to protect the inviolability and sanctity of Rome from the warring European powers and make it 'the sanctuary of the arts of peace'.[49]

Implemented by means of a revived large-scale patronage, Clement XI's cultural programme was not a mere reaction to the new universalistic ambitions of the great foreign monarchies, which were by then competing in equipping their capital cities with modern scientific institutions and splendid monuments.[50] It was shaped by the aspiration to prove the pope's prerogatives beyond doubt, document the history of Rome and of the Catholic Church, and display them in their indisputable materiality. Accordingly, an obsession with proof loomed in ecclesiastical history, in antiquarianism and in all other disciplines, in reaction to the sceptical arguments of libertines and secular jurisdictionalists. The investigation into sudden death happened in the same years that astronomer and antiquarian Francesco Bianchini built a meridian in order to amend the Gregorian calendar by means of well-grounded experiments (*certis experimentis*). These took place in St Mary of the Angels, the Roman basilica situated in the ancient baths of Diocletian and steeped in the solemnity of the ancient Romans and the sanctity of Christian martyrs.[51] At that time, Roman men of letters and antiquarians undertook the systematic study of the material testimonies to the

---

[47] I borrow the definition from Paul Hazard's influential book *The European Mind, 1680–1715*, trans. J.L. May, London, 1953.

[48] G. Ricuperati, 'Francesco Bianchini e l'idea di storia universale "figurata"', *Rivista storica italiana*, 117, 2005, pp. 872–943, quotation at p. 909; V. Ferrone, *Scienza, natura, religione: mondo newtoniano e cultura italiana nel primo Settecento*, Naples, 1982, pp. 57–95, 366–94.

[49] As stated by F. Bianchini, *De kalendario et cyclo Caesaris ac ... descriptio, et explanatio basis in Campo Martio nuper detectæ sub columna Antonino Pio olim dicata*, Rome, 1703, p. 2.

[50] J.E. McClellan, *Science Reorganized: Scientific Societies in the Eighteenth Century*, New York, 1985; F. Waquet, *Le modèle français et l'Italie savante: conscience de soi et perception de l'autre dans la république des lettres, 1660–1750*, Rome, 1989; D. Roche, 'Académies et académisme: le modèle français au XVIIIe siècle', *Mélanges de l'École française de Rome: Italie et Méditerranée*, 108, 1996, pp. 643–58; C. Charle, ed., *Le temps des capitales culturelles: XVIIIe–XXe siècles*, Seyssel, 2009. On the artistic rivalry associated with the myth of the universal monarchy, see D. Erben, *Paris und Rom: die staatlich gelenkten Kunstbeziehungen unter Ludwig XIV*, Berlin, 2004.

[51] J.L. Heilbron, *The Sun in the Church: Cathedrals as Solar Observatories*, Cambridge, MA, 1999.

past, such as medals and bas-reliefs. The same Bianchini, appointed prefect of the antiquities of Rome, promoted the first ban on the export of archaeological artefacts and artworks in 1701 and 1704. He then also began working on the creation of a Museum of Sacred History in the Vatican, which would host the material sources of that indisputable history of the Roman Church based on 'monuments' set out by Bianchini himself in his *Istoria universale provata con monumenti, e figurata con simboli degli Antichi* (1697). It is the period, in short, when something close to a 'scientific gaze' was first cast on the past and on Nature, a time marked by the coexistence of revived apologetic aims and a new critical stance.[52] The quest for evidence and the pursuit of irrefutable proofs are a common thread in the cultural patronage of Pope Albani in defence of the Apostolic See, the Roman magisterium and the pontifical government.

The medical inquest on sudden death, extraordinary as it was, can be read as yet another facet of Albani's patronage of science and must be set against the background of the quest for evidence in contemporary culture. If specimens of material culture such as archaeological finds and works of art did not lie, neither did corpses opened up before an audience of trustworthy witnesses and experts. In Lancisi's words, dissections were indeed *tuta ac solida experimenta*. Accordingly, the anatomo-pathological inquest of 1706 was not solely a policing action, a demonstration of power in the management of public security, nor was it a generic instance of scientific patronage. It was just as much the expression of this precise intellectual tendency.

Moreover, upon this same intellectual stance rested the conception of medicine as rational experimental science upheld by the moderns that underpinned the Roman medical investigation. It should not be overlooked that, although by the early eighteenth century necropsy was commonly acknowledged as useful, it still met with some opposition. Insistence on the truthfulness of dissected bodies was a distinctive tenet of 'neoterics' or modern rationalists, who viewed normal and morbid anatomy as the foundation of the knowledge of the body and the understanding of illness. However, there were still many advocates of a medicine based on observation and induction, who upheld the traditional separation between theoretical and practical medicine and voiced scepticism about the real benefits of morbid anatomy for medical practice.

---

[52]   C.M.S. Johns, *Papal Art and Cultural Politics: Rome in the Age of Clement XI*, Cambridge, 1993, pp. 24, 196; F. de Polignac and J. Raspi Serra, eds, *La fascination de l'Antique, 1700–1770 Rome découverte, Rome inventée*, Lyon, 1998; V. Kockel and B. Sölch, eds, *Francesco Bianchini und die europäische gelehrte Welt um 1700*, Berlin, 2005 (particularly relevant here is C.M.S. Johns, 'Pope Albani and Francesco Bianchini: Intellectual and Visual Culture in Early Eighteenth-Century Rome', pp. 41–55). For the scientific and religious antecedents to these intellectual developments, see B. Neveu, *Érudition et religion aux XVIIe et XVIIIe siècles*, Paris, 1994.

It is worth remembering that, only a few years prior to the Sapienza investigation, the 'rationalists' and the 'empiricists' had violently clashed over the usefulness of anatomy and of microscope observations for practical medicine. The conflict crystallised around the celebrated anatomist Marcello Malpighi and his colleague and opponent at the University of Bologna, Girolamo Sbaraglia.[53] The appointment of the former as chief physician to Pope Innocent XII in 1692 marked a great symbolic victory for the moderns. Nevertheless, the controversy continued, and became entrenched with the suspicions of heterodoxy associated with atomism. Atomism was the more or less overt postulate at the basis of the 'subtle anatomy' of the moderns, understood as the study of the basic components of all physical objects, including the human body. In the final decade of the seventeenth century, the defenders of scholasticism and, most importantly, the Inquisition launched a violent attack against atomistic philosophy, which involved a number of prominent physicians in Rome and elsewhere.[54] After Malpighi's death in 1694, Giorgio Baglivi, now professor of practical medicine in Rome, took over the defence of normal, morbid and comparative anatomy (*De Praxi Medica*, 1696). Baglivi and Lancisi, who taught anatomy in the same university at the time, collaborated on the edition of Malpighi's *Opera posthuma*, which included his most significant methodological writings.[55] The conflict was, however, not over. In the first years of the eighteenth century, while Sbaraglia responded to Malpighi posthumously, others in Rome wrote against the use of the microscope in anatomy as inconsistent, useless for medical practice and, moreover, theologically suspect.[56] Proponents of modern rational medicine reacted in 1705 with a caustic *Epistola*, written under a pseudonym by Giovan

---

[53]   M. Cavazza, 'The Uselessness of Anatomy: Mini and Sbaraglia versus Malpighi', in *Marcello Malpighi: Anatomist and Physician*, ed. D. Bertoloni Meli, Florence, 1997, pp. 129–45. The two coteries drew their names and a number of contentious topics from the ancient medical sects, recently discussed in V. Nutton, *Ancient Medicine*, London, 2004. On the controversies surrounding the use of the microscope, see C. Wilson, *The Invisible World: Early Modern Philosophy and the Invention of the Microscope*, Princeton, 1995.

[54]   L. Osbat, *L'inquisizione a Napoli: Il processo agli ateisti, 1688–1697*, Rome, 1974; P. Galluzzi, 'La scienza davanti alla Chiesa e al Principe in una polemica universitaria del secondo Seicento', in *Studi in onore di Arnaldo d'Addario*, ed. L. Borgia et al., vol. 4, Lecce, 1995, pp. 1317–44.

[55]   In particular Malpighi's *Risposta* to Sbaraglia's pamphlet *De recentiore medicorum studio dissertatio*, now in *Opere scelte di Marcello Malpighi*, ed. L. Belloni, Turin, 1967, pp. 493–631.

[56]   For instance, B. Ciccolini, *Via brevis ad veram naturalis phylosophiae et medicinae scientiam perducens ... contra atomistarum dogmata*, Rome, 1696; P.A. Papi, *Sacra authorum recentiorum critica in philosophia, chimia, et medicina*, Rome, 1706; M. Poli, *Il Trionfo degli Acidi Vendicati dalle Calunnie di molti Moderni ... contro il sistema, e prattica delli moderni Democritici, et Epicurei riformati*, Rome, 1706. On this medical debate in relation to the Inquisition's activity, see M.P. Donato, 'Scienza e teologia nelle congregazioni romane: la

Battista Morgagni, dedicated to none other than the papal Secretary of State, Cardinal Fabrizio Paolucci, and published in Rome with the support of Lancisi, who in the meantime had become chief physician to the pope.[57]

At the time of the sudden death investigation, therefore, neoterics had already penetrated principal Roman medical institutions: Sapienza University, the College of Physicians and the papal court. But they had not been able to put an end to disputes, or gain a solid supremacy over all medical philosophies competing for hegemony in the professional and scientific arena. To them, most particularly, not solely for the medical profession in general, the investigation of 1706 offered at one and the same time an unexpected opportunity and a form of definitive legitimation.

A Pope and his Physician

Unquestionably, the papal physician Giovanni M. Lancisi was one of those who firmly believed that autopsies provided the 'experimental' evidence on which medical knowledge must be based, and unfailingly led to uncovering the 'true causes of evil' and to successfully dealing with public health emergencies. It is hard to imagine the investigation at La Sapienza without Lancisi, who presumably advised Clement XI on how to proceed. As personal physician to the pope, he had direct access to the sovereign (and indeed the relations between the two men transcended their respective positions),[58] and at the same time he could lay claim to a prominent role in the management of public health. Lancisi's personality and his prerogatives as court physician do in fact provide a further key to understanding the political and medical response to the sudden death crisis in early eighteenth-century Rome. Once again, peculiar intellectual and political circumstances enhanced long-term institutional trends and made Rome into a laboratory of innovation.

---

questione atomista, 1626–1727', in *Rome et la science moderne: entre Renaissance et Lumières*, ed. A. Romano, Rome, 2008, pp. 595–634.

[57] [G.B. Morgagni], *Epistola in qua plus centum, et quinquaginta errores ostendetur in recenti libro inscripto Oculorum, et mentis vigiliae*, Rome, 1705, on which see M. Cavazza, 'L'impegno del giovane Morgagni per la riforma dell'Accademia degli Inquieti e in difesa della tradizione malpighiana', and A. Dini, 'La difesa della "medicina razionale" e il giovane Morgagni', in *De sedibus et causis: Morgagni nel centenario*, ed. V. Cappelletti and F. Di Trocchio, Rome, 1986, pp. 91–103 and 147–54.

[58] The distinction between the personal and professional relationships of monarchs and their personal physicians is discussed by C. Jones, 'The Médecins du Roi at the End of the Ancien Régime and in the French Revolution', in *Medicine at the Courts*, ed. Nutton, pp. 214–67.

The figure of the papal personal physician or secret archiater ('secret' as he was one of the members of the pope's *camera segreta*, the inner circle of his personal servants) had emerged between the fifteenth and sixteenth centuries, when papal court ceremonial was substantially codified. It was further defined in the following century, when a clearer separation between the pope's personal physician and those attending the personnel of the apostolic palaces (*medici di palazzo*) was established in the wake of the restructuring of the papal household.[59] Usually, the pope chose his chief physician from among his own compatriots and clients, or sometimes appointed the most renowned professionals of the moment. These included some great names of the history of early modern medicine, such as Girolamo Accoramboni, physician to Leo X and Paul III; the physician of Julius III, Ippolito Salviani; Andrea Bacci, archiater of Sixtus V; and Malpighi, chief physician to Pope Innocent XII. Papal archiaters were usually admitted to the Roman College of Physicians and, although they did not follow the normal *cursus honorum*, their enrolment granted the College a sizeable increment in visibility and authority.[60]

As the health of the head of the Church was the concern of the entire Christian world, popes' personal physicians had never been entirely private persona. However, their status changed from court officers to real public figures towards the end of the sixteenth century, in parallel with the strengthening of the papal monarchy. Since they derived their authority from the sacred person of the sovereign pontiff, they gained precedence over all other physicians, including the protomedicus.[61] On occasions, papal physicians were consulted on issues of the greatest relevance for the community and on other health hazards. One such instance occurred during the plague of 1656, when Matteo Naldi, physician to Alexander VII, dedicated to the people of Rome a volume replete with 'advice for prevention'.[62] As he was, strictly speaking, simultaneously inside and outside the corporative professional order, the pope's physician often played a decisive role in solving delicate issues for the medical profession as a whole. For instance,

---

[59] G. Moroni, *Dizionario di erudizione storico-ecclesiastica*, vol. 44, Venice, 1847, pp. 111–22. Paravicini Bagliani, *The Pope's Body*, p. 186, traces back to 1213 the first mention of a *medicus pape*. See also M.A. Visceglia, 'Denominare e classificare: familia e familiari del papa nella lunga durata dell'età moderna', in *Offices et papauté: XIVe–XVIIe siècle: charges, hommes, destins*, ed. A. Jamme and O. Poncet, Rome, 2005, pp. 159–95.

[60] The rolls of papal archiaters are established in G. Marini, *Degli archiatri pontifici*, Rome, 1784. Among the members of the College who were also papal archiaters, only 19 per cent came from Rome (my calculation on the basis of the colleagues' list appended to the *Statuta* of 1676 (see Chapter 1, n. 103)).

[61] Balsarini, *Memorie della Sapienza*, fol. 238. On the political implications of the secret archiater's office, see Paravicini Bagliani, *The Pope's Body*, pp. 194–8; Palmer, 'Medicine at the Papal Court'.

[62] M. Naldi, *Regole per la cura del contagio*, Rome, 1656.

in 1673, archiater Florido Salvatori overcame the internal resistance to the establishment of the register of all licensed practitioners.[63] The physician to Pope Innocent XII, Luca Tozzi, oversaw the reform of the assistance to the poor by the Office of Papal Charities.[64] The first history of papal physicians was published in 1696, hinting at the increasingly prominent public role played by archiaters.[65]

One eager to take on a prominent public role was surely Lancisi, who at the time of the sudden death 'epidemic' had already distinguished himself as an eminent man of science and a staunch defender of modern medicine. In truth, he was the real architect of the moderns' favour with Pope Albani, and the figure behind the symbolic and concrete revival of the medical establishment in early eighteenth-century Rome.

Lancisi's biography unfolds throughout all relevant institutions and practices for medicine and science in early modern Rome. Born in 1654, he studied at the Roman College, where he received the traditional Jesuit late humanist education. The centre of Jesuit orthodoxy, the Roman College was nevertheless home to a lively group of professors of mixed mathematics who were engaged in the renewal of Aristotelianism and who brought innovative scientific elements into Lancisi's education.[66] He then began attending the philosophy and medicine course at the University of Rome, and entered that 'two-speed' microcosm that was La Sapienza at the end of the seventeenth century, where Galenist senior professors taught alongside younger 'neoteric' scholars such as Paolo Manfredi, Giacomo Sinibaldi, Lucantonio Porzio and Francesco Nazari, editor of the *Giornale de' Letterati* and reader of a second chair of philosophy from 1669 to his death.[67]

---

63   Ms ASR, Università di Roma, b. 75, fols 126–34.

64   Ms VL, Vat. lat. 8635; *Lettera venuta di Roma all'Altezza Serenissima di Cosimo III Gran Duca di Toscana, sopra l'elemosine pontificie*, Florence, 1699.

65   I refer to P. Mandosio, *Theatron in quo maximorum christiani orbis pontificum archiatros*, Rome, 1696.

66   M. Torrini, 'Giuseppe Ferroni gesuita e galileiano', *Physis*, 90, 1973, pp. 411–23; A.R. Capoccia, 'L'insegnamento della filosofia cartesiana nel Collegio Romano agli inizi del XVIII secolo', *Roma moderna e contemporanea*, 7, 1999, pp. 499–535; P. Findlen, 'Living in the Shadow of Galileo: Antonio Baldigiani (1647–1711), a Jesuit Scientist in Late Seventeenth-Century Rome', in *Conflicting Duties*, ed. Donato and Kraye, pp. 211–54.

67   F.M. Renazzi, *Storia dell'università di Roma detta comunemente la Sapienza*, vol. 3, Rome, 1805, pp. 189–93; J.-M. Gardair, *Le 'Giornale de' letterati' de Rome (1668–1681)*, Florence, 1984; F. Favino, 'Mathematics and Mathematicians at the University of Rome "La Sapienza" (XVII–XVIII Centuries)', *Science and Education*, 15, 2006, pp. 357–92; C. Carella, *L'insegnamento della filosofia alla "Sapienza" di Roma nel Seicento: le cattedre e i maestri*, Florence, 2007. On Porzio, a Neapolitan Cartesian, see A. Dini, *Filosofia della natura, medicina, religione: Lucantonio Porzio*, Milan, 1985. On Manfredi, who was an active anatomist and among the first physicians in Rome to experiment with blood transfusion, see M.P. Donato, 'Manfredi Paolo', in DBI, vol. 65, 2010, pp. 157–60.

After gaining his doctorate in 1672, Lancisi joined various medical circles and academies: the *Accademia dei Risoluti*, led by the already mentioned archiater and protomedicus Salvatori, the anatomy academy *ad indagandas morborum sedes*, headed by surgeon Guglielmo Riva,[68] and the scientific coterie of Queen Christina of Sweden's mathematician, Giordano Vitale.[69] According to his first biographer, Mario Crescimbeni,

> Among his [Lancisi's] many toils, he pursued with great solicitude that of anatomy and the dissection of cadavers, attending to it in all of the city's hospitals with assiduity, much attention and fervour.[70]

In 1676 Lancisi entered the hospital of Santo Spirito as assistant physician to one of the four primary doctors, Giovanni Tiracorda. A model and symbol of the pope's charity towards the sick and the poor, this grandiose hospital functioned as a point of encounter between the court and the medical profession.[71] The opportunities for promotion that it could afford worked to perfection in Lancisi's case, not least because of his ability to stand out in intellectual circles and become acquainted with eminent colleagues. He became one of the leading personalities of another academy, Girolamo Brasavola's *Congresso Medico*, which he attended 'without intermission' for many years, and he greatly contributed to the academy's reputation as the meeting point of medical *novatores*. In the *Congresso Medico* he read a few of his early dissertations inspired by chemical-mechanical and corpuscularian theories.[72] When the chair of anatomy and surgery at La Sapienza became vacant in 1683, Lancisi won the appointment to the post over several celebrated surgeons who had been his colleagues at the

---

[68]   The goal of Riva's anatomy academy is stated in the introduction to the *Statuta* of the Roman College of Physicians of 1676; on its founder Riva, see P. Savio, 'Ricerche sull'anatomico Guglielmo Riva', *Bollettino storico-bibliografico subalpino*, 66, 1968, pp. 229–67, and Chapters 3 and 4 of this book.

[69]   Years later, when Giordano applied for the lectureship of mathematics at Sapienza University, he recalled Lancisi as one of his former students in his presentation letter; see ms Rome, Biblioteca dell'Accademia Nazionale dei Lincei, Corsiniano 1379, fol. 220. On Giordano, see M. Torrini, *Dopo Galileo: una polemica scientifica 1684–1711*, Florence, 1979, pp. 85–118.

[70]   G.M. Crescimbeni, 'Vita di monsignor Gio. Maria Lancisi', in *Vite degli arcadi*, p. 186.

[71]   S. De Renzi, '"A Fountain for the Thirsty" and a Bank for the Pope: Charity, Conflicts, and Medical Careers at the Hospital of Santo Spirito in Seventeenth-Century Rome', in *Health Care and Poor Relief in Counter-Reformation Europe*, ed. O.P. Grell, A. Cunningham and J. Arrizabalaga, London, 1999, pp. 102–31.

[72]   *Congressus Medico-Romanus habitus in aedibus D. Hieronymi Brasavoli die lunae 21. septembris 1682*, Rome, 1682; *Congresso medico-romano tenuto in casa del sig.r dr. Girolamo Brasavoli a di 4 ag. 1687*, Rome, 1687.

hospital of Santo Spirito.[73] As a lecturer, he attempted to give new impetus to this discipline in the wake of his predecessor Paolo Manfredi. In the prolusion to his first public dissection in 1683, Lancisi outlined a programme of mechanical anatomy, describing the body as a 'machine that is not solely mobile, but also self-propelled, consisting of many different *machinulae* of solids ... with the fluids flowing therein'.[74] In subsequent years, he delivered the anatomy lessons in rotation with those *de tumoribus* and *de vulneribus capitis*, alternating between an openly mechanical approach focused on bodily machinulae and filters, and a chemical-corpuscular stance.[75] In addition, according to his biographer, 'in order to give better demonstrations, and more appropriately welcome the noble audience who were wont to appear, he did all that was in his power to build the large theatre constructed which is still in existence'.[76] The biographer is perhaps too generous to be entirely trusted, but it is certain that a new anatomical theatre 'praised for being very comfortable' – the one used for the autopsies in 1706 – was built to Lancisi's specifications, although his duties in the care of Pope Innocent XI then often kept him too busy to deliver his teaching in it.[77]

In fact, the real turning point for Lancisi's career came in 1688, once again with the help of the connections that he had formed at the hospital of Santo Spirito. Upon the untimely demise of the archiater in office, Francesco Santucci, Lancisi's old master Tiracorda was offered the prestigious appointment but declined because of age and recommended his former assistant. Lancisi was eventually appointed secret archiater at the young age of 34. Needless to say, the office of court physician was a most coveted one, although not entirely free from inconveniences or risks. As was customary, Lancisi was also made secret remunerated chamberlain (*cameriere segreto partecipante*) and canon in San

---

[73]   Among the candidates were Ippolito Magnani, previously chief surgeon at the hospital of Consolazione, San Giacomo and finally at Santo Spirito, and Bernardino Genga, chief surgeon at Santo Spirito (both were actually graduate physicians but worked as surgeons); see ms Rome, Biblioteca dell'Accademia Nazionale dei Lincei, Corsiniano 1379, fols 217–32.

[74]   G.M. Lancisi, 'Anatomica humani corporis synopsis prolusio', in his *Opera varia*, vol. 2, Venice, 1739, pp. 78–84.

[75]   Ms BLR, Lancisi 153, *Prolusiones et orationes variae*, in which see especially the dissertations of the years 1685 and 1686, fols 11–20, on surgery, and *de partibus corporis humani*, and that of 1692, fols 41–4, on glands, in honour of Malpighi, who had just arrived in Rome to take up the post of archiater to Innocent XII.

[76]   Crescimbeni, *Vita*, p. 187.

[77]   Ms Rome, Biblioteca Alessandrina 60, P. Balsarini, *Memorie della Sapienza*, fol. 33. Sketches for the new anatomical theatre are in ms ASR, Università di Roma, b. 69, fasc. 1. However, from the janitor's notes (ms ASR, Università di Roma, b. 85, fol. 112) we learn that, in 1688, 'Mr Lancisi, Professor of Surgery and Anatomy, after having been appointed secret physician ... only lectured one more time.'

Lorenzo in Damaso. Like many unmarried papal physicians before him, he moved into the apostolic palace. Residing in the Vatican gave secret archiaters the tremendous privilege of easy access to the person of the pope (usually old and in need of constant medical care), and consequently the invaluable opportunity to occasionally act as a discreet but influential adviser. Soon after his court appointment, Lancisi was also duly admitted to the College of Physicians.

As already mentioned, the palatine appointment depended on the pope's choice. However, it was forfeited with the holy patient's death, and the former archiater might not enjoy the same favour with the faction supporting the new pope.[78] Hence, in 1689, following Pope Odescalchi's death, Lancisi had to revert to his private practice and former occupations, but not before performing the autopsy on Innocent XI's venerable corpse, as was the secret archiater's duty with the assistance of the papal surgeon. Years later, Lancisi would relate the results of this dissection in a manuscript, *Giornale dell'ultima infermità di Innocenzo XI* (*Journal of the last illness of Innocent XI*), written in view of the beatification process of Pope Odescalchi. It has been claimed that, through this memoir, Lancisi aimed to clear himself of any potential allegations regarding the cure of the dying pope,[79] but on closer examination his writings bear witness to his aspiration to stand comparison with his great Renaissance predecessors. Similarly to Realdo Colombo – who had performed the post-mortem examination on the body of Ignatius of Loyola and described Ignatius's enormous kidney stones in *De re anatomica* (1559) – Lancisi described how he had found in Pope Innocent's body stones so large as to be considered evidence of a miracle. In Lancisi's view, not only had God providentially chosen Odescalchi as his earthly vicar, but 'at a time of greatest need for the church, He also administered to him the manner [that is, the strength] by which he could long survive such a grave disease'.[80] Lancisi's portrait of Innocent XI as the pope who 'broke the chains of barbaric slavery', was prepared to suffer martyrdom 'to defend even the smallest liberty of the holy inheritance transmitted to his hands' and demonstrated how 'a pope free of personal interests could act',[81] was in reality a spiritual and political manifesto for the intended recipient of his tract, the newly elected Pope Clement XI, whom the physician urged to pursue reforms and to remain independent from the European monarchies.

It is true, however, that shortly after losing his court appointment, Lancisi was targeted by the Inquisition. In the last decade of the seventeenth century,

---

[78]   Palmer, 'Medicine at the Papal Court', calculated that no more than 20 physicians out of 118 retained their appointment for more than one pope. Cardinals also elected a physician and a surgeon for the time of the conclave.

[79]   C. Preti in DBI, vol. 53, 2004, pp. 360–64.

[80]   Ms BLR, Lancisi 149, fol. 217. On Ignatius's autopsy, see Andretta, 'Anatomie du vénérable'.

[81]   Ms BLR, Lancisi 149, fol. 1 and fols 295v–296r.

the Holy Office engaged in a wave of repression against proponents of heterodox ideas. Some members of the Congresso Medico (Brasavola, the founder, Giacomo Sinibaldi, Sulpizio Antonio Mazzuto and Lancisi himself) were denounced for their alleged adherence to Epicurean and libertine doctrines as well as atomic theories of the universe.[82] The ensuing investigation ended in a reprimand. The academy was forbidden to debate metaphysical topics and was eventually discontinued. After his Inquisition trial, and presumably as a response to it, Lancisi prepared for the academy of Fisiocritici in Siena a dissertation, *Sul modo di filosofar nell'arte medica* (*How to philosophise on the art of medicine*), setting out the principles of modern medicine as a rational science grounded in experiments and in 'certain geometric and mechanical principles'. Furthermore, in answer to persistent criticism addressed to neoterics, he defended the usefulness of anatomy and chemistry for the understanding of the body and medical practice.[83]

His prosecution by the Holy Office did not really hinder Lancisi's advancement, either in his work as a lecturer or that as a medical practitioner. Judging from the surviving manuscripts of his courses, he continued to teach medicine according to the principles of mechanical philosophy.[84] In 1696 he published the report of the post-mortem he had performed on his former colleague Malpighi in 1694 in the Parisian journal *Progrès de la médecine* and in the *Philosophical Transactions*, which marked his debut on the international scene.[85] In the same year, he became professor of theoretical medicine. In the winter of 1695, an epidemic of petechial fever in the area around the Vatican pushed him to turn his interests to public health. According to his own testimony, as he was then serving as treating physician to the Cardinal Chamberlain (*Camerlengo*) Altieri, he made suggestions for the containment and prevention of similar calamities.[86]

In 1700, at the still relatively young age of 46, Lancisi regained the post of chief physician to the pope, now Giovan Francesco Albani, Clement XI. The two men were almost peers, had known each other for years and had much in common: they had both studied at the Roman College, attended the literary Academy of the Arcadia and been canons at the basilica of San Lorenzo in

---

[82]   They were accused of 'discussing the doctrine of the atoms following the teachings of Descartes, Gassendi and Epicurus'; see M.P. Donato, 'L'onere della prova: il Sant'Uffizio, l'atomismo e i medici romani', *Nuncius*, 18, 2003, pp. 69–87.

[83]   'Del modo di filosofar nell'Arte medica, e si prova che per la medicina razionale è meglio servirsi della filosofia sperimentale che di qualunque altra', *Galleria di Minerva*, 4, 1700, 3, pp. 33–5.

[84]   See, in particular, Lancisi's inaugural lecture of 1693 on subtle anatomy, now in ms BLR, Lancisi 153, fols 45–50.

[85]   *Philosophical Transactions*, 19, 1695–97, pp. 467–71.

[86]   G.M. Lancisi, *De noxiis paludum effluviis, eorumque remediis libri duo*, Rome, 1717, p. 156; A. Corradi, *Annali delle epidemie occorse in Italia dalla prime memorie fino al 1850*, vol. 2, Bologna, 1973, pp. 280–84.

Damaso. The year 1700 marked the beginning of a solid partnership between the pope and his physician that would last for two decades. The following year, Lancisi was knighted and moved up to the more prestigious university chair of practical medicine. It is worth mentioning that in those years, for his lessons on *morbis capitis* (diseases of the head), Lancisi focused his research on the brain and especially on the vascular system and the meninges. Conducted in parallel to those of other anatomists in Rome, these studies would be the source of new ideas when the physician came to deal with sudden death.[87] It is true, though, that his attendance at the university was affected by his duties at the apostolic palace, 'not only', as he would write, 'to attend to the tireless care of an ailing prince, but for his endless visiting and consulting ... for all the most prominent gentlemen of this great city and of the whole state'.[88] His court appointment implied further responsibilities. After the Tiber flood in December 1702, Lancisi engaged in the sanitation of the city, threatened by stagnant waters and dead bodies floating in the river.[89] Three years later, he followed the course of a pernicious 'verminous fever' in Orvieto (a town that Albani had once ruled as governor in his early career) and drew up a list of sanitary measures, which the pontiff agreed to implement.[90]

In the meantime, the relationship between the pope and his doctor was cemented by several missions in which Lancisi was able to prove his skills as a physician as well as an antiquarian and a panegyrist, as he did in his trip to Urbino, the hometown of the Albani family, in 1703 to attend the graduation of the pope's nephew, Annibale.[91] In 1705 Lancisi was invited by Ludovico Antonio Muratori, under his pseudonym Lamindo Pritaneo, to preside over a nascent Accademia d'Italia, meant to renew 'good taste' in Italian letters and sciences, but unfortunately the project was wrecked by the War of the Spanish Succession.[92] However, in 1706 Lancisi gained admission to the Royal Society of London, to which he had long aspired. It was then that he came up against the sudden death crisis, at a particularly delicate moment for both the Catholic Church and his patient and mentor Clement XI.

As we have already seen, thanks to the papal archiater's direct involvement, the emergency was addressed in an innovative way through an investigation in

---

[87]   Ms BLR, Lancisi 306.

[88]   *Lettere inedite scientifico-letterarie di Lodovico Muratori, Vitaliano Donati, Gio. Maria Lancisi, Daniele Le Clerc*, ed. A. Roncetti, Milan, 1845, p. 214, letter to Antonio Vallisneri of 30 May 1716.

[89]   Lancisi, *Dissertatio de nativis et adventitiis romani coeli qualitatibus (cui accedit historia epidemiae rheumaticae)*, Rome, 1711, pp. 118–21.

[90]   Lancisi, *De noxiis paludum effluviis*, pp. 185–201.

[91]   Ms BLR, Lancisi 147, and Lancisi 171, on a further trip to Urbino in 1705.

[92]   A. Vecchi, 'La nuova accademia letteraria d'Italia', in *Accademie e cultura: aspetti storici tra Sei e Settecento*, Florence, 1979, pp. 39–72.

the style of the moderns. The investigation's final outcome was in fact Lancisi's book *De subitaneis mortibus* in which he could definitively prove, by virtue of the 'anatomist's knife', that no real danger loomed over the citizens of Rome. Thanks to the successful management of the crisis, he further strengthened his professional position and his personal power. Elected to the permanent magistrature of the College of Physicians at the end of 1706, over the following years Lancisi held the office of protomedicus numerous times, always retaining that of secret archiater. Cumulating these various positions and operating inside and outside the corporate apparatus by virtue of his direct relationship with the pope, Lancisi became a self-defined 'minister for momentous affairs' during the ambitious and yet constantly troubled pontificate of Clement XI.[93] In his tireless activities as a public official, the pope's trusted servant and a reputed author and editor, Lancisi was able to take full advantage of Clement XI's programme of political and ideological revival of Rome.[94] He was, in short, the key player in an unprecedented, though instable, balance between the ambitions of the medical profession and the needs of the papal monarchy; the corporate organisation of society and absolutism; the traditional values of hierarchy and authority and the modernisation of medicine. Precisely this balance set the conditions for the anatomo-pathological investigation of sudden death of 1706 and fostered, as we shall see in the next chapter, a more active public role for physicians.

---

[93]   Lancisi's self-description in a letter to Morgagni, also quoted in Brambilla, 'La medicina del Settecento', p. 54.

[94]   M. Conforti, 'The Biblioteca Lancisiana and the 1714 Edition of Eustachi's Anatomical Plates, or: Ancients and Moderns Reconciled', in *Conflicting Duties*, ed. Donato and Kraye, pp. 303–18; A. Cunningham, *The Anatomist Anatomis'd: An Experimental Discipline in Enlightenment Europe*, Aldershot, 2010, pp. 73–5.

Chapter 3

From the Dead to the Living: Medicine and Public Health in the Early Eighteenth Century

Experts on Death Protecting the Living

Lancisi's book *De subitaneis mortibus* was published in 1707, a year after the wave of unexpected 'accidents' that had terrorised Rome. It bore all the hallmarks of an official publication, not least because it was published by the printer Buagni, whose workshop had been recently installed in the hospice of San Michele a Ripa by order of the pope.[1] Clement XI rewarded the author with the sum of one hundred *scudi* from his personal endowment.[2] The book, 'admirable for the solidity of its doctrines, the abundance of medical learning and the clarity of its style and order', was very well received. It was reviewed in scholarly journals such as *Galleria di Minerva*, *Giornale de' Letterati d'Italia*, *Journal des Savants* and *Acta Eruditorum*; both foreign periodicals especially underscored that Lancisi's study had been commissioned by the pope.[3] It was immediately reprinted in Lucca, and a revised edition, prepared with the help of the young, talented anatomist Giovan Battista Morgagni, appeared in Venice the following year.[4] The alliance between the sovereign pontiff and his doctors in the defence of the people of Rome was thus widely disseminated throughout war-torn Europe.

Before the papal archiater's tract had even left the printing press, the pope made plain his satisfaction with the brilliant management of the sudden death

---

[1] S. Franchi, *Le impressioni sceniche: dizionario bio-bibliografico degli editori e stampatori romani e laziali di testi drammatici e libretti per musica dal 1579 al 1800*, Rome, 1994, pp. 97–8.

[2] Ms ASV, Fondo Albani, vol. 7, fol. 258.

[3] Quotation from *Galleria di Minerva*, 1706 (but 1707), p. 302; *Giornale de' Letterati d'Italia*, 1710, pp. 397–417; *Acta eruditorum*, 1708, pp. 174–9; *Journal des Sçavans*, 1709, *Supplément*, pp. 81–4.

[4] *Typis & sumptibus Peregrini Frediani*, Lucca, 1707; *sumptibus Andreae Poleti*, Venice, 1708, followed by another edition *sumptibus Jo. Firedrich Gleditsch*, Rome [that is, Leipzig], 1709 (also mentioned in *Acta eruditorum*, 1709, pp. 466–7). On the preparation of the amended Venetian edition, see *Lettere di Lancisi a Morgagni e parecchie altre dello stesso Morgagni, ora per la prima volta pubblicate*, ed. A. Corradi, Pavia, 1876.

mystery by consulting his physicians on issues that had previously been outside the sphere of competence for medical practitioners. As early as December 1706, the pope asked the College of Physicians for advice on burials and a plan for cemeteries. Authorities had been concerned with the issue of burials for some time, though only out of religious concerns and especially with regard to the conservation of early Christian relics. Now, their objective was to 'abolish or curb the custom of church burials that are most dangerous for public health'.[5]

Lancisi himself examined the matter on behalf of the College. In the memorandum he prepared, he categorically regarded a reform in burial practices to be an absolute necessity. Church interments had to be relinquished and new cemetery sites implemented. As for these new cemeteries, graves dug in the ground were preferable to stone burial vaults. The latter were costly and, more importantly, dangerous because they slowed the decomposition of corpses. In a city like Rome, where there were

> at least twenty dead every day, viz six to seven thousand in a year, this creates
> in each tomb a most noxious mass of rotting parts, which, when the tombs are
> opened, disperses in the air and infects nearby places, from which it spreads to
> other areas.

Instead, when burying in the ground 'the alteration of putrid parts does not occur, provided one proceeds in a proper method'. After assessing the needs of the population on the basis of 'ordinary' mortality – let us remember incidentally that the cardinal vicar had only recently begun to record births and deaths in Rome – Lancisi advised that no less than four new cemeteries were necessary. These were to be located outside the city but 'not too far removed', in places carefully chosen for their position and the direction of the winds at the four cardinal points. These sites were then further indicated as being between Porta del Popolo and Porta Angelica, between Porta San Giovanni and Porta Latina, between Porta Pia and Porta Salaria and finally outside Porta Portese.

Each facility was to be given 'an area of forty thousand square [Roman] architectural palms' and would accommodate a suitable number of tombs which could be reused not before two years 'as a precaution'. Altogether they would process 8,000 bodies a year – a number above what constituted 'present annual mortality'. Naturally, every cemetery should be equipped with a 'suitable, comfortable vestry chapel ... with an annexed tomb that may adequately contain

---

    5   Ms Madrid, Archivo Historico Nacional, Consejos, leg. 3151, exp. 48, n. 5, the folios from which I am quoting are unnumbered. Lancisi's memorandum is in a collection of documents about cemeteries gathered in conjunction with Charles III of Spain's reforms of burial practices. I am grateful to M.C. Giannini for his help in obtaining a copy of the document.

the bones which gradually must be excavated out of the graves'. The graves were to be 'shaped in the most regular fashion, and the ground divided in so many equal portions', all uniformly at the same distance from one another, in keeping with an austere penitential spirit. Finally,

> in filling the grave with soil, it must be procured that it be well compacted, and that hayseeds be scattered over it which will soon make grass grow. A small wooden cross will indicate the occupied spaces, and the date, with painted numbers and letters.

Moreover,

> It could be commanded that the parishes of St Lorenzo outside the Walls, St Agnese, St Lorenzo and Urbano in Prima Porta, of St Paolo and St Sebastiano, St Angelo alle Fornaci, St Lazaro, and St Francesco on Monte Mario form their own small cemeteries, with the same precautions as the other four localities, for the reason that they are all outside Rome, and have land annexed, [and this would] limit the inconvenience of transportation.

In his project, Lancisi also detailed ways of dealing with corpses and bones. 'With this method, public health is in great part provided for', he concluded. Drawing on a notion of papal absolutism as a leveller and reformer of privileges, at least in the hour of death, Lancisi also provided Clement XI with arguments to overcome the resistance and objections that ecclesiastical dignitaries and 'those who have noble tombs' might raise against such a revolutionary project. He accordingly conceded that the regular clergy be given the liberty to build small cemeteries in convent precincts, 'but with the aforesaid precautions ... to be strictly observed'; secular clergy, on the other hand, might be allowed a church burial,

> but with many precautions to be agreed upon, such as entombing their coffins in every available space in the church crypt, as is now done for persons of ecclesiastical dignity.

As for members of the nobility and their 'need for eternity',[6] Lancisi unhesitatingly asserted that 'also those who have their own sepulchre can be

---

    [6]   I borrow this expression from M.A. Visceglia, *Il bisogno di eternità: i comportamenti aristocratici a Napoli in età moderna*, Naples, 1988, esp. on sepulchres pp. 107–39; C. Franceschini, 'Ricerche sulle cappelle di famiglia a Roma in età moderna', *Archivio italiano per la storia della pietà*, 14, 2001, pp. 345–413.On the choice of burial places, see also V. Harding, *The Dead and the Living in Paris and London*, Cambridge, 2002.

compelled to apply more diligence'; however, he added cautiously that 'these measures can be considered at a later time, and must not hinder the realisation of His Holiness' noble idea'.

To my knowledge, the 1706 plan is the first to deal with an issue which, in the second half of the eighteenth century, would motivate experts and rulers of many European countries and eventually lead to the creation of modern extra-urban cemeteries.[7] And it is clearly connected with the sudden death 'epidemics'. Ever since antiquity, decaying corpses had been thought to corrupt air, and all available texts on sudden death listed proximity to such decay as a possible cause.[8] Despite the reassuring conclusions reached both by the archiater and the protomedicus at the end of their investigation, neither of them had ruled out the possibility that corrupt air might have played a role in the anomalous spate of deaths. Incidentally, in his *De subitaneis mortibus*, Lancisi warned that opening tombs would inevitably release toxic particles into the air.[9] As we have seen, air was no longer considered an element that could be corrupted in its essence; according to modern natural philosophy, air was composed of different chemical substances and was a vehicle for corpuscles and particles that 'corrupt' it in the sense that they alter its right composition. Such revisited theories on air, however, did but conceptually reinforce the idea that sources of contamination could actively be removed – hence the Roman College of Physicians' request that the dead be dislodged to protect the living.[10]

In more general political and cultural terms, the medico-legal investigation into sudden death in Rome had introduced death as a legitimate issue in the

---

[7]   M. Jenner, 'Death, Decomposition and Dechristianization? Public Health and Church Burial in Eighteenth-Century England', *English Historical Review*, 120, 2005, pp. 615–32, points at criticisms of interments in churches in Britain in the 1720s, which bear strong similarities to Lancisi's plan in Catholic Rome. Jenner rightly highlights the importance of religious considerations in this debate and the impact of ecclesiastical antiquarianism aimed at restoring the uses of the primitive Church. On the Enlightenment campaign against burial in churches and the creation of *extra muros* cemeteries, see P. Ariès, *The Hour of Our Death*, trans. H. Weaver, London, 1981, chs 10 and 11; R.A. Etlin, *The Architecture of Death: The Transformation of the Cemetery in Eighteenth-Century Paris*, Cambridge, MA, 1984; G. Tomasi, *Per salvare i viventi: le origini settecentesche del cimitero extraurbano*, Bologna, 2001.

[8]   P. Grassi, *Mortis repentinae examen ... cum brevi methodo praesagendi et praecavendi*, Modena, 1612, pp. 61–2; G. Terilli, *De causis mortis repentinae tractatio in qua etiam disputatur quid sit mors et vita in genere et quae mortis causae communes, singula vero quae de causis mortis repentinae enarrantur*, Venice, 1615, p. 60; G. Baglivi, *Opere complete medico-pratiche ed anatomiche*, Florence, 1842, p. 608.

[9]   SM, p. 14.

[10]   J.C. Riley, *The Eighteenth-Century Campaign to Avoid Disease*, Basingstoke, 1987, underscores the difference between early modern and modern Hippocratism; see further L. Brockliss and C. Jones, *The Medical World of Early Modern France*, Oxford, 1997, pp. 730–69.

public debate. Through it, physicians appropriated an event that up until then had been the preserve of families and of the Church, made it a matter of public health and established themselves as experts on death. The plan for cemeteries represented the immediate effect of the invasion of medicine in previously unexplored territories.

Clement XI's 'noble idea', however, remained just a blueprint 'because of the declamations of the clergy and of popular superstition, as well as because of the government's weakness'.[11] After all, notwithstanding its early success, medicine failed to actually arrogate to itself the management of death in papal Rome and break the boundary between medicine and religion. The living rather than the dead remained the focus of the government's care, and in a rather traditional way: parish churches and rural vicariates were erected in the suburban areas indicated in the plan, so that the inhabitants would not be deprived of spiritual assistance and the holy sacraments in their last hour.[12] Except for the small cemetery designed by architect Ferdinando Fuga and built in 1745 next to the hospital of Santo Spirito (one of the first of its kind in Europe), the dead lay forgotten until 1809. In that year the newly established Napoleonic administration began construction of two cemeteries in the areas indicated by the College in the original 1706 plan, Verano and Monte Mario. But construction was disrupted again at the Restoration and it took no less than the recurring outbreaks of cholera in the 1830s to convince the papal government to complete the Verano cemetery, still in use today.[13]

---

[11] This quotation concerning the failure of the Roman plan for cemeteries – an issue that would be progressively invested of wider political and social implications – is drawn from the late eighteenth-century anonymous note attached to the plan in the archival folder concerning cemeteries; see above, n. 5. Among other things, this later note describes methods of transportation and interment of dead bodies in the Roman parish churches and hospitals that were still in use in the second half of the eighteenth century.

[12] G.F. Rossi, 'Erezione di parrocchie rurali e modalità pastorali di avvicinamento dei lavoratori nella campagna di Roma nel Sei-Settecento', in *L'uomo e la storia: studi storici in onore di M. Petrocchi*, ed. R. Chiacchella and G.F. Rossi, vol. 1, Rome, 1983, pp. 183–221.

[13] O. Montenovesi, *Il Campo santo di Roma: storia e descrizione*, Rome, 1915 (it is noteworthy that the architects Camporesi and Stern then thought it advisable to built vaulted tombs rather than graveyard burials, not to overtly upset popular sensibilities); L. Bertolaccini, *Città e cimiteri: dall'eredità medievale alla codificazione ottocentesca*, Rome, 2004. In the meantime, the non-Catholic cemetery near Caius Cestius's pyramid on the Via Ostiense had been built. The anonymous note annexed to Lancisi's plan considered it exemplary of a correct dislocation for cemeteries. On this cemetery, also called the 'English cemetery', see A. Menniti Ippolito, 'Il "vecchio recinto" del Testaccio: agli inizi della sepoltura degli acattolici in Roma', in *The Protestant Cemetery in Rome: The 'Parte Antica'*, ed. A. Menniti Ippolito and P. Vian, Rome, 1989, pp. 15–90.

Early Medical Police and the Containment and Prevention of Epidemic Disease

It can be argued on the basis of the 1706 medical investigation and plan for cemeteries that Rome contributed to the birth of the *medizinische Polizey* that would later be developed in some European states during the eighteenth and nineteenth centuries as an instrument of health and demographic control.[14] The term medical police, however, implies that, in the name of public welfare and prosperity, medical authorities are invested with direct decisional and executive powers over the spheres of individual and collective life that were previously the preserve of religious authority. Such empowerment of medicine by the state could not really take place in the Papal States, where the spiritual and the temporal realms coincided. Indeed, the double nature of the papal monarchy set connatural, stringent limits to the practice of absolutism and to any substantial reform of temporal government. This did not fail to curb Clement XI's ambitions altogether. The constitutive terms of the subordination of medicine to religion, nonetheless, underwent some degree of change in favour of the former.

The positive outcome of the sudden death emergency was reflected in a novel activism of the Roman medical body. Guided by their magistrates and led by the influential papal archiater Lancisi, physicians sought to benefit from Clement XI's patronage to claim a more compelling role in the public arena and consolidate their authority. Public health thus became an intrinsic part of pope Albani's paternalistic pontificate.[15]

---

[14]   R. Taiani, *Il governo dell'esistenza: organizzazione sanitaria e tutela della salute pubblica in Trentino nella prima metà del XIX secolo*, Bologna, 1995; C. Pancino, ed., *Politica e salute: dalla polizia medica all'igiene*, Bologna, 2003. More specifically on the management of death, see M. Canella, 'La gestione della morte nel Milanese tra età moderna e contemporanea: l'intervento dello stato dall'indagine conoscitiva all'azione legislativa', in *Specchio della popolazione: la percezione dei fatti e problemi demografici nel passato*, ed. A. Menzione, Udine, 2003, pp. 55–80. However, the implementation of efficient systems of data collection and classification regarding causes of mortality took nearly two centuries, due to the complex underlying theoretical issues and the competing claims of different institutions (the state, treating physicians, medical experts, city councils and so forth). See G.C. Alter and A.H. Carmichael, 'Reflections on the Classification of Causes of Death', *Continuity and Change*, 12, 1997, pp. 169–73.

[15]   On the increased activism of the protomedicus concerning infringement of residual autonomous medical jurisdictions and exertion of a firmer control over healing practitioners, see ms ASR, Università di Roma, b. 59 and 62. Nevertheless, the Protomedicate's recent empowerment was rapidly invalidated under Benedict XIII and Benedict XIV, who restored several privileges to local colleges and universities. See further A. Kolega, 'Speziali, spagirici, droghieri e ciarlatani: l'offerta terapeutica a Roma tra Seicento e Settecento', *Roma moderna e contemporanea*, 4, 1998, pp. 311–48. For a comparison with other contexts, see J. Geyer-Kordesch, 'Court Physicians and State Regulation in Eighteenth-Century Prussia: The

In truth, the recurrent epidemics that hit the Papal State at the beginning of the eighteenth century provided the medical profession with plenty of occasions to play an active role. Epidemics were traditionally within the sphere of competence of medicine and offered, as we have seen, exceptionally good professional opportunities. Now, new arguments and procedures were introduced, and resulted in a shift of emphasis from individual to collective health.

One such instance was a pandemic of catarrhal fevers that hit the cities of Ferentino, Anagni and Frosinone, and reached the capital in the winter of 1709. Compared to the beginning of the century, the situation had further worsened. The War of the Spanish Succession had escalated into an open conflict between the Apostolic See and Emperor Joseph I of Austria. In 1708, the Imperial army occupied Comacchio, near Ferrara, and the pope's declaration of war ended in a brief, disastrous military campaign, which eventually forced the pope to accept a disadvantageous armistice; the ill-fated military adventure was then inevitably compounded by food shortage and a dire financial crisis.[16] The following year, the alleged author of a satirical pamphlet against the pope, Filippo Rivarola, was decapitated in Rome in an attempt to curb the population's open discontent with the court, held responsible for 'having brought all these calamities upon themselves'. It was to no avail, and according to French observers even the exceptionally bad weather and cold temperatures were imputed to the government.[17]

The epidemic appeared extremely serious from the very outset. In a few weeks, the number of victims rose to such a high number that the tolling of bells was forbidden so as 'not to grieve the sick'.[18] At first, the government agreed to the measures recommended by the protomedicus and the papal archiater, such as the moderation of Lent fasting rules and extraordinary street cleaning.

Emergence of Medical Science and the Demystification of the Body', in *Medicine at the Courts of Europe, 1500–1837*, ed. V. Nutton, London, 1990, pp. 155–81; A. Lunel, *La maison médicale du Roi: XVIe–XVIIIe siècles. Le pouvoir royal et les professions de santé (médecins, chirurgiens, apothicaires)*, Seyssel, 2008, pp. 201–34.

[16] L. von Pastor, *History of the Popes from the Close of the Middle Ages*, trans. E. Graf, vol. 33, London, 1957, pp. 61–9; S. Tabacchi, *Il Buon Governo: le finanze locali nello Stato della Chiesa (secoli XVI–XVIII)*, Rome, 2007, pp. 374–84.

[17] *Correspondance des directeurs de l'Académie de France à Rome avec les surintendants des bâtiments*, ed. A. de Montaiglon, vol. 3, Paris, 1889, pp. 250–52.

[18] Valesio, vol. 4, p. 240; A. Corradi, *Annali delle epidemie occorse in Italia dalle prime memorie fino al 1850*, vol. 2, Bologna, 1973 pp. 304–13; S. Jarcho, 'The "Epidemia Rheumatica" Described by Lancisi (1711)', in *Healing and History: Essays for George Rosen*, ed. C.E. Rosenberg, New York, 1979, pp. 51–8. G. Olagüe de Ros, 'La epidemia europea de gripe de 1708–1709', *Dynamis*, 1, 1981, pp. 51–86, analyses Lancisi's, Ramazzini's and Hoffmann's contributions. Sanitary measures in the Papal States are reported in ms BLR, Lancisi 172, fols 378–421; Lancisi, *Dissertatio de nativis et adventitiis romani coeli qualitatibus (cui accedit historia epidemiae rheumaticae)*, Rome, 1711, pp. 125–70.

Then, a special *peritorum conventus* (experts' meeting) was summoned to tackle the worsening situation. Its composition was in itself a novelty, as it featured the prelate chief governor (commendatore) of the hospital of Santo Spirito, the lay administrators (custodi) of the hospital of San Salvatore, Protomedicus Tomassini with the College of Physicians' counsellors, the four chief physicians at Santo Spirito, the head surgeon at San Salvatore, Antonio Pacchioni, and, of course, the ubiquitous Lancisi as secretary. The doctors' *consilium* dictated the sanitation programme. Some of the actions it urged included cleaning the streets and clearing away stagnant water, improving the people's food provision, transferring sick farm workers and labourers to the hospital of Santo Spirito in order to give them adequate care, calling on local doctors to lend immediate assistance to sick poor and allowing the consumption of meat during Lent. After all, the doctors wrote with an apparent lack of self-interest, 'the poor and the sick are the dearest friends of the Redeemer and His most accomplished image'. By helping them, the pope would make himself dear to God and to the people, since, in his position as a prince and as a pontiff, he had a 'stronger obligation' than any other monarch to be his subjects' 'common Father'.[19]

Physicians were also part of the special congregation created in 1711 to confront an outbreak of cattle plague which spread rapidly over the whole of Italy, killing thousands of animals. Once again, the pope and his ministers availed themselves of the novel alliance of piety and science. While processions and vigils were staged to beg God to put an end to the calamity,[20] the Sacra Consulta asked Lancisi and other physicians to police livestock quarantine. Drastic measures were devised for the segregation, culling and interment of infected animals, and the use of any food cut from their meat strictly forbidden.[21]

In 1712, the epizootic seemingly spread to horses. The Sacra Consulta and Apostolic Chamber once again sent for Lancisi and the incumbent protomedicus Michelangelo Paoli accompanied by the College of Physicians' magistrates. Despite their reassuring findings on the nature of the horse sickness, a large number of diseased beasts had to be culled. Doctors provided instructions on how to dispose of the carcasses, as these might contaminate other animals as well

---

[19]   Ms BLR, Lancisi 301, *Epidemia delle febbri e dei mali di petto vagata particolarmente in Roma nei mesi di gennaro, febbraro e marzo del MDCCIX*, quotations at fols 353–4.

[20]   Ms ASV, Fondo Albani, vol. 28, fols 8–41.

[21]   G.M. Lancisi, *Dissertatio historica de bovilla peste, ex Campaniae finibus anno 1713 Latio importata, deque praesidiis ... ad avertendam aeris labem, et annonae caritatem opportune adhibitis*, Rome, 1715; Corradi, *Annali delle epidemie*, pp. 318–25; C.A. Spinage, *Cattle Plague. A History*, New York, 2003, pp. 105-14, points at the fact that Roman sanitary police served as a model elsewhere, especially France; S. Zanier, 'Dalla paura alla prova: la relazione manoscritta, i trattati medici e le decisioni istituzionali durante la gestione dell'epizootia degli anni 1711–15 nel Nord Est dell'Italia', *Medicina e storia*, 6, 2006, pp. 51–85.

as fields and cities.[22] Dead animals, not only human remains, were a danger to life and health, but in this case, medical police did not run the risk of clashing with any 'superstition' and could be fully enforced.

Again, in 1713, the government resorted to medical experts when the sale of a forest near Cisterna, in the south of Latium, was debated, thus bringing to the fore the issue of the salubrity of the marshes occupying the ancient *Ager romanus*. The affair had wide economical and political repercussions. The forest was one of a few in a large area that otherwise hosted a prosperous, if hardly salubrious, marshland economy. Furthermore, the woodland belonged to the powerful Caetani family. The Caetanis' decision to sell it raised the issue of the barons' prerogatives over feudal communities, which Clement XI had recently placed under the supervision of the congregation of Buon Governo (1704). In the case in point, moreover, the baron was no less than Duke Gaetano Francesco Caetani, whose siding with the Empire during the War of the Spanish Succession had already cost him the duchy of Sermoneta in 1702 by virtue of a papal act of confiscation that would be the last of its kind in the history of the Papal States.[23] The legal suit went on for two years in front of an ad hoc congregation presided over by the cardinal Camerlengo. It was punctuated by an array of petitions, in which more and more ink was spent on arguments concerning the salubriousness of the region, the well-being of the population and the preventative measures to ensure both. The defence 'of public health, of the life and safety of inhabitants' was upheld against the commercial designs of the duke, who eventually lost the legal suit.[24]

These instances of sanitary interventionism in early eighteenth-century Rome were aligned with the tendencies underlying papal absolutism that, at that time, strove to impose a firmer central control at the periphery. This was

---

[22] A.M. Borromeo, *Istoria dell'epidemia de' buoj accaduta nel Padovano l'anno MDCCXI ... aggiuntovi un altro ragionamento di Monsig. Lancisi, intorno all'epidemia de' cavalli*, Naples, 1712, particularly pp. 192–3; ms BLR, Lancisi 264, fols 615–18, *Parere dato in risposta al cardinal Sacripante circa i mali che nascono in vicinanza dello scorticaro de cavalli*.

[23] It was not until 1710 that the lordship of Sermoneta was returned to Gaetano's son Michelangelo Caetani, who then came back to Rome from his exile in Vienna; see G. Delille, 'Sermoneta e il Lazio meridionale nell'età moderna', in *Sermoneta e i Caetani: dinamiche politiche, sociali e culturali di un territorio tra medioevo ed età moderna*, ed. L. Fiorani, Rome, 1999, pp. 109–23; D. Armando, 'Assetto territoriale e dinamiche dei poteri nel ducato di Sermoneta (1586–1817)', in *Bonifacio VIII, i Caetani e la storia del Lazio*, Rome, 2004, pp. 143–74.

[24] Quoted from Cardinal Corradini's *votum* on the affair, now in ms ASV, Fondo Albani, vol. 18, fols 244–57, here at fol. 250r. The final papal chirograph of 15 September 1715 ratified restrictions to the felling of trees as recommended by medical experts. Lancisi's and other expert reports can be found in ms ASV, Fondo Albani, vol. 18; mss BLR, Lancisi 264, fols 675–715 and 739–47; Lancisi 295, fols 116–19, 144–64; ms ASR, Università di Roma, b. 61, fasc. 9.

not peculiar to the Papal States. At the turn of the seventeenth and eighteenth centuries, other capitals witnessed similar developments, and it has been argued that a common trend underpins what can be viewed as early Enlightenment reforms. Hence early instances of medical police in this period resulted from the converging strategies of municipal elites and central governments.[25] In Rome, medical policing reflects the revival of the notion of papal 'good rule', whose variegated policies all aimed at limiting the customary liberties of social bodies without breaking the corporative pact altogether, while shifting the balance of power towards the centre. Within this framework, a concern for public health became a wise political move for the sovereign pontiff, the 'common Father', as it potentially was a matter that required both rational policies and discipline. Medical doctors – particularly their corporative organisations in the capital city – were an integral part of this evolution and drew legitimation from their connections with political power in the wake of the sudden death investigation. Of course, their authority was still subject to the limits of a traditional hierarchy of values and prerogatives, which made them at one time major players and at other times mere involuntary beneficiaries of the government's concern for public safety.[26] Their role was still that of consultants, and nevertheless their surveillance of public health now tended to extend across the perimeter of the traditional corporate organisation of medicine.

---

[25]   There is general agreement in historiography that these measures, despite their questionable impact on the incidence of epidemics, did improve urban sanitary conditions. But whereas specialists of urban history underscore the role played by municipal elites – for example, M.S.R. Jenner, 'Curare l'ambiente senza dottori? Igiene pubblica a Londra nella prima età moderna', and R. Sansa, 'Le norme decorose e il lavoro sporco: l'igiene urbana in tre capitali europee: Londra, Parigi, Roma tra XVI e XVIII secolo', *Storia urbana*, 29, 2006, pp. 39–64 and 85–112 respectively – historians of medicine regard such developments as early instances of medical police. See G. Rosen, *From Medical Police to Social Medicine: Essays on the History of Health Care*, New York, 1974; M. Raeff, *The Well-Ordered Police State: Social and Institutional Change Through Law in the Germanies and Russia, 1600–1800*, New Haven and London, 1983, pp. 119–35.

[26]   This is evident especially in hospitals, which had always been points of convergence and conflict between Roman civic elites and the papal central government. The administration of hospitals and other charitable institutions was subjected to several reforms between the seventeenth and eighteenth centuries to curb the autonomy of municipal elites, reorder the financial management and improve the spiritual and bodily care of the sick. Motivations for such neo-Tridentine reforms were religious and political – that is, reforms mainly aimed at limiting the lay governors' power – but by and large they promoted the role of medical staff. See S. Dominici, 'Il governo dell'ospedale di Santo Spirito e dei suoi annessi nel secolo XVII: Continuità e riforme', *Il Veltro*, 5–6, 2001, pp. 239–51; D. Rosselli, 'Tra Campidoglio e luoghi pii: elites romane di età barocca', in *Gruppi ed identità sociali nell'Italia di età moderna: percorsi di ricerca*, ed. B. Salvemini, Bari, 1998, pp. 143–98. On the Congregazione della Visita apostolica, see Chapter 7.

On all occasions, at any rate, the medical profession's contribution to the welfare of the Papal States was extolled by the indefatigable Lancisi. Over the course of many years, the archiater readily turned the achievements of papal health policies to the advantage of both the government and the physicians, inflating each one's increased authority and prestige.

Just as he had done in 1706 for sudden death, he published the proceedings of the commission instituted in 1709 to deal with the catarrhal fever epidemic in a tract that delved into the problem of Roman air in the style of Hippocrates. The book was divided into three parts. The first part analysed the air, water and weather conditions to be expected in Rome in ordinary times. It drew upon a variety of classical and modern sources, and abounded in medico-topographical and climate observations as well as chemical experiments. The second part examined the factors that altered the naturally optimal conditions, leading to periods of 'morbid constitution'; Lancisi imputed insalubrity to human action such as, for instance, neglect of sanitation in cities and land abandonment. Finally, the third part detailed all the initiatives that had been undertaken to fight the 1709 epidemics,

> so that not only doctors ... but also princes and magistrates may learn how to usefully avoid and correct such illness from the charity, vigilance and providence of our most Holy Lord Clement XI.[27]

Again, at the end of the epizootic outbreak in 1715, following the model of Cardinal Girolamo Gastaldi's widely celebrated tract on the 1656 plague *Tractatus de avertenda et profliganda peste politico-legalis*, Lancisi collected all medical and administrative records (expert reports, edicts, regulations) in a *Dissertatio historica de bovilla peste*.[28] Two years later, in 1717, he published the proceedings of the legal suit on the forest of Cisterna in a wide-ranging study about marshland effluvia and tertiary fevers, *De noxiis paludum effluviis, eorumque remediis*.[29] The publication featured a wealth of epidemiological observations, post-mortem reports, therapeutic experiments

---

[27] Lancisi, *Dissertatio de nativis*, p. 124. Lancisi's tract is dedicated to Clement XI's nephew and newly promoted cardinal Annibale Albani.

[28] Lancisi, *Dissertatio historica de bovilla peste*. Cardinal Gastaldi's plague tract was published in 1684 by Manolessi in Bologna, and can be deemed an instance of late seventeenth-century papal absolutism. Interestingly, though, it also shed light on the subordination of the medical profession to religious authority, which was now challenged; see M.P. Donato, 'La peste dopo la peste: economia di un discorso romano (1656–1720)', *Roma moderna e contemporanea*, 14, 2006, pp. 159–74.

[29] G.M. Lancisi, *De noxiis paludum effluviis, eorumque remediis libri duo*, Rome, 1717, pp. 86–133. On this famous treatise on malaria, see R. Sallares, *Malaria and Rome: A History of Malaria in Ancient Italy*, Oxford, 2002, pp. 46–7; M. Conforti, S. Marinozzi and

and sanitation measures adopted over time to combat epidemics in various towns in the Papal States (Civitavecchia, Bagnorea, Pesaro, Ferentino). Since 'singular [clinical] observations, even though they be frequent, can only form a confused mass of examples' and do not lead to a real understanding of illness, the author's intention in combining various forms of medical knowledge was to produce an 'accurate history of epidemics ... to discern the real causes of things'.[30] Lancisi's was in fact the Roman version of comparable environmental medical research that was then being undertaken in other parts of Europe by renowned physicians such as Thomas Sydenham, Bernardino Ramazzini and Friedrich Hoffman. Each claimed to follow the teachings of Hippocrates, which urged investigation into the connections between environment, climate, lifestyle and illness. Among other things, Lancisi described in his book how, in 1695, the Tiber had flooded the tombs in the church of Santa Maria, near Porta Angelica, dragging away the buried remains which contaminated its waters. Then he detailed how, shortly afterwards, an outbreak of petechial fever degenerating in apoplectic accidents had hit the city districts closest to the river.

Morbi causas investigandas, emendandas et avertendas: More on Public Dissections and the Physician's Authority

It should not be overlooked that a more active role of physicians in public affairs did not – could not – imply a change in current medical practices for the prevention and containment of epidemics. Theories of air had been modernised in corpuscularian or atomist terms, but sanitary responses still rested on a fairly traditional ideal of good environment, and measures implemented for its improvement remained very much the same over the early modern period. Eighteenth-century Hippocratism would still resort to very similar conceptual categories and tools.[31] However, willingness to protect public health was made

---

V. Gazzaniga, 'Delle arie, acque e luoghi: igiene e sanità pubblica a Roma nell'opera di Giovanni Maria Lancisi', *Roma moderna e contemporanea*, 13, 2005, pp. 115–32.

[30]   Lancisi, *De noxiis paludum effluviis*, p. 147.

[31]   Riley, *The Eighteenth-Century Campaign*; G. Miller, 'Airs, Waters, and Places in History', *Journal of the History of Medicine*, 17, 1962, pp. 129–40; C. Hannaway, 'The Société Royale de Médecine and Epidemics in the Ancien Régime', *Bulletin of the History of Medicine*, 47, 1972, pp. 256–73; J.P. Desaive et al., *Médecins, climat, et épidémies à la fin du XVIIIe siècle*, Paris, 1972. Arguments were still the same in the eighteenth-century debate on cemeteries, see Tomasi, *Per salvare i viventi*, pp. 233–91. The association of predisposing causes (food, lifestyle, climate) and triggering causes in epidemics was revived in the nineteenth century in regard to cholera, as analysed by C. Hamlin, 'Predisposing Causes and Public Health in Early Nineteenth-Century Medical Thought', *Social History of Medicine*, 5, 1992, pp. 43–70. See

more explicit. This entailed the adoption of novel investigative methods, such as the systematic collection of epidemiological observations, and the development of medical topographies and studies of climate. Such methods followed in the wake of early eighteenth-century Hippocratic medicine and were already at work in Lancisi's 1717 tract on marshland exhalations.[32] More interestingly from our viewpoint, pathological anatomy came to occupy a prominent role as the empirical foundation of medical authority too.

Indeed, in terms of the medico-political function of dissection, the 1706 Roman investigation can be viewed as the beginnings of something of a 'public health policy through corpses', which would later become established, albeit in a discontinuous manner, as part of modern medical policing.[33] None of the theoretical and practical aspects of autopsy were entirely new; what was unprecedented was their use in validating the physician's knowledge and action in society. We shall deal later with the anatomo-pathological method from the viewpoint of medical science, and focus instead on how physicians exploited it in their relationship with political power and the public. The aim is to assess how the peculiar configuration of powers and knowledge in early eighteenth-century papal Rome produced significant innovation, though precarious and destined to find better application in other contexts.

On more than one occasion, Roman physicians dealing with health emergencies in the first half of the eighteenth century used and presented autopsies as the preliminary operation *ad morbi causas investigandas, emendandas et avertendas* (in order to investigate, correct and prevent the causes of disease). Post-mortems were mostly performed in the main city hospitals, and their results were increasingly often being introduced in the discourse on the proper, effective ways of understanding and containing the maladies of the people, both endemic and epidemic. In truth, already in the late seventeenth century corpses had been occasionally dissected in connection with the outbreak of pestilential fevers.[34] Dissections were arguably encouraged by the widespread practice of post-mortem in Roman hospitals. However, it is a fact that the increased relevance given to morbid anatomy in guiding medical debate and justifying health policies was principally due to the investigation of 1706

---

further S. Barles, *La ville délétère: médecins et ingénieurs dans l'espace urbain (XVIIIe–XXe siècles)*, Seyssel, 1999.

[32] According to Riley, *The Eighteenth-Century Campaign*, pp. 31–47, and I. Golinski, *British Weather and the Climate of Enlightenment*, Chicago, 2007, pp. 140–50, British medicine was particularly concerned with climate, while medical topographies were mainly developed in continental Europe.

[33] J.P. Frank, *System einer vollständigen medizinischer Polizey*, vol. 6, Vienna, 1816; F. Freschi, *Sulle cause della morte improvvisa e sulla loro maniera di agire*, Florence, 1850 (reference to Lancisi at pp. 10–13).

[34] Lancisi, *De noxiis paludum effluviis*, pp. 160–62.

and the positive solution of that particular crisis. Thus, in the immediate wake of that event, during the influenza pandemic of 1709, physicians referred in their *consilium* to necropsies that were being carried out in the city's hospitals, which were overflowing with patients.[35] The same method was applied in the provinces. Dr Giuseppe Fieschi was sent to Bagnorea in 1707 along with two apprentice surgeons of the hospital of Santo Spirito at Lancisi's suggestion to tackle the strange pestilential fevers that had resulted in the patients' sudden deaths and performed a number of autopsies and reported them to Rome to decide on a course of action.[36] Public dissections were also performed on animals, when emergency arose. During the 1711 cattle plague, several infected cattle were dissected before doctors gave their expert opinion. Although such procedures were not unheard of (similar initiatives were also taken in Venice and Ferrara), the relevance given to them in public discourse as the basis for discerning the nature of veterinary diseases was unprecedented.

When the infection seemed to spread to horses, dissections received even greater publicity. In April 1712, surgeon Vincenzo Fuini carried out the dissection of a dead horse and the vivisection of a dying one in Castel Sant'Angelo, in the presence of the secretary to the cardinal chamberlain, the Capitoline Conservators (that is, the civic magistrates), court dignitaries and 'many other Roman knights'; all of the city farriers were also summoned. Supervised by the ever-present Lancisi, the examination was conducted on the animals' whole body, including the head and internal organs, and revealed inflammation of the intestines and of the brain, with an alteration of the blood. Incidentally, vivisection confirmed that there were no polyps in the horse's blood, 'whence it can be deduced that the stagnations in the heart for the most part occurred during [the animal's] agony'.[37]

It is noteworthy that the 1711 epizootic fuelled yet another confrontation between Aristotelians and 'neoterics' on the usefulness of dissection as a means of identifying diseases. The Theatine priest Antonio Maria Borromeo lent his pen to the views of empiricists, who were doubtful of this method. There were too many differences in the reports, Borromeo wrote, too contrasting views among the sects of the moderns – in short, there was too much uncertainty.[38] Lancisi in person took pains to counter such arguments. Though he conceded that 'in the case of pestilent disease, since the poisonous fermentation produces

---

[35]   Lancisi, *Dissertatio de nativis*, p. 129.

[36]   In several cases, Fieschi detected alterations in the cerebral meninges, similar to those reported in Rome in 1706; see Lancisi, *De noxiis paludum effluviis*, pp. 228–34. Lancisi's involvement and directive role is recorded in ms BLR, Lancisi 172, fols 3–156.

[37]   Borromeo, *Istoria dell'epidemia de' buoj*, p. 201.

[38]   Ibid., pp. 14–124. A brief biographical sketch on Borromeo can be found in G. Vedova, *Biografia degli scrittori padovani*, vol. 1, Padua, 1832, pp. 142–4.

a thousand stagnations and mutations during the death throes, we can draw but little profit ... through opening corpses', he added vexedly that

> the so-called rational medicine, of which I am a proud practitioner, owes great part of its proficiency to subtle anatomy, and the true knowledge of the manners by which our diseases are produced.[39]

In the first decades of the eighteenth century, other medical practitioners besides Lancisi (who was, after all, in many ways a rather extraordinary figure) adopted the same approach. The truth of the dissected body now proved a valuable asset to reinforce the health magistrates' authority in the face of real or presumed dangers to public health, and assumed greater value in the economy of medical public discourse.

A perfect representative of such attitude is, for instance, Domenico Gagliardi. Born not far from the capital, in the small town of Marino, Gagliardi graduated in Rome in 1676. He gained some renown thanks to his 1689 study *Anatomes ossium*, in which he extended to bone formation the theory of phytogenesis advanced in the book *Anatomes plantarum* by Malpighi (whom Gagliardi saluted as the 'Columbus of the microcosm' for his studies of microscopic anatomy).[40] Assistant and subsequently head physician at Santo Spirito, Gagliardi was admitted to the Roman College of Physicians around 1695. In 1707, he replaced in the perpetual magistrature his colleague Antonio Piacenti, who had died unexpectedly during the sudden death 'epidemic'; unfortunately, he was soon forced to vacate his college seat in favour of Lancisi, who had just triumphed over that same emergency. Re-admitted to the perpetual magistrature in 1712, Gagliardi held the protomedicus office for the first time in 1714, and in this capacity he intervened in the legal suit concerning the forest of Cisterna. Protomedicus again in 1718, Gagliardi published *L'idea del vero medico fisico e morale* (*The mirror of the true doctor in physics and morals*), a treatise on medical ethics and a modern *ratio studiorum* (plan of studies) for medical students in which he defended the usefulness of post-mortems for medical education and practice.[41] He then undertook an ambitious programme of popularising modern

---

[39] Borromeo, *Istoria dell'epidemia de' buoj*, pp. 155, 129. It should not be overlooked that acute infectious diseases are the most difficult to be detected by means of an autopsy.

[40] D. Gagliardi, *Anatomes ossium novis inventis illustratae*, Rome, 1689, republished in Le Clerc and Manget's *Bibliotheca anatomica*, 2nd edn, vol. 2, Geneva, 1699, pp. 1207–22, and further mentioned by J.J. Manget, *Bibliotheca scriptorum medicorum*, Geneva, 1731, p. 367.

[41] D. Gagliardi, *L'idea del vero medico Fisico, e Morale, formata secondo li documenti, ed operazioni d'Ippocrate*, Rome, 1718, p. 37. Students were advised to 'be in attendance [of post-mortems], and the more so if you have observed the illness of the poor deceased ...

medicine.[42] When the plague struck Marseille in 1720, Gagliardi happened to be chief physician once again. He immediately sent to the printing press a book of reassuring *Consigli preservativi e curativi in tempo di contagio* (*Preservative and curative advice in time of contagion*) in which he explained contagion in corpuscularian terms.[43]

Mercifully, the plague never crossed the borders of the Papal States. That same year in winter, however, Rome was hit by a spate of 'chest disease' that showed several characteristics in common with the influenza epidemic of 1709. It was a further opportunity for Gagliardi to extol the modernity of both his own approach and that of the institutions he represented. In the *Relazione de' mali di petto che corrono presentemente* (*Report on the chest afflictions occurring at present*), he compared recent and past outbreaks of equivalent illnesses on the basis of clinical observations and anatomo-pathological reports.[44] His medical inquiry pivots around autopsies – 'very many' of which, Gagliardi states, were performed at the hospital of Santo Spirito in 1713 and in 1720 at his request, and a few of which he related in the appendix to his volume. In this work post-mortems are presented as the true 'experimental' foundation in devising the right prophylaxis and treatment for each affliction.[45] Incidentally, Gagliardi took the time to rebut by means of authority, logic and experience, any criticism of dissection for medical purposes, dismissing all sterile doubts that 'those

---

since by manner of such inspections you will gain better knowledge of the affected parts, and furthermore of the causes of disease'.

   [42]   D. Gagliardi, *Dell'infermo istruito*, Rome, 1720, and *L'educazione de' figliuoli morale e medica*, Rome, 1722.

   [43]   Printed in Rome in 1720, about which see Donato, 'La peste dopo la peste'.

   [44]   D. Gagliardi, *Relazione de' mali di petto che corrono presentemente ... ove mediante reiterate aperture de' cadaveri, ed esperienze fatte ... si mostrano le cause, cura, e preservativi*, Rome, 1720, analysed by G. Olagüe de Ros, 'La "Relazione de' male di petto" (1720) de Domenico Gagliardi (ca. 1660–ca. 1735) en el ambiente anatomoclinico romano', *Dynamis*, 3, 1983, pp. 289–302.

   [45]   Gagliardi, *Relazione de' mali di petto*, pp. 6–10. Despite a certain number of analogies, Gagliardi underscores the differences found in the post-mortems. While in 1713 no recurrent or noteworthy lesions in the organs had been observed on the dissecting table, in 1720 many deceased patients showed hepatisation of the lungs, which presented 'a lobe with the aforesaid gangrene, and the other with phlegmon; moreover in some corpses a propagation of this disease to the other viscera was found, that is, in the heart and pericardium, or in the liver, spleen, kidneys or intestines, and even more frequently in the pleura and the transverse septum, with most notable extravasation in scirrhous swellings ... We observed in most of the corpses very hard and considerably large polypous concretions in the heart, and in some of them, which were supposedly affected by angina, we did not find any alterations in their fauces, but rather abundance of pus in the lungs.'

gangrenes or rots that are discovered upon the opening of corpses might be the product of cadaveric putrefaction'.[46]

Obviously, a doctor of medicine and philosophy like Gagliardi would seek to establish the universal causes of the epidemic of chest afflictions on the basis of sound reasoning and would speculate about causes beyond the specific cases that he had examined. His conceptual framework is the familiar corpuscularian notion of air corruption. While differing from the 'celebrated author' who had studied the 1709 flu epidemic – that is, Lancisi – Gagliardi echoes some of the philosophical tenets as well as the epidemiological and environmental argumentations of his more prominent colleague. In the end, he delivers an all too familiar account of earthquakes and volcanic eruptions diffusing 'putrefactive and corrosive' particles in the atmosphere. 'Being material and ponderous molecules', noxious particles produce 'the fixation of the [bodily] lymphs and corruptions of the blood' and eventually provoke the hepatisation of the lungs as observed on the dissecting table. Obviously, damage is especially severe for ailing bodies 'devoid of vigour because of malnutrition', 'without clothes' or weakened by 'a medicine improperly prepared'. Accordingly, Gagliardi proposed to extend medical surveillance to the quality of food (usually under the control of the pope's paternalistic government through the congregations of the Annona and of the Grascia), since

> it is ascertained that, when weak constitutions reign, the greatest benefit that can be given to the people is to examine in great detail all those things from which they take nourishment, to seek out whether there may be any defects to correct.[47]

Hence, the truth of the dissected bodies underpins medical counsel with empirical evidence and facilitates physicians in their duty to advise and reassure the people in the face of sanitary emergencies. It allows them to stress their own political role. In short, in order to protect the living, medicine must gain knowledge of the dead. We thus need to return to the corpse – how to view it, interpret it and make it the foundation of medical rationality – and explore the 'taming of death' in eighteenth-century medical theory.

---

[46] Ibid., pp. 12–13.
[47] Ibid., pp. 38–9, 41, 51.

PART II
Sudden Death in Medical Theory and Practice

Chapter 4

A New Stance on Death:
The Mechanical Medicine of Lancisi's
De subitaneis mortibus (1707)

Sudden Death in the Hippocratic-Galenic Medical Tradition

So far we have dealt with sudden death mainly as a social and political issue, analysing how physicians repositioned themselves in society and reformulated their authority by confronting an unprecedented emergency in a novel way. We shall now consider sudden death from the viewpoint of medical knowledge and practice, looking specifically at Lancisi's *De subitaneis mortibus*. This text was not only an investigation into death – in fact, the first modern scientific work on death[1] – but also a report on public health, an account of the autopsies performed 'at the pope's command' and a treatise of mechanical medicine. Each aspect of Lancisi's work raises questions. What characterises mechanical medicine in theory and in practice? What does it contribute to the understanding of the phenomenon of sudden death and of death in general? And to what extent did the context in which Lancisi's book originated – that is, early eighteenth-century Rome – determine its content?

Obviously, Lancisi was not the first to explore the subject of sudden death. To medical professionals, it was a standard problem associated with apoplexy and syncope (that is, heart failure), which had been described in many *loci* of the great medical authors of classical antiquity. Unexpected death was in fact a calamitous event that a good physician was expected to anticipate by means of the observation of a complex network of signs (the pulse and breath, above all) and his insight into the individual dispositions of his patients.

The main concern with sudden death in the Hippocratic corpus (for instance in *Aphorisms* II, 41 and 44) is precisely the identification of at-risk individuals such as the obese, athletes and the elderly. The theme is associated with apoplexy (a term meaning being struck all of a sudden, as if by lightning) and epilepsy.[2]

---

[1]   E.H. Ackerknecht, 'Death in the History of Medicine', *Bulletin of the History of Medicine*, 42, 1968, pp. 19–23.

[2]   E. Clarke, 'Apoplexy in the Hippocratic Writings', *Bulletin of the History of Medicine*, 37, 1963, pp. 301–14; H. Bruun, 'Sudden Death as an Apoplectic Sign in the Hippocratic

Although diagnosis and localisation of the affected part of the body are of secondary importance in Hippocratic medicine, apoplexy is attributed to a flux of cold humours towards the head that refrigerates the blood abruptly and thus deprives the body of its vital heat. Hippocratic texts disagree as to which of the four humours is the prime cause. Some *Aphorisms* indicate black bile, while *Diseases II* points to phlegm: phlegm is attracted to the head by a warming of the vessels of the head but it then cools the brain too rapidly. Phlegm is also associated with epilepsy in *On the Sacred Disease*, while *Airs, Waters and Places* comments on the role of climate and winds. Furthermore, by way of offering guidance for practitioners, several texts in the Hippocratic corpus hint at the signs by which an attack can be anticipated.[3]

Aretaeus of Cappadocia, another Greek physician famous for his careful clinical observations, associates sudden death with syncope and apoplexy, and treats the former as an acute disease of the heart and the latter as a disease of the nerves similar to paralysis.[4] In the same vein, reviving the teachings of the leader of the Greek Methodic School Soranus of Ephesus, Caelius Aurelianus classifies apoplexy as an acute deadly disease and gives a description of the prodromal signs (that is, the signs between the appearance of the first symptoms and the actual crisis) which would remain standard for all subsequent authors.[5]

Corpus', *Classica et mediaevalia*, 50, 1999, pp. 5–24; B. Gundert, 'Soma and Psyche in Hippocratic Medicine', in *Psyche and Soma: Physicians and Metaphysicians on the Mind-Body Problem from Antiquity to Enlightenment*, ed. J.P. Wright and P. Potter, Oxford, 2000, pp. 13–36.

[3]   Among the prodromic signs are sudden headache, aphonia, weakness, hypovision and sleepiness. Some of these symptoms can also prelude an epileptic attack, which can be of an apoplectic kind and cause a swift death; see O. Temkin, *The Falling Sickness: A History of Epilepsy from the Greeks to the Beginnings of Modern Neurology*, Baltimore, 1971, pp. 40–56.

[4]   I have used René Laënnec's translation of Aretaeus's *Des causes et des signes des maladies aiguës et chroniques*, ed. M.D. Grmek, Geneva, 2000, p. 44 on syncope, p. 80 on paralysis, in relation to which apoplexy is treated as a chronic illness of the nerves.

[5]   Caelius Aurelianus, *On Acute and Chronic Diseases*, ed. and trans. I.E. Drabkin, Chicago, 1950, pp. 332–5. According to the principles of the Methodic school, apoplexy is a 'constrictory' illness (*status strictus*). Methodical doctrines enjoyed a revival in the seventeenth and eighteenth centuries when the pathology of the solids prevailed on the traditional pathology of humours. On the interpretations concerning diseases of the *kardias* (the area between the stomach, the oesophagus and the heart), sometimes mistaken for syncope, see R. Siegel, 'Descriptions of Circulatory Collapse and Coronary Thrombosis in the Fifth Century AD by Caelius Aurelianus', *American Journal of Cardiology*, 7, 1961, pp. 427–31; C.R.S. Harris, *The Heart and the Vascular System in Ancient Greek Medicine, from Alcmaeon to Galen*, Oxford, 1973, pp. 432–50.

In the vast body of writings by Galen, the most influential physician of the Roman imperial age, sudden death is treated both as an issue of general physiology and as a practical medical topic. In the wake of Aristotle, Galen considers the hierarchy of vital functions (those organs that are necessary for life) and imputes swift death to impeded respiration and, ultimately, to heart failure, the heart being the primary seat of innate heat and the vital faculties. Even in brain diseases like apoplexy, death in fact only occurs if the vital faculties are affected.[6] From a strictly medical standpoint, however, Galen describes apoplexy as a rapid, sudden affliction with deprivation of sense and motion nearly always entailing immediate death, and considers it a 'cold disease' of the brain, mostly caused by phlegm, sometimes by blood or black bile. Galen clearly derives his doctrine and prognostic pessimism from Hippocrates, on whose writings he commentated extensively, but he provides a fuller account based on a more sophisticated anatomical and physiological doctrine.[7] His teachings are further systematised by the Persian physician and philosopher Avicenna in his immensely influential *Canon of Medicine*. With the stated aim of reconciling Galen and Aristotle on the subject of vital faculties, Avicenna sets the seat of vital heat and *spiritus* in the heart. He accordingly distinguishes syncope from apoplexy, though both potentially entail swift death, and provides an ordered exposition of the various types of both afflictions with their specific diagnosis,

---

[6] A. Debru, *Le corps respirant: la pensée physiologique chez Galien*, Leiden, 1996; J. Rocca, *Galen on the Brain: Anatomical Knowledge and Physiological Speculation in the Second Century AD*, Leiden, 2003, pp. 432–55. As is well known, while Aristotle considers the heart the only and foremost vital centre (the first to form and the last to die), Galen attributes the natural functions (digestion, reproduction), vital functions (maintenance of heat) and animal functions (sensation and motion) to the liver, the heart and the brain respectively. However, he accepts that death is always brought about by the impairment of vital faculties. See Harris, *The Heart*, pp. 267–396; P. Manuli and M. Vegetti, *Cuore, sangue e cervello: biologia e antropologia nel pensiero antico*, Milan, 1977.

[7] In Galen's physiology, the vital spirits in the blood are filtered into animal spirits by the network of arteries known as the *rete mirabile* which lies at the basis of the cranium. The animal spirits are perfected in the cerebral ventricles where the nourishing venous blood from the liver is also available, with the help of inhaled air. Spirits are finally diffused through the nerves to produce motion and sensation. According to this paradigm, there are two types of apoplexy: from local unbalance, when viscous matter obstructs the flowing of animal spirits, and from plethora, if a superabundance of blood overheats the vessels and thus cools the brain; see A. Karenberg, 'Reconstructing a Doctrine: Galen on Apoplexy', *Journal of the History of the Neurosciences*, 3, 1994, pp. 85–101. The differential diagnosis of sudden loss of consciousness is based on respiration: when breathing is laborious, there is apoplexy, otherwise there is *stupor*.

prognosis and treatment.[8] Avicenna's presentation of syncope and apoplexy in connection to sudden death would then pass to scholastic medicine.[9]

Late Renaissance Galenism produced renewed interest in the problem. Sixteenth-century authors dealing with apoplexy and syncope blended Aristotelianism with modern anatomical awareness. They strove to define the essence of life and to inquire into the human body's faculties, as was appropriate for learned professors of philosophy and medicine, and elaborated on Aristotle's natural philosophy and Galen's medical theory at length. However, as their knowledge of human anatomy increased, adjustments had to be made and new questions arose.[10] To choose but one example, Annibale Albertini's *De affectionibus cordis libri tres* aptly illustrates how sudden death is dealt with in early modern Galenism.[11] After a long, scholarly presentation of Aristotle, Galen and other ancient and modern authorities on the natural and vital faculties and a complex classification of all preternatural states of the heart, Albertini defines syncope as a sudden impairment of innate heat, an unanticipated and swift 'unnatural cooling of the natural heat of the heart and of the whole body' caused by humours of opposite – that is, cold – quality, poisons or other pernicious 'occult qualities',[12] or by disordered motions of the soul.[13]

---

[8]   S. Jarcho, *The Concept of Heart Failure: From Avicenna to Albertini*, Cambridge, MA, 1980, pp. 1–16; A. Karenberg and I. Hort, 'Medieval Descriptions and Doctrines of Stroke 2. Between Galenism and Aristotelism: Islamic Theories of Apoplexy (800–1200)', *Journal of the History of the Neurosciences*, 7, 3, 1998, pp. 174–85; for a more general appraisal, see B. Kisch, 'What Keeps Men Alive? A Survey of the History of Thoughts About Life and Death', in *The Historical Development of Physiological Thought*, ed. C. McC. Brooks and P.F. Cranefield, New York, 1959, pp. 309–34.

[9]   A. Karenberg and I. Hort, 'Medieval Descriptions and Doctrines of Stroke 3. Multiplying Speculations: The High and Late Middle Ages (1000–1450)', *Journal of the History of the Neurosciences*, 7, 3, 1998, pp. 186–200.

[10]   See, for example, J. Fernel, *Universa medicina*, Paris, 1554, *Pathologia*, on apoplexy p. 133, on syncope p. 159, where Fernel echoes Avicenna nearly to the letter but adds three post-mortem observations. On the views of apoplexy held by the French Hippocratics Hollier, Duret and Baillou, see I.M. Lonie 'The "Paris Hippocratics": Teaching and Research in Paris in the Second Half of the Sixteenth Century', in *The Medical Renaissance of the Sixteenth Century*, ed. A. Wear, R.K. French and I.M. Lonie, Cambridge, 1985, pp. 155–74. Jarcho, *The Concept of Heart Failure*, pp. 28–83, analyses Girolamo Capivaccio's acclaimed book *Practica medicina* (1594).

[11]   A. Albertini *De affectionibus cordis libri tres*, Venice, 1618, esp. pp. 295–310. See also F. Bartoletti, *Methodus in dyspnoeam seu de respirationibus libri quatuor*, Bologna, 1633.

[12]   On the doctrine of occult qualities (occult in the sense that they are not perceived by the senses or reason, unlike the essential and manifest qualities such as colours and tastes), of great significance in Renaissance medicine, see L.D. Richardson, 'The Generation of Disease: Occult Causes and Diseases of the Total Substance', in *The Medical Renaissance*, ed. Wear, French and Lonie, pp. 175–94.

[13]   S. Cavallo and T. Storey, *Healthy Living in Late Renaissance Italy*, Oxford, 2013, pp. 179–85.

Occasionally, cases of sudden death that might also include post-mortem examination are incorporated in the collections of *historiae* and *curationes* that emerged as a specific genre of medical literature from the sixteenth to seventeenth century with the aim of connecting individual cases to the general medical doctrine, for instance in Amatus Lusitanus' *Curationum medicinalium centuriae* (1560)[14] or in Rembert Dodoens's *Medicinalium observationum* (1581).[15] Case histories, especially if complete with an autopsy report, would then be reprinted together with similar ones in late seventeenth-century compilations of medical observations, such as Théophile Bonet's *Sepulchretum*, which assembled observations from various sources and rearranged them into an ordered scheme *a capite ad calcem* (from head to toe).[16]

In addition, a specific medical literature on sudden death began to appear at the end of the sixteenth century, along with works on apoplexy and diseases of the heart, despite the traditional reluctance of Hippocratic-Galenic medicine to go beyond the relationship with the living patient and address death.[17] One such tract is *Mortis repentinae examen* by Paolo Grassi, court physician in Novellara and Correggio. The book begins with a learned disquisition on the essence of life and death, which is understood as a 'corruption of the innate heat' and drying up of radical moisture. Grassi is aware of discrepancies among *auctoritates* in explaining vital heat and spirit, as well as in defining natural and violent death, but he nevertheless indicates three ways in which a 'violent' depletion of life might occur: 'by sudden suffocation, or unanticipated dissolution, or sudden corruption.'[18] The direct cause of sudden death is humoral plethora, which can

---

[14]   Lusitanus was the first to describe death by myocardial infarction with coronary occlusion according to J.O. Leibowitz, *The History of Coronary Heart Disease*, Berkeley, CA, 1970, p. 62. On the flourishing literature of *observationes*, see G. Pomata, 'Praxis Historialis: The Uses of Historiae in Early Modern Medicine', in *Historia: Empiricism and Erudition in Early Modern Europe*, ed. G. Pomata and N.G. Siraisi, Cambridge, MA, 2005, pp. 105–46.

[15]   R. Dodoens, *Medicinalium observationum exempla rara, recognita et aucta*, Cologne, 1581, pp. 19–24, 227; see also P. van Foreest (Forestus), *Observationum medicinalium libri tres, de capitis et cerebri morbis ac symptomatis*, Leiden, 1602, pp. 580–606.

[16]   T. Bonet, *Sepulchretum, sive Anatomia practica*, vol. 1, Geneva, 1679, pp. 76–123 for apoplexy; pp. 693–710 for *mors repentina*; pp. 678–92 for syncope; T. Bonet, *Medicina septentrionalis collatitia*, Geneva, 1686, p. 496 on sudden death. See further H.S. Schutta and H.M. Howe, 'Concepts of "Apoplexy" as Reflected in Bonet's "Sepulchretum"', *Journal of the History of the Neurosciences*, 15, 2006, pp. 250–68.

[17]   Of course, in Graeco-Roman medicine death is one of the possible events that a physician might foretell to his patient, as J. Pigeaud underscores in 'La question du cadavre dans l'Antiquité gréco-romaine', *Micrologus*, 7, 1999, pp. 43–71.

[18]   P. Grassi, *Mortis repentinae examen una cum brevis methodo praesagiendi et praecavendi omnes, qui subeunt illius periculum*, Modena, 1612, p. 29. On Grassi, see G. Cosmacini, 'Sulle morti improvvise', in *Il medico di fronte alla morte (secoli XVI–XXI)*, ed. G. Cosmacini and G. Vigarello, Turin, 2008, pp. 23–32.

incur various types of *dyscrasia* (disequilibrium) and affect different organs. Grassi does not fail to confront the classic question of life functions and advances an interpretation that would reconcile Aristotle (through Avicenna) and Galen, since he states that both heart and brain can cause sudden death.[19] As for the remote causes of humoral dyscrasia, they include a long list of factors related to lifestyle, environment and accidental circumstances. Efficacious treatment, Grassi continues, consists mainly of bloodletting as well as a strict regulation of the non-naturals with the main objective of protecting the heart.

A further instance of late Aristotelian Galenism is *De causis mortis repentinae tractatio* by the Veronese physician Domenico Terilli.[20] Quoting Aristotle's *Parva Naturalia*, Terilli identifies life with the 'subsistence of natural heat in the vegetative soul' and he then settles on a definition of sudden death as the 'extinction of innate heat that spreads from the heart throughout the body, which originates from an internal or external cause, and acts with the greatest and most violent swiftness'.[21] Unexpected death results from a rapid deprivation of innate heat. Since innate heat can be altered 'by an opposite quality' (that is, cold, for instance if one drinks an excessively cold drink), suffocated by a rush of humours (like a flame that is put out), dispersed or dissolved, Terilli distinguishes various kinds of sudden death, which might in fact ensue from a variety of natural (related to the bodily constitution) or non-natural (external or pathological) causes such as the rupture of great vessels, the dispersion of animal spirits through an excess of activity, suffocation of the uterus or poisonous exhalations from earthquakes and cemeteries.

Arguments similar to Grassi's and Terilli's recur in the work of other sixteenth- and seventeenth-century medical writers, for instance in the brief medico-practical tract *De morbis subitaneis* by François Ranchin, a physician from Montpellier and one of the most famous practitioners in France at the time. Notably though, Ranchin deals with sudden onset of illness rather than with

---

[19]   The heart, which is 'the source and the origin of natural heat and the seat of life itself' can be damaged, for instance, by unruly emotions that provoke a sudden movement of vital spirits and blood which 'suffocate' innate heat; also a brain ailment such as the obstruction of the ventricles or *rete mirabile* by an excess of humours or dense vapours can impede breathing, which regulates vital heat and, consequently, life. A plethora of blood might also hinder the renewal of vital heat, which runs out or suffocates if 'the superfluous elements thick with vapours and smut are not expelled and the air substance that refrigerates and ventilates is not inhaled'. Finally, an opposite quality (cold) can extinguish innate heat and an occult quality (such as the plague) can corrupt it.

[20]   D. Terilli, *De causis mortis repentinae tractatio in qua etiam disputatur quid sit mors et vita in genere et quae mortis causae communes, singula vero quae de causis mortis repentinae enarrantur*, Venice, 1615.

[21]   Ibid., p. 14.

death.[22] In fact, in late Galenic medicine, although sudden death is the stated object of a few writings, it is never characterised except by means of tautology, nor is it precisely explained. In most cases, age and ageing, rather than death, are the true topic of medical discourse, and a few writers explicitly point to this ambiguity when they recall that ancient authorities did not agree whether there was such a thing in nature as violent or sudden death.[23]

Matter and Motion in Giovanni M. Lancisi's Interpretation of Life and Death

A considerable distance separates Lancisi's *De subitaneis mortibus* from early seventeenth-century literature on the subject. Nearly a century of circulatory physiology had followed Harvey's discovery of the circulation of the blood (1628), during which time systematic anatomical studies on the main organs as well as on the 'subtler' corporal parts, underpinned by mechanical, atomist and corpuscularian natural philosophy, had dramatically altered the image of the human body.

Right from his preliminary definition of life, Lancisi abandons the Aristotelian heritage in favour of a clear mechanistic option. Thus, he defines life, 'according to the anatomists and the chemists', 'due not merely to one, but to a combination of several principles, and chiefly of two – to the organic structure of the solid parts of major function, and at the same time to a corresponding mixture, to the fluidity and mass of liquid parts of like function'.[24] There is no place in Lancisi's treatise either for vital heat and its dissipation/suffocation, or for the vapours and vitalist principles of Galenic medicine. The body is now perceived, conceived and analysed as an organised aggregation of machines of different sizes and functions, whereas the rational soul is mentioned once at

---

[22]   In F. Ranchin, *Opuscula medica*, Lyon, 1627, pp. 593–669.

[23]   F. Fedeli, *De relationibus medicorum libri quatuor*, Palermo, 1602, pp. 345–9; M. Flacius, *Commentariorum physicorum de vita et morte libri IIII*, Frankfurt, 1584, pp. 86–9. The association of death and old age is described by Grassi, *Examen mortis repentinae*, p. 29: 'Animated beings age because they become desiccated either through the passing of time or due to the continuous loss of substance, while innate heat, operating on the radical moisture and consuming it by feeding on it, attacks the bodies and desiccates them, which further provokes the draining away of the entire vital substance, until the subject becomes unfit for life.' On this particular issue, see M.D. Grmek, *On Ageing and Old Age: Basic Problems and Historic Aspects of Gerontology and Geriatrics*, The Hague, 1958, and below, Chapter 6.

[24]   SM, p. 3. For a general overview on early modern and modern biological models, see W. Bernardi, 'Fisiologia e mondo della vita', in *Storia della scienza moderna e contemporanea*, ed. P. Rossi, vol. 1, Milan, 2000, pp. 375–400; F. Duchesneau, *Les modèles du vivant de Descartes à Leibniz*, Paris, 1998.

the beginning, as being 'in control' of the bodily machine, and twice briefly as 'departing' from the dying body.

Three major organs of the human machine (trachea and lungs; heart and blood vessels; brain and the nervous system) are considered by Lancisi to be indispensable for the conservation of life, jointly with three fluids: air, blood and 'nerve juice', which is secreted by the brain 'with its membranes' and propelled 'in a wavelike fashion' through the nerves. Lancisi gives the circulation of these fluids a central role in 'animal economy' (that is, physiology), following William Harvey, whom he considered to be the inventor of modern medicine and whose teachings he extended to respiration and cerebral-neural functions. In truth, neural circulation was a cornerstone of post-Harveyan and post-Cartesian physiology, which was informed by a principle of natural uniformity and unity.[25]

Hence, life can be considered a 'constant flow and reflow, more or less perceptible, of air, blood, nerve juice through and from the organs of major function sufficiently well disposed'; these fluids are stirred 'mutually and alternatively, more or less perceptibly', with the help of a myriad other organs throughout the body (glands, ducts, muscles).[26] Lancisi's definition echoes the teachings of, on the one hand, the ancient Methodics and, on the other hand, Galileo, Descartes and their disciples.[27] Conversely, death is understood as the disintegration of the ordered and continuous movements of solids and liquids. These obey physical laws that are known by means of reason and experiment. This 'natural necessity' represents the background against which clinical

---

[25]   E. Clarke, 'The Neural Circulation: The Use of Analogy in Medicine', *Medical History*, 22, 1978, pp. 291–307.

[26]   SM, p. 4.

[27]   According to G.A. Borelli, *On the Movements of Animals* (1680–1681), trans. P. Maquet, Berlin and Heidelberg, 1989, p. 319, 'the life of the animals or their vital operations consists of continuous and uninterrupted movement. The limbs and all solid, fluid and spirituous elements are activated by the blood when the body is in movement or is displaced from one place to the other, when it eats, digests, makes chyle and transforms food into blood, when it feeds and repairs lost elements, when it expresses sensations. In summary, nothing remains stable in an animal as long as it is alive.' Similar definitions of life are to be found in several contemporary Italian medical works, printed either in Rome or elsewhere; see, for example, G. Lanzoni, 'Dissertatio de vita et morte', *Appendix: Ephemeridum medico-physicarum Academiae ... Naturae Curiosurum*, 1699–1700, pp. 113–19; A. Pascoli, *Delle febbri teorica e pratica*, Perugia, 1699, p. 53; A. Pacchioni, *De durae meningis fabrica et usu disquisitio anatomica*, Rome, 1701, p. 90; G. Baglivi, *Specimen quatuor librorum de fibra motrice et morbosa*, Rome, 1702, p. 260. F. Hoffman, *Idea fundamentalis universae medicinae ex sanguinis mechanismo*, Halle, 1704, also put forward a mechanistic definition of life, though he emphasised the role of blood. For a general overview, see T.S. Hall, *Ideas of Life and Matter: Studies in the History of General Physiology: 600 B.C.–1900 A.D.*, Chicago, 1969; A. Pichot, *Histoire de la notion de vie*, Paris, 1993.

and anatomo-pathological observations must be set in order to formulate explanations and conjectures.

Lancisi differentiates himself from his less prominent colleagues in Clement XI's Rome who dealt with sudden death as yet another endemic malady and he seizes the opportunity to pronounce on life and death in general. He devotes the initial pages of his work to clarifying the notion of sudden death. Be it premature, violent or natural, abrupt death is always caused by an obstacle blocking the motion of the major fluids and solids, and 'if one of these, or several, or all have been impaired, either separately or together, to an extreme degree and most persistently, then an unexpected death is likely to threaten.'[28] A truly unanticipated demise is a rare event, and in most cases death is preceded by some kind of ailment. Pre-mortem pathological conditions, however, might be undetectable, which is the reason why sudden death sometimes strikes people who are in apparent good health, and the reason why it is so frightening and horrifying. In the rest of the treatise Lancisi develops a practical medicine that is consistent with a mechanical and hydraulic vision of the human body.

The content of Book One is organised 'by reason of the cause and of the manner, of the disease which causes death',[29] proceeding from the three fluids to the three major organs rather than by 'artificial definitions' – that is, without taking into account the medical entities traditionally associated with sudden death such as syncope and apoplexy. Lancisi examines the various combinations of defects that eventually produce unexpected death. He begins with fluids, more precisely with air, and this represents both an homage to Hippocrates and Galen, given the importance they attributed to breathing,[30] and an assertion of modernity, given the enormous interest the topic elicited in seventeenth-century science.[31] Air is not discussed as an Aristotelian element but as an elastic corpuscular fluid, and Robert Boyle is the first author cited to support the argument that excessive, rapid rarefaction or condensation of air might cause death. Of course, air also commonly brings about death by carrying noxious fumes and poisons that enter the body through the airways or skull fissures.[32] As regards ailments of the blood, Lancisi points to alterations of its mass and pressure provoking an arterial collapse, cardiac valve regurgitation or vessel lacerations. Accordingly, he reassesses that form of sudden death which followed

---

[28]   SM, pp. 14–15.

[29]   SM, p. 7.

[30]   Harris, *The Heart*, pp. 346–65; Debru, *Le corps respirant*, p. 129.

[31]   Hall, *Ideas of Life and Matter*, vol. 1, pp. 267–78; R.G. Frank, *Harvey and the Oxford Physiologists: A Study of Scientific Ideas*, Berkeley, CA, 1980.

[32]   Air penetrating the brain through the sutures of the cranium is a Galenic tenet, translated in chemical corpuscular terms as regards apoplexy by C. Fracassati, *Dissertatio epistolica responsoria de cerebro*, in [M. Malpighi and C. Fracassati], *Tetras anatomicarum epistolarum*, Bologna, 1665, pp. 258–429.

strong emotions. This had traditionally been attributed to a sudden plethora of humours which extinguished the innate heat in the heart; rather, 'the hearth and its vessels do not have an unlimited capacity to contain blood, nor sufficient power to propel it'.[33] Blood pathologies can also be of a chemical nature, the blood then lacking its natural viscosity and fermentation. Lancisi does not describe in detail the fermentative process, so familiar had the theory of Frans de La Boë Sylvius, Willis and their followers become, as we saw in Chapter 1. If so, lethal quantities of serum would ooze through the tissues, in the lungs and in the brain. Lancisi argues that this is what happens in the so-called 'serous apoplexies', which is confirmed by post-mortem detection of serum in the brain.[34] Finally, Lancisi examines the anomalies of fluids in the nerves.

At the time when the papal archiater was writing his tract, the brain was probably the most extensively studied organ. As the Danish anatomist Niels Stensen explained, it was 'the most renowned anatomical problem of the century'.[35] Hitherto, knowledge of the brain had been more or less limited to the gross anatomy described by ancient and Renaissance anatomists (Vesalio, Varolio, Casserio, Spigelius). Attention had been focused on the ventricles, as consensus was nearly unanimous that it was there that the vital spirits were distilled into the animal spirits. These were necessary to the so-called 'animal functions' of sense and motion, although there was no agreement as to how the distillation process worked, what the residual humours of such distillation were (catarrh or phlegm) or what the precise consistency of animal spirits was or how they were produced. In the mid-seventeenth century, however, most of the old established notions on the brain and the nervous system came under scrutiny. Modern theories basically displaced the distillation of animal spirits (now understood as a material substance, albeit 'most subtle') from the ventricles to the cortex. The cortex underwent micro-anatomical research based on the assumption that neural circulation was analogous to the circulation of the blood and that the brain functioned as a gland or filter like other organs.[36]

---

[33]   SM, p. 19.

[34]   SM, p. 20. The distinction between sanguineous and serous apoplexies, which refers indirectly to Galen, is already found in Daniel Sennert and Théophile Bonet. It would also be purported by Giovan Battista Morgagni.

[35]   N. Stensen [Steno], *Discours sur l'anatomie du cerveau*, Paris, 1669, p. 4.

[36]   Let us recall the milestones of post-Harveyan neurology. J.J. Wepfer, *Observationes anatomicae ex cadaveribus eorum, quos sustulit apoplexia*, 1658, offered a more precise description of the cerebral arteries refuting once and for all the existence of *rete mirabile* at the base of the skull; F. de la Boë Sylvius, *Disputationum medicarum*, 1660, moved the production of animal spirits from the ventricles to the cortex; N. Stensen, *Observationes anatomicae*, 1662, demonstrated that tears are secreted by specific glands, thus striking a deadly blow to the ancient notion of cerebral excretion that had already been disputed by K.V. Schneider, *De osse cribriforme*, 1655; T. Willis, *De cerebri anatome*, 1664, distinguished

Consequently, new ideas about cerebral pathologies emerged too, starting with the work of the first post-Harveyan writer on apoplexy, the Swiss physician Johann Jakob Wepfer. Through autopsies Wepfer demonstrated a connection between haemorrhages and apoplexy and thus refuted the old understanding of apoplexy as an obstruction of the brain ventricles by viscous matter. Immediately afterwards, the Italian physician Carlo Fracassati reinterpreted the old notion that nerves were blocked in apoplexy as the obstruction of the medullar fibres of the white matter.[37] According to Lancisi, weaknesses in neural circulation (such as insufficient quantity of blood from which the fluid is distilled in the cortex or haemorrhages compressing the cortex) or the abnormal chemical composition and fluidity of the nervous juice are all liable to provoke sudden death.[38]

---

voluntary and involuntary nervous systems and put forward a scheme of the brain's localised functional specialisation; M. Malpighi, *De viscerum structura*, 1664–65, launched micro-anatomic studies of the cerebral substance, which he considered to be glandular (grey matter) and medullary (white matter and medial structure) in nature: grey matter filters the blood through its meatus (which Malpighi compares to glands in analogy with kidney follicles),while white matter is composed of an infinite number of *fibrae albae* which transmit impulses to those nervous filaments that originate in them. Not to be omitted from this list is Stensen, *Discours sur l'anatomie du cerveau*, 1666, which challenged Descartes's theory postulating the pineal gland as the organ connecting the immaterial soul/mind and the material brain. For an introduction to the history of neurology, see G. Scherz, ed., *Steno and Brain Research in the Seventeenth Century*, Oxford, 1968, especially L. Belloni, 'Die Neuroanatomie von Marcello Malpighi', pp. 193–206; E. Clarke and C.D. O'Malley, *The Human Brain and Spinal Cord: A Historical Study Illustrated by Writings from Antiquity to the Twentieth Century*, Berkeley, CA, 1968; R.G. Mazzolini, 'Schemi e modelli della macchina pensante (1662–1762)', in *La fabbrica del pensiero: dall'arte della memoria alle neuroscienze*, Milan, 1989, pp. 68–143.

[37] See, respectively, Wepfer, *Observationes anatomicae*; Fracassati, *Dissertatio epistolica*. Because of new empirical evidence, several alternative hypothesis concerning apoplexy circulated in late seventeenth-century medical culture, and F. Bayle, *Tractatus de apoplexia*, Toulouse, 1677, summed them up in five main groups: presence of thick, viscous matter in the ventricles; compression at the base of the brain whence nerves originate; disruption of blood flow to the brain; morbid softness of the brain; and inflammation of cerebral matter. It should be recalled incidentally that apoplexy was not the only affection undergoing revision, and that many other cerebral and neurological pathologies began to be viewed as 'psychiatric' in a modern sense; see R.G. Frank, 'Thomas Willis and His Circle: Brain and Mind in Seventeenth-Century Medicine', in *The Languages of Psyche: Mind and Body in Enlightenment Thought*, ed. G.S. Rousseau, Berkeley, CA, 1990, pp. 107–46.

[38] Lancisi largely draws the idea that acidity of the nervous fluid triggers convulsions and epilepsy and eventually leads to apoplexy from the Galilean Florentine anatomist and physician Lorenzo Bellini, *De urinis et pulsibus. De missione sanguinis. De febribus. De morbis capitis et pectoris*, Bologna, 1683, on whom see G. Weber, *L'anatomia patologica di Lorenzo Bellini, anatomico (1643–1704)*, Florence, 1998, esp. pp. 24–43.

The following chapters of *De subitaneis mortibus* delve into the defects of the solid organs of the body. A primary condition for the healthy functioning of the human body is the integrity of tissues, which need to be 'structurally in a perfect and natural condition, and ... continually engaged in the alternate movement of contraction and dilatation'.[39] Dilatability and contractibility are considered to be intrinsic characteristics of human tissues, and more specifically of fibres. In truth, fibres play an important role within mechanical anatomy as the smallest component of the bodily machine, very like the anatomo-medical equivalent of physical atoms. Those anatomists who followed Galilean natural philosophy like Borelli, Baglivi and Lancisi himself resorted to considering fibres as a key element in their mechanical explanation of involuntary motion. This kind of structural analysis contributed even further to the disappearance of immaterial and metaphysical principles from accounts of animal physiology.[40]

Retaining the tripartite division adopted in discussing fluids, Lancisi examines the three major solid organs responsible for life – that is, the trachea and lungs (which contemporary medicine no longer considered to be an appendix to the heart), the heart and great vessels, the brain and nerves. For each of these functional units he enumerates several instances of wounds, mechanical impediments, lacerations and obstructions that can lead to sudden death. Concerning the brain and nerves, Lancisi especially insists on the role

---

[39]   SM, pp. 25, 8.

[40]   Duchesneau, *Les modèles du vivant*, pp. 182–90, characterises Italian seventeenth-century physiology as microstructuralism. On the 'anatomical' or 'structurist method' (function is modelled on structure, the study of which reveals the function) and its cultural and religious implications, see W.F. Bynum, 'The Anatomical Method, Natural Theology, and the Functions of the Brain', *Isis*, 64, 1973, pp. 444–68. The physiology of muscles also attracted much attention from seventeenth-century anatomists and natural philosophers like Willis, Mayow, Croone, Stensen and Borelli. Within such a framework, in his 1702 treatise *De fibra motrice*, Baglivi put forward a general theory of fibres as the microstructure responsible for the transmission of motion. He distinguishes fibres into *muscularis sive motricis* that are insensitive and originate from tendons and ultimately from bones, and membranaceous that are made up of countless extremely thin filaments produced by the meninges and that in turn form other viscera; fibres have an intrinsic elastic strength – that is, the ability to re-assume their original shape after impetus, unlike fluids, which are elastic but merely passively. On Baglivi's mechanical physiology, see J. Jimenez Girona, *La medicina de Baglivi*, Madrid, 1955; M.D. Grmek, *La première révolution biologique*, Paris, 1990, pp. 159–88; F. Duchesneau, *La physiologie des Lumières: empirisme, modèles et théories*, The Hague, 1982, pp. 116–26; N. Zurak, 'Nervous System in the Fibrillar Theory of Giorgio Baglivi', *Medicina nei secoli*, 12, 2000, pp. 147–58. For a general overview of seventeenth-century research on muscles, see E. Bastholm, *The History of Muscle Physiology*, Copenhagen, 1950. On further developments of fibre theory as the key element for the secularisation of the body in British medicine, see now H. Ishizuka, 'Fibre Body': The Concept of Fibre in Eighteenth-century Medicine, c.1700– 40', *Medical History*, 56, 2012, pp. 562–84.

of the meninges for the healthy economy of the neural system. According to the teachings of Thomas Willis and Marcello Malpighi, further elaborated by Giorgio Baglivi and Antonio Pacchioni in Rome, the meninges 'squeeze' the cerebral cortex (deemed to be glandular in composition) and thus propel the nerve fluid through the nerves.[41] Hence, if blows, wounds or contusions harm the meninges, the ensuing accumulation of serum, pus and tumours oppress the cerebral mass, turn acid and subvert the entire economy of the organ.

In other words, in that 'extraordinarily delicate and fine and ingeniously interwoven and divided structure of fluids and solids' that is life,[42] pathology most frequently results from a mutual impairment of fluids and solids. Except for congenital malformations, the morbid state of air, blood and nerve fluid corrodes, lacerates or obstructs the corresponding organs which, in turn, are no longer able to filter and propel the right quantity of fluids and let them disperse or amass pathologically. Therefore, 'the abnormalities of the two orders [of fluid and solid parts] necessarily proceed together',[43] although they mainly originate from the fluids, as these are not elemental substances but corpuscular compounds subject to rapid transformations. The corpuscle composing fluids are described by Lancisi in both chemical and mechanical terms. For instance, he speaks of 'wedge-like' eroding salts gradually tearing apart the fibrous connection, but on the following page he refers to chemical reactions between acrid and sulphurous particles.[44] His definitions remain vague and alternate between what seems to be an essentialist qualitative (chemical) perception and a more mechanistic view of the properties of minimal particles, depending on the scale of observation. In this respect, Lancisi's approach is not dissimilar to Boyle's, Malpighi's and, not less importantly, Borelli's in the second book of his influential *De motu animalium*.[45]

Thus, following the tripartite division of fluids and organs 'of most use', Lancisi reformulates the ancient notions of suffocation (asphyxia), syncope and

---

[41]   Baglivi, *Specimen quatuor librorum de fibra*; Pacchioni, *De durae meningis*; and see M. Neuburger, *The Historical Development of Experimental Brain and Spinal Cord Physiology before Flourens*, ed. and trans. E. Clarke, Baltimore, pp. 71–96; M.P. Donato, 'Il normale, il patologico e la sezione cadaverica in età moderna', *Quaderni Storici*, 136, 2011, pp. 75–98.

[42]   SM, p. 6.

[43]   SM, p. 25.

[44]   SM, pp. 141–2, where Lancisi speaks of 'percussionis, ac repercussionis vi ... energia cunei erodentium salium', which is a clear allusion to Giovanni Alfonso Borelli's *De vi percussionis liber*, Bologna, 1667.

[45]   M. Hunter, ed., *Robert Boyle Reconsidered*, Cambridge, 1994; J. Salem, ed., *L'Atomisme aux XVIIe et XVIIIe siècles*, Paris, 1999; A. Clericuzio, *Elements, Principles and Corpuscles: A Study of Atomism and Chemistry in the Seventeenth Century*, Dordrecht, 2000. S. Gomez Lopez, 'Marcello Malpighi and Atomism', in *Marcello Malpighi: Anatomist and Physician*, ed. D. Bertoloni Meli, Florence, 1997, pp. 175–89, underscores the theoretical differences between Borelli's and Malpighi's corpuscularianism.

apoplexy, already unsystematically evoked in previous works on unexpected death, linking them more firmly to the corresponding affected organ (lungs, heart or brain). Post-mortem evidence is introduced in the course of Book One to support the general theory. In addition to the autopsies conducted in the anatomy theatre at the university in Rome in 1706, Lancisi presents as examples a number of cases of apparently unanticipated deaths from his personal professional experience that were preceded by migraine, melancholy and loss of consciousness. He describes morbid alterations of the meninges and the cortex detected in post-mortems and endeavours to connect them to clinical signs reported in the living patient. One case in particular he discusses in detail. Cavalier dal Pozzo had suffered from migraine in the left side of the head and melancholy leading to a first epileptic seizure, which was followed by amnesia and repeated losses of consciousness up to the final attack; dissection then revealed hardened meninges and a big tumour in the right-side frontal lobe expanding in the cortex and the encephalic trunk. Post-mortem findings thus confirm for Lancisi, on the one hand, the centrality of meninges in the economy of vital and sensory-motor functions and, on the other hand, the fatal impact of abnormal secretion of fluids in these tissues.

It is important to bear in mind that *De subitaneis mortibus* is intended to serve practical purposes and is largely devoted to clinical issues. Considering sudden death from the medical practitioner's standpoint, Lancisi first discusses how to ascertain death and then classifies the ailments leading to swift, unanticipated death into curable and incurable ones. A few chapters are devoted to those premonitory signs that a good clinician must be capable of detecting. Foretelling the end is a physician's critical (and most difficult) task, even if he will not be able to find a cure. Lancisi remarks that

> sudden deaths usually happen to those who, because they have become familiar with certain diseases, regard them as of no consequence, either due to the light nature of their symptoms or because they have become accustomed to them and hope that their illness will either mend with the help of Nature alone, or that they would die only after a prolonged agony.[46]

He enumerates a long list of signs and symptoms in the patient's respiration, voice, pulse, posture, breath, sight and neuro-vegetative functions (convulsions, fainting, loss of memory) which hint at ailments probably affecting internal parts.

In Lancisi's medicine, manifest signs are considered to point at the 'hidden truth' – that is, the true cause of death that dissection would eventually reveal. This is at least in theory; in practice, Lancisi's is not too distant from established

---

[46]   SM, p. 64.

medical semeiotics. In line with the traditional practice of learned Western medicine, he endeavours to formulate clinical teachings in such a way as to be consistent with statements by Hippocrates and Galen, considered as insuperable masters of clinical insight. Some simply reproduced old habits of bedside observation, slightly modified to fit into a new physiological theory, such as the suppressed evacuations to which Lancisi often calls attention. Spontaneous evacuations (nose bleeds, sputum, expectorations) eliminating peccant matter were essential in humoral medicine, and retain their significance within the new conception of the body machine.

It is true, however, that Lancisi's semeiotic traditionalism is mitigated by the clearer distinction he introduces between signs of disease and causes. Sometimes, he argues, substances that are no longer evacuated can gather, become toxic and damage organs (typically, the lungs), but in most cases they are 'but signs' hinting at the overall deterioration of an organism. Indeed, 'since the autopsies on human bodies have become more common', they have revealed that actual lesions such as aneurysms do cause death.[47] At any rate, Lancisi is aware that many diseases 'originate from internal but hidden causes that provide no indications ... as they lie buried in cavities, [and] indeed do rarely come to the notice of physicians',[48] and that only the 'anatomist's knife' would ultimately bring them to light on the dissecting table. In Lancisi's treatise, therefore, clinical external signs oscillate between pertaining to prognosis in the Hippocratic tradition (in that they reveal something of the course of the disease) and pertaining to diagnosis (in that they reveal something of the nature and the seat of the disease, at least retrospectively through autopsy). The importance of post-mortem evidence – the truth of the corpse – is the underlying theme of *De subitaneis mortibus* as a whole, and a key feature of the book, and we shall come back to this point in greater detail.

In compliance with its practical purpose, *De subitaneis mortibus* also delves into therapeutics. Lancisi shares a hygiene-oriented approach to health and illness with the vast majority of his contemporaries, but he sets out its mechanistic rationale more explicitly. Regimen (together with moderate physical exercise to strengthen tissues) constitutes the best prophylactic and curative strategy since it reduces the mass and pressure of the blood. For this same reason, phlebotomy can be a valuable treatment. Besides, Lancisi prescribes several medicinal remedies, which are mainly meant to sweeten and fluidify the blood and neural juice in order to contrast potential damage on solid tissues. Not surprisingly, drugs are very much the same as Galenic therapeutics, but their rationale is

---

[47] SM, p. 77. Jarcho, *The Concept of Heart Failure*, pp. 270–72, expresses scepticism as to whether Lancisi makes a real distinction between signs and causes in his analysis. On the conceptualisation of the two terms during the Renaissance, see N.G. Siraisi, 'Disease and Symptom as Problematic Concepts in Renaissance Medicine', in *Res et Verba in the Renaissance*, ed. E. Kessler and I. Maclean, Wiesbaden, 2002, pp. 217–39.

[48] SM, p. 62.

different as they are now selected on the grounds of their supposed mechanical and chemical action upon the particles of bodily fluids and microcomponents (fibres, microscopic glands). The same course of therapy had been previously adopted by other mechanical physicians such as Malpighi and Lorenzo Bellini, and, incidentally, it represented an indirect response to Galenists and empiricists, who dismissed the 'subtle anatomy' of neoterics as useless for medical practice.[49]

The Certain Principles of the Moderns and the Enduring Teachings of the Ancients, or: How to Write a Masterpiece on Mechanical Medicine in Catholic Rome

Lancisi's book is a mature example of seventeenth-century mechanistic and corpuscularian medicine. Drawing on Boyle, Borelli, Willis, Malpighi, Bellini and further back in time Galileo and Descartes, he elaborates his particular synthesis of contemporary medical culture. The fact that those authors advanced differing views of physiology is of little significance.[50] Since he writes a treatise encompassing theory and practice, Lancisi can enunciate general Galilean and Cartesian philosophical principles but then endeavour to reconcile mechanical medicine and experimental corpuscularian (rather than Paracelsian or 'metaphysical') chemistry, forsaking neither those masters of observation Hippocrates and Galen nor morbid anatomy. He also systematises half a century of studies on respiration, the brain and circulatory pathology – that is, the three fields that had undergone the most development in the second half of the seventeenth century. *De subitaneis mortibus* is arguably one of the works that best exemplifies what historian of medicine Giorgio Cosmacini has described as 'the contradictions ... of the Italian medical vanguard', hesitating between a new, forward-looking scientific approach to the human body and an empirical medicine which puts observation, description and clinical experience at its heart.[51]

In light of the diffidence with which many members of the Roman curia and Church still regarded modern physics and Cartesian biology, one might wonder how such an explicit manifesto of mechanical medicine could appear in Rome with such great solemnity and under the enthusiastic protection of the pontiff, whose coat of arms was emblazoned on the frontispiece. Descartes had already been suspended *donec corrigatur* by the congregation of the Index of Prohibited Books in 1663 and for decades, the Inquisition and the Index had been indicting

---

[49]   D. Bertoloni Meli, 'Mechanistic Pathology and Therapy in the Medical Assayer of Marcello Malpighi', *Medical History*, 51, 2007, pp. 165–80.

[50]   A. Guerrini, 'The Varieties of Mechanical Medicine: Borelli, Malpighi, Bellini, and Pitcairne', in *Marcello Malpighi*, ed. Bertoloni Meli, pp. 111–28.

[51]   G. Cosmacini, *Storia della medicina e della sanità in Italia*, Rome and Bari, 1995, p. 173, referring to Baglivi.

men and books that challenged scholastic hylomorphism and crossed the boundaries of metaphysics when treating physics or medicine. Hence, attacks against the proponents of mechanistic and atomist theories were periodically revived.[52] Thus, as late as 1711 a short dissertation on the soul of animals by Alessandro Pascoli, Lancisi's successor to the chair of anatomy, was forbidden by the Holy Office after a fierce polemic between Pascoli and another Roman physician.[53] The Roman curia, however, was a polycentric and plural institution in the corridors of which those skilled and knowledgeable enough could always find the right interlocutor.[54] As we saw in Chapter 2, there were many learned prelates in Pope Albani's entourage who were abreast of developments in contemporary natural philosophy, supported Clement XI's patronage of science and thought that the credit and power of the Roman Catholic Church and curia would be better defended through an alliance with modern science, provided that it steered clear of metaphysical speculation and a few particularly delicate subjects.

What is more, a scientific work like *De subitaneis mortibus* did not appear in a void. A slow scientific and ideological accretion of mechanical philosophy and medicine had already taken place. I have outlined in Chapter 2 the interweaving of cultural issues, political motivations and institutional processes that led to a reappraisal of the role of medicine in society, as well as to an overall modernisation of medical culture. In this regard it is most notable that, from the 1660s onwards, mechanistic physiology attracted growing interest not only within the medical profession but in a wider learned audience. Guglielmo Riva's public demonstration of human and animal lymphatic vessels and Paolo Manfredi's blood transfusions, for instance, fascinated Roman *virtuosi*.[55] In the

---

[52] M.P. Donato, 'Scienza e teologia nelle congregazioni romane: la questione atomista, 1626–1727', in *Rome et la science moderne: entre Renaissance and Lumières*, ed. A. Romano, Rome, 2008, pp. 595–634.

[53] Ms ACDF, S. Offitii, Censurae librorum 1711–14, n. 7. I am referring here to [A. Pascoli] *Sofilo Molossio pastore arcade perugino, e custode degli armenti automatici in Arcadia*, Rome, 1706.

[54] M. Caffiero, M.P. Donato and A. Romano, 'De la catholicité post-tridentine à la République romaine: splendeurs et misères des intellectuels courtisans', in *Naples, Rome, Florence: une histoire comparée des milieux intellectuels italiens*, ed. J. Boutier, B. Marin and A. Romano, Rome, 2006, pp. 171–208. The role played by the court in fostering intellectual innovation was, of course, not peculiar to Rome; see H. Trevor Roper, 'The Court Physician and Paracelsianism', in *Medicine at the Courts of Europe, 1500–1837*, ed. V. Nutton, London, 1990, pp. 79–94; H.J. Cook, 'Living in Revolutionary Times: Medical Change under William and Mary', in *Patronage and Institutions: Science, Technology, and Medicine at the European Courts 1500–1750*, ed. B.T. Moran, Woodbridge, 1991, pp. 111–35.

[55] Riva's diagrams were only published posthumously (see *La prima tavola anatomica sui vasi chiliferi dimostrati nell'uomo ... opera di Guglielmo Riva*, Rome, 1936), but the popularity of his anatomical demonstrations among *virtuosi* and learned prelates is attested in a letter from mathematician and theologian Michelangelo Ricci to Leopoldo de Medici of 29 June

last decades of the seventeenth century, Rome was indeed the foremost centre of philosophical and scientific debate in the entire Italian Peninsula. While anti-scholastic *novatores* fought to assert the compatibility between religion and modern atomistic and corpuscularian natural philosophy,[56] mechanical medicine broke through. It was in Rome that Christina of Sweden fostered and financially supported the publication of such a masterpiece of mechanism as Borelli's *De motu animalium*. Moreover, as we have seen, mechanical anatomy and medicine was taught *ex cathedra* at Sapienza University by Lancisi with the court's approval and by his successors to the chair of anatomy at the beginning of the eighteenth century.[57]

Around about the same time, the practice of dissecting human corpses became more frequent and accessible. I have already mentioned the new university anatomical theatre built in the 1670s, a facility where anatomy demonstrations could be performed before a large audience of experts and laymen and in the presence of several cardinals.[58] In hospitals, the teaching programme for apprentice surgeons was also reorganised and more time was reserved for practising dissection, while medical autopsies on deceased patients

---

1665, now in MS Florence, Biblioteca Nazionale, Galileiano 277, fol. 197. As for blood transfusions, see P. Manfredi, *Ragguaglio degl'esperimenti fatti ... circa la nuova operatione della trasfusione del sangue da individuo ad individuo, et in bruti et in huomini*, Rome, 1668; P. Manfredi, *De nova et inaudita medico-chyrurgica operatione sanguinem transfundente de individuo ad individuum; prius in brutis deinde in homine Romae experta*, Rome, 1668.

56   J.-M. Gardair, *Le "Giornale de' Letterati" de Rome (1668–1681)*, Florence, 1984; A. Romano, 'I problemi scientifici nel "Giornale de' Letterati" (1668–1681)', in *Dall'erudizione alla politica: Giornali, giornalisti ed editori a Roma tra XVII e XX secolo*, ed. M. Caffiero and G. Monsagrati, Milan, 1997, pp. 17–38; M.P. Donato, 'L'onere della prova: il Sant'Uffizio, l'atomismo e i medici romani', *Nuncius*, 18, 2003, pp. 69–87; M.P. Donato, 'Seventeenth-Century "Scientific" Academies in Rome and the Cimento's Disputed Legacy', in *The Accademia del Cimento and its European Context*, ed. M. Beretta, A. Clericuzio and L.M. Principe, Sagamore Beach, MA, 2009, pp. 151–64.

57   A. Pascoli, *Il corpo-umano, o breve storia, dove con nuovo metodo si descrivono in compendio tutti gli organi suoi, e i loro principali ufizi*, Perugia, 1700; Ms London, Wellcome Library, 4612–13, *Institutiones medicae* by Pascoli and Giacomo Sinibaldi; Ms BNR, Varia 96, Pascoli's lessons in anatomy and theoretical medicine.

58   Since its first appearance and especially during anatomical demonstrations, the university anatomical theatre had become a place where medical culture was transmitted to a larger audience and where scientific, ethical and religious issues related to medicine intermingled; see G. Ferrari, 'Public Anatomy Lessons and the Carnival: The Anatomy Theatre of Bologna', *Past and Present*, 117, 1987, pp. 50–106. On anatomical theatres as places for the formulation and dissemination of new discoveries, see J. Rupp, 'Matters of Life and Death: The Social and Cultural Conditions of the Rise of Anatomical Theatres, with Special Reference to Seventeenth Century Holland', *History of Science*, 28, 1990, pp. 264–87.

were made easier for attending physicians.[59] These circumstances led to the wider acceptance of anatomo-pathological methods as well as the revival of anatomical and physiological research. Moreover, several works by Roman authors appeared in print, which were well received in the Republic of Letters thus adding to the prestige of Roman science.[60]

If the context was favourable for such work as *De subitaneis mortibus* – or at least not hostile to it – the text itself suited it. It would not be incorrect to say that Lancisi's mechanical medicine verges on materialism. No principle apart from the material 'animal economy' is brought into play. The term animal spirits is used as a synonym for nervous fluid and denotes a real liquid flowing in specific vessels and performing distinctive tasks. The 'pulsative faculty' of the heart and arteries is mentioned once; but it appears to be a generic designation of their movement (active for the heart and passive for the arteries). It is equally true, however, that Lancisi is extremely cautious in dealing with metaphysical topics and writes along the lines enunciated in his methodological essay *Del modo di filosofar nell'arte medica* after his 1690 Inquisition trial. After a few introductory remarks, he avoids formal and general statements about matter and about the relationship between the mind and the body; nor does he take a position on the subject of the ultimate nature of material corpuscles. He remains in the field of *medicina practica* and, in addition, draws on a few Renaissance authors who were at odds with mechanism, introducing contradictory ideas but also moderating the ideological outlook of his work. This 'conciliatory' approach was consistent with the specific habits of practical medicine, which differed from those in anatomy and physiology and were more inclined to eclecticism. After all, the physician's foremost task, in the final analysis, was to cure and to give counsel, rather than to philosophise about the nature of things, and to that purpose some useful indications could always be gathered from past masters.

This does not mean, however, that Lancisi refrained from generalisations, or that he considered medicine to offer merely probable knowledge. His book proceeds in an authoritative mode, presenting his new ideas about sudden death in the manner of a classical, deductive exposition, for which all the basic principles had already been ascertained by a century of modern physiology. The whole treatise rests on assumptions such as the centrality of autopsy, the mechanistic appraisal of 'animal economy' and the corpuscular interpretation of matter. What is more, the mechanical and mildly materialistic approach of *De subitaneis*

---

[59]   M. Conforti and S. De Renzi, 'Sapere anatomico negli ospedali romani: formazione dei chirurghi e pratiche sperimentali (1620–1720)', in *Rome et la science moderne*, ed. Romano, pp. 433–72.

[60]   I refer to works such as, for instance, P. Manfredi, *Novae circa oculum observationes*, Rome, 1674; P. Manfredi, *Novae circa aurem observationes*, Rome, 1674; D. Gagliardi, *Anatomes ossium novis inventis illustratae*, Rome, 1689; Baglivi, *Specimen quatuor librorum de fibra.*

mortibus did offer new insight into sudden death. With their spirits and innate heat, Aristotelian-Galenic medical authors defining death only *a contrario* (death as the exhaustion of life) had failed to clarify the abruptness of sudden death. In contrast, mechanistic explanations insisting on the laceration of the solid parts by fluids could modulate the succession of events in time, distinguishing the slow, at times imperceptible morbid process and its breaking point. Lancisi is thus able to defend his notion that sudden death, notwithstanding the surprise and sensation it creates when it hits seemingly healthy people, actually only strikes bodies that are already plagued with undetected disease.

This original reinterpretation of death over time – which we will discuss further in greater detail – informs Lancisi's general theory, as well as the analysis of individual cases, enabling him to provide a rational, natural and reassuring explanation of the lethal events. In his account of an 'apoplexy with epileptic and syncopal affliction', for instance, he puts forward his hypothesis as to how the blood vessels of the pia mater and of the lungs had been

> thinned by the acidity of the liquids that circulated herein and due to the lacerating force ... of the convulsions ... [the vessels and meninges] broke in the end in a final epileptic attack, and there was blood extravasation in the brain ... whence the sudden death.[61]

Again, referring to a 'sudden death from syncopal apoplexy', he warns that ulcers 'for sure do not become ensculptured upon the viscera by an eroding liquid in one single moment of time', but in time pressure gets to a point when all of a sudden it brings on 'a stroke of the fluids and solids within the brain'.[62] Every autopsy report features a chronological account of the disease from the onset of the initial morbid condition to the final crisis, which is, Lancisi adds, sometimes accelerated by marginal external factors that turn out to be lethal for subjects poised between life and death.

The three main theoretical enunciations – mechanism, corpuscularianism, probing value of dissection – connect the general theory of Book One of *De subitaneis mortibus* with Book Two, which, in the manner of Hippocrates, deals with sudden deaths and their causes, as they occurred in Rome in 1705 and 1706. The papal archiater dismisses the hypotheses that had circulated during those frightful months through simple deduction: for example, that exhalations were caused by earthquakes was disproven by the fact that the populations near the epicentres had not been affected. Other suggestions included the abuse of chocolate, the use of rotten tobacco and the presence of an 'unknown poison in the air', no traces of which were ever found in the dissected bodies. Contagion

---

[61] SM, p. 126.
[62] SM, p. 137.

was also ruled out on account of the fact that physicians and surgeons treating or dissecting the unfortunate patients had not been infected. Indeed, on the contrary, autopsies proved that the deaths in Rome were the result of 'a particular concourse of causes in each individual case'.[63]

However, the increase in the cases of sudden death in a particular time and place required an explanation. In imitation of Hippocrate's *Airs, Waters and Places* and *Epidemics I*,[64] Lancisi prefers to take into consideration abrupt temperature changes, air pressure and winds. Bad weather had raged in Rome throughout the two years preceding the wave of unanticipated deaths, interfering with bodily fluids. An excessively hot summer dehydrates the body and destroys the oily, balsamic components of blood, he argues, and then autumnal rain insinuates vitriolic ferments in it, while the cold winter winds impede transpiration and, together with bad diet, aggravate the conditions of sick people.

In this section of his treatise, Lancisi draws more explicitly on fermentation pathology, and refers to Sylvius when discussing the accumulation of fermentative particles in the blood resulting in coagulation and separation of serum.[65] But Hippocratism also grows stronger. In particular, the papal physician insists on the dangerous association between weather and lifestyle in order to corroborate his statement that diverse, individual circumstances have brought about death in each case. Social conditions (rich people prone to excessive eating and drinking, and the poor poorly nourished and deprived of medical assistance) and gender do in fact matter. Why were women less affected than men, asks Lancisi. Was it because women 'constantly cleansed by their menstruations, are protected from acquiring the disease afflicting mechanism to the fullness of its irritative and suffocative power', or instead because 'women, also those from among the common stratum, do for the most part lead a more temperate life and are thus less inclined to the accumulation of injurious fluids'?[66] On this basis, Lancisi refutes the idea of an 'epidemic' of sudden deaths in Rome, where at any rate the number of deaths was not altogether above average. He therefore conclusively states that 'the cause of those unforeseen deaths was not one that was absolutely common to all'.[67]

---

[63]   SM, p. 113.

[64]   On the reception of these Hippocratic collections in the eighteenth century, see T. Vetter, 'Essai sur la littérature hippocratique au dix-huitième siècle', in *La Collection hippocratique et son rôle dans l'histoire de la médecine*, Leiden, 1975, pp. 347–67.

[65]   F. de La Boë (Sylvius), *Opera medica, hoc est, Disputationum medicarum decas, Methodi medendi libri duo, Ideae novae praxeos medicae libri tres*, Geneva, 1681; insistence on the separation of haematic components derives from Malpighi's *De polypo cordis* (1666), now in *Opere scelte di Marcello Malpighi*, ed. L. Belloni, Turin, 1969, pp. 191–216; M. Conforti, 'Il "moto fermentativo prima origine della vita": dibattiti sulla natura del sangue in Italia tra Sei e Settecento', *Medicina nei secoli*, 15, 2003, pp. 269–90.

[66]   SM, p. 120.

[67]   SM, p. 112.

The correlation between reasoning, observation and post-mortem findings is woven into a coherent discourse; with the aid of authoritative references to Hippocrates throughout, the rationality of medicine is constructed from the combination of mental image (reasoning), history (case studies, environmental records) and physical data (autopsy).[68] So, Lancisi discloses the underlying methodological principles of his modern rational medicine:

> Even though I had easily come to this conclusion by reasoning from the signs, in the end I was only then truly satisfied when I saw that the internal perception of my mind had been proven by external testimony of the things themselves and by the positive evidence of the post-mortem examinations.[69]

On the dissecting table, the proper cause of death can be traced back to or conjectured from the visible lesions. Dissection provides a form of medical experience which, although moving backward from death towards life, ultimately serves the clinician.

The bulk of Book Two is devoted to *historiae*. Only three cases concern successful treatments, and the rest of the chapters deal with deceased people whose history can nevertheless provide valuable insight. One regards a prelate who had died abruptly in autumn 1706 after a long and apparently harmless illness, and five refer to the autopsies performed at La Sapienza that same year. Their detailed exposition, complete with case history, description of the dissected body and a final explanation (*scholium*), supplies the empirical foundation of Lancisi's theory, while calling the reader to be a virtual witness and elevating the autopsies to the definitive status of public facts.[70]

The defects ascertained on the dissecting table are principally located in the heart and in the brain of the deceased. Lesions in the cardiovascular system particularly are described with a wealth of details. Lancisi accompanies the reader

---

[68]   E. Hamraoui, 'L'oeuvre d'Hippocrate revisitée par la pensée médicale des Lumières: l'exemple des traités médicaux de G.M. Lancisi (1654–1720)', in *Hellénisme et hippocratisme dans l'Europe méditerranéenne: autour de D. Coray*, ed. E. Andréani, H. Michel and E. Pélaquier, Montpellier, 1996, pp. 101–19. On the 'invention' of Hippocratism as a method of observation, see R. Rey, 'Les anamorphoses d'Hippocrate au XVIIIe siècle', in *Maladie et maladies: histoire et conceptualisation. Mélanges en l'honneur de Mirko Grmek*, ed. D. Gourevitch, Geneva, 1992, pp. 257–76.

[69]   SM, p. 112.

[70]   S. Schaffer and S. Shapin, *Leviathan and the Air-Pump: Hobbes, Boyle and the Experimental Life*, Princeton, 1985, p. 55; G. Cantor, 'The Rhetoric of Experiment', in *The Uses of Experiment: Studies in the Natural Sciences*, ed. D. Gooding, T. Pinch and S. Schaffer, Cambridge, 1989, pp. 169–73; in regard to medicine, see N.G. Siraisi, 'Segni evidenti, teoria e testimonianza nelle narrazioni di autopsie del Rinascimento', *Quaderni Storici*, 36, 2001, pp. 719–44, esp. pp. 728–30.

step by step in discovering injuries and abnormalities, as in the case of Stefano Ascieri, a cobbler struck down by an aneurysm in the aorta in March 1706:

> Right behind the pericardium lay hidden an aneurysm of the aorta. Then, when the knife was brought into play, we encountered immediately a bony lamella, oval in shape, which had taken hold of the external part of the dilated artery, by means of which it adhered to the sternum and the ribs. Underneath that lamella and around the cavity of the first part of the ascending aorta, we found a polyp-like substance, very similar to lard, encrusted with great neatness into an arch ... This body ... did not allow itself to be pulled apart into multiple laminas, like so many sheets (as is everywhere usual). ... Meanwhile the cavity of the aneurysm turned out to be so wide that it would easily have admitted a fist ... at the base of the heart within the pericardium and at the lower side of the aneurysm, some certain dark striae, indications perhaps of larger, future apertures, had been observed. ... As we were examining the pericardium, which was extremely swollen and nevertheless soft ... when cut, it yielded an immense quantity of blood ... which had been discharged and turned into clots ... This blood, indeed, had poured out, when within the vestibule of the vena cava next to the right auricle, a hole of about one inch in diameter had been opened.[71]

In spite of their variety, however, the interpretation of pathological findings is mostly dependent on Willis's and Sylvius's idea of blood pathologies as excessive or defective fermentation and on a rather schematic hydraulic perception of the body-as-machine. The emphasis is on fluids – blood which is too dense or too soluble, or too acrid, nervous fluid which is too irritating. The mutual action of fluids and solids is given careful attention, according to Lancisi's main (mechanistic) tenet that diverse, mutual impairments develop together:

> The abnormalities of both types necessarily work together ... for that reason you do not find any defect of the solids that is likely to kill suddenly, unless it blocks the movement of the body liquids, nor do you find in turn any lethal defects of the fluids without some injuries to the solids.[72]

Although each individual death has its own specific cause, they have something in common, namely the progressive deterioration of one of the three main circulatory systems which, over time, is transmitted to other organs. Moreover, in the majority of cases, adverse congenital predisposition or pathological conditions

---

[71] SM, p. 164. On narrative techniques in early modern medicine and science, see P. Dear, 'Totius in verba: Rhetoric and Authority in the Early Royal Society', *Isis*, 76, 1985, pp. 145–61; G. Baroncini, *Forme di esperienza e rivoluzione scientifica*, Florence, 1992, pp. 145–73.

[72] SM, p. 25.

are exacerbated by reckless behaviour as regards food, drink or sex, as the pope's physician reminds the reader with gravity, quoting in his concluding pages nothing less than the Gospel of Luke (21.34–5): 'And take heed to yourselves, lest at any time your hearts be overcharged with surfeiting, and drunkenness, and cares of this life, and so that day [of judgement] come upon you unawares'.[73]

In the light of the general theory of Book One and the particular facts of Book Two, Lancisi is able to conclude reassuringly that not only do unexpected incidents rarely occur, but that they 'attacked the Romans because of the particular disposition of each individual body'.[74] Nothing can be attributed to extraordinary circumstances of any kind. It was a conclusion similar to that reached by his colleagues, but it was based on new arguments and on the empirical evidence yielded by the dissected bodies. In any event, the papal physician took care to distance himself both from the ancients, since they were not aware of blood circulation, and from his contemporaries because of 'the scantiness of their observations and their utterly inadequate investigation of causes'.[75]

What in fact distinguishes Lancisi from his colleagues is that while the latter sought to establish consistency between the events and the doctrine, the former investigates the phenomenon of sudden death as such. He does not proceed from the doctrine to facts, but from facts to a new doctrine that would follow the principles of modern experimental and mechanical natural philosophy. Facts include autopsy findings, first of all, and environmental and epidemiological observations according to the teachings of the ancient, sublime masters of observation such as Hippocrates and Galen.

Hence, the mechanistic approach of *De subitaneis mortibus*, corroborated by the anatomo-pathological method, offered a coherent, credible explanation, as well as a naturalistic interpretation, of the strange, disturbing phenomena that had terrorised Rome. Lancisi accomplished the task the pope had assigned to him and fulfilled his public role by reassuring frightened people, but nevertheless exhorting them to live a sober (Christian) life. In doing so, he legitimated mechanical medicine and morbid anatomy in an official publication under the pope's aegis. As for what it meant for an early eighteenth-century rational doctor to actually examine a dead body in order to understand disease and explain death we shall explore in the next chapter.

---

[73] SM, p. 79.
[74] SM, p. 115.
[75] SM, *Occasio scribendi*, unpaginated.

Chapter 5

The Pathological Gaze: The Problematic Status of Post-mortem Evidence in Early Eighteenth-Century Medicine

Visible and Invisible in Lancisi's Pathological Anatomy

Lancisi's *De subitaneis mortibus* has been the object of contrasting appraisals. For some it is a relic of humoral medicine superficially updated through the use of modern notions and terms;[1] to others it is a modern interpretation of illness and death by means of systematic use of necropsy.[2] The attempt to correlate pre-mortem symptoms with post-mortem results is undeniably a key feature of the book. Accordingly, it can be argued that *De subitaneis mortibus* is an early instance of modern anatomo-localistic medicine which was to be codified in Giovan Battista Morgagni's *De sedibus et causis morborum per anatomen indagatis* (1761) and later developed by the celebrated Parisian School into a more sophisticated tissular pathology. In anatomo-localistic pathology, diseases have a precise localisation (morbid localisation) and must therefore be studied prevalently through necropsy, drawing systematic comparisons between clinical and post-mortem observations and correlating symptoms to specific lesions. If such an interpretation of Lancisi's work is correct, some chronological and geographical assumptions underpinning the history of eighteenth-century medicine should be modified, and early eighteenth-century Rome deservedly reassessed as one centre from which this modern 'pathological paradigm' radiated. It should also be seen as one of the first places in which post-mortem findings were postulated and used as the main empirical foundation of medical knowledge.

---

[1]   M. Hoffmann, *Die Lehre vom plötzlichen Tod in Lancisis Werk De subitaneis mortibus*, Berlin, 1935, esp. p. 59; S. Jarcho, *The Concept of Heart Failure: From Avicenna to Albertini*, Cambridge, MA, 1980, pp. 257–74.

[2]   K. Sprengel, *Versuch einer pragmatischen Gesichte der Arzneikunde*, vol. 5, Halle, 1803, p. 533; M. Calabresi, 'J.M. Lancisi and "De subitaneis mortibus"', in *Essays in the History of Medicine Presented to Professor Arturo Castiglioni, Bulletin of the History of Medicine*, Supplement 3, 1944, pp. 48–54; 'He laid the foundations of a true understanding of the pathologies of the heart', according to E.R. Long, *A History of Pathology*, New York, 1965, p. 67; G. Cosmacini, *Storia della medicina e della sanità in Italia*, Rome and Bari, 1995, p. 217.

Still, such a reassessment raises several questions. What did looking into the body actually mean in early eighteenth-century rational medicine? What material and intellectual resources made an ancient practice like autopsy into an indispensable validation of medical theory and practice? How did empirical knowledge and medical theory combine to make death become the standpoint from which disease could be understood and life acted upon? What did this entail in practice?

As I have indicated, Book Two of *De subitaneis mortibus* is composed of *historiae*, which Lancisi calls 'physico-medical observations'. This was innovative in itself, although post-mortem reports were commonplace in contemporary practical medicine literature and were gathered in special anthologies, such as the already mentioned *Sepulchretum* by Bonet.[3] Lancisi narrates cases of sudden death detailing their clinical history, post-mortem examination and a final *scholium* or interpretation, the purpose of which is 'to make the particular cause of each sudden death stand forth, disentangled, and in clear light'.[4] This structure of post-mortem reports was already codified in medical literature, and explicitly recommended by Joseph Konrad Peyer in his *Methodus historiarum anatomico-medicarum* (1678) as the most suitable for 'weaving the thread of true pathology'.[5] It allowed the description of both the symptoms in the living patient and the state of their dissected corpse, which were then to be considered against the background of the general theory. On the whole, it corroborated the centrality of anatomo-pathological observations as the demonstrative core of each *historia*. 'Nothing teaches us more clearly than the dissection of bodies which bring to the light of day the hidden causes of death' is a credo Lancisi often reiterated.[6]

Certainly, the late Galenic literature on sudden death attests to the fact that the opening up of bodies was not new *per se*. In his *Mortis repentinae examen*, for instance, Grassi reported on the post-mortem of a monk who had died suddenly after an asthma attack, though the report was an excerpt from another book.[7] In Terilli's *De causis mortis repentinae*, autopsies are more numerous and are variously drawn from other texts, the author's own medical practice or his colleagues' reported experience. These forms of experience were in fact

---

3   Cosmacini, *Storia della medicina*, pp. 54 ff.; H. Chiari, 'Geschichte der pathologischen Anatomie des Menschen', in T. Puschmann, *Handbuch der Geschichte der Medizin* (1903), vol. 2, Hildesheim and New York, 1971, pp. 473–559.

4   SM, p. 174.

5   Now in G. Weber, *L'anatomia patologica di Lorenzo Bellini, anatomico (1643–1704)*, Florence, 1998, pp. 135–52.

6   SM, p. 157.

7   P. Grassi, *Mortis repentinae examen una cum brevis methodo praesagiendi et praecavendi omnes, qui subeunt illius periculum*, Modena, 1612, p. 47; the case is excerpted from the widely renowned *De morbis internis* by J. Houllier (1571).

equivalent to the extent that they all provided empirical knowledge as distinct from theory; all were facts – or, at least, factoids – regardless of their origin. After all, university-trained doctors had accepted the authority of the ancients as an incontrovertible fact for centuries.[8]

It is important to bear in mind that although Graeco-Roman, medieval and Renaissance medicine were focused on humours, none of them discounted the importance of lesions to organs and fleshy parts, which could be ascertained either by chance (in wounds) or intentionally, by opening up the corpse. Nonetheless, in the Hippocratic-Galenic tradition, disease was mainly conceived as a dysfunction or imbalance, the 'lesion' affecting a faculty rather than a part. Hence, traditional medical semeiotics (that is, the complex of signs and symptoms which point to and at the same time constitute the dysfunction, since a disease is in fact a syndrome of signs) was a self-referential system, and had no real need of autopsy.[9] When post-mortems were performed, anatomo-pathological findings merely confirmed humoral physiology. Terilli, for instance, invariably ascertained a great quantity of phlegm or putrefied blood in the heart or lungs of patients who had died unexpectedly, and this confirmed his view that the vital faculty had been affected so severely as to extinguish life. Observations on the connection between external signs and internal localised ailments were posited by Terilli and other late Galenic medical writers but were absolutely marginal within the dominant notion of disease. Sixteenth- and seventeenth-century medico-practical literature in the observational empirical vein of *observationes* and *curationes* made no exception. To mention just one Roman work, Domenico Panaroli's *Observationes medicinales* contains several post-mortem observations, and yet these did not contradict the physiology of qualities and faculties. Thus, for instance, Panaroli recounted the case of a girl who had died unexpectedly and was dissected at the hospital of Santo Spirito, and whose blood-filled heart he considered as the unmistakable proof that an abrupt extinction of innate heat had occurred.[10] When autopsies were performed in the framework of legal

---

[8]   C. Crisciani, 'Fatti, teorie, *narratio* e i malati a corte: note su empirismo in medicina nel tardo-medioevo', *Quaderni Storici*, 36, 2001, pp. 695–718. On textual factoids, see A. Blair, 'Humanist Methods in Natural Philosophy: The Commonplace Book', *Journal of the History of Ideas*, 53, 1992, pp. 541–51.

[9]   J. Bylebyl, 'The Manifest and the Hidden in the Renaissance Clinic', in *Medicine and the Five Senses*, ed. W.F. Bynum and R. Porter, Cambridge, 1993, pp. 40–60; M.D. Grmek, 'The Concept of Disease', in *Western Medical Thought from Antiquity to the Middle Ages*, ed. M.D. Grmek, trans. A. Shugaar, Cambridge, MA, 1998, pp. 241–58. It must be borne in mind that there has never been in history any nosology responding to a single criterion, and that some pathological entities identified in antiquity (for instance, diabetes) remained over the centuries regardless of medical theories and anatomo-pathological findings.

[10]   D. Panaroli, *Iatrologismorum, seu medicinalium observationum pentecostae quinque*, Rome, 1652, pp. 72–4; on this topic, see N.G. Siraisi, 'Segni evidenti, teoria e testimonianza

proceedings, they were aimed at recognising traces that were compatible with the alleged immediate cause of death such as wounds or poison.

For Lancisi, on the contrary, post-mortem dissections took on a rather different role. His work came after decades during which dissecting had become an increasingly widespread practice. By the end of the seventeenth century, post-mortem reports were no longer occasionally inserted among medical observations as instances of 'curious' anomalies but systematically assembled in what had become a *practical anatomy* based on a vast number of case histories.[11] Accordingly, autopsy was now not just a fact among others, but *the* fact on which medical truth should rest. The accurate examination of organs – which were carefully extracted, incised, weighed and manipulated – provided the empirical evidence that confirmed or disproved hypotheses and unveiled the 'true causes' of disease and death.

Moreover, when an early eighteenth-century rational doctor looked into an open corpse on the dissecting table, he saw it in a different way from his Galenist predecessors. Within the circulatory physiology to which Lancisi referred, fluids were no longer as ubiquitous as Galenic humours but were channelled into specific somatic systems; consequently, lesions affecting solids and tissues acquired greater significance.[12] If nothing other than fluids and solids interact in a body, and life itself can be viewed as the 'continual flux' of material components, then an autopsy reveals real physical damage, rather than an unnatural condition that is loosely compatible with the standard definition of a disease (itself based on the signs and symptoms in the living patient). A lesion is the *locus* of disease and the last stage of a morbid process that can be conjectured from the localisation and type of lesion itself. Materialisation, localisation and the increasing importance of dissection are indissociable. In other words, whereas Galenists ordinarily assigned pathological details observed in the corpse to ubiquitous, immaterial and metaphysical elements such as faculties and spirits, mechanistic medicine regarded physio-pathological phenomena as the outcome of material elements; consequently, the tangible knowledge yielded by cadaveric dissection provided its own rationale unrelated to metaphysics.

---

nelle narrazioni di autopsie del Rinascimento', *Quaderni Storici*, 36, 2001, pp. 719–44.

[11]   A. Cunningham, *The Anatomist Anatomis'd: An Experimental Discipline in Enlightenment Europe*, Aldershot, 2010; M.P. Donato, 'Il normale, il patologico e la sezione cadaverica in età moderna', *Quaderni Storici*, 136, 2011, pp. 75–98.

[12]   N. Mani, 'Neue Konzepte der Pathologie im 17. Jahrhundert', *Gesnerus*, 40, 1983, pp. 109–17; M.D. Grmek, 'Il concetto di malattia', in *Storia del pensiero medico occidentale*, ed. M.D. Grmek, vol. 2, *Dal Rinascimento all'inizio dell'Ottocento*, Rome and Bari, 1996, pp. 259–89; J. Konert and H.G. Dietrich, 'Giovanni Battista Morgagni und der Beginn der pathologischen Anatomie', in *Anatomie: Sektionen einer medizinischen Wissenschaft im 18. Jahrhundert*, ed. J. Helm and K. Stukenbrock, Wiesbaden, 2003, pp. 127–38.

This does not mean that modern mechanical medicine never brought into play invisible realities, but rather that the polarity between visible and invisible was recast in a novel and problematic way.[13] In Lancisi's view, what has only been guessed at in life can be *seen* in death, when 'a priori conjectures find their confirmation in what has clearly occurred in the body'.[14] But what did he look at, what did he *see* in the dissected body?

In the first place, in mechanical medicine there was a wide margin of ambiguity in post-mortem visible findings that depended on the central pathogen role still assigned to fluids. Not by chance the main objection raised by empiricists and sceptics against the usefulness of autopsies concerned the instability of liquids, since they pointed at the fact that it was impossible to establish whether alterations revealed on the dissecting table were the cause or, on the contrary, the effect of death. In response, rational doctors admitted the difficulties they faced in ascertaining the movements of fluids, but nevertheless insisted on their fundamental intelligibility, as did Lancisi himself in the heated debate surrounding the use of animal dissections during the 1711 cattle plague.[15] What cannot actually be seen can be conjectured on the grounds of reason and experience by means of analogy, he claimed. Such a claim was rooted in the assumption of Nature's regularity, a central one in Galilean natural philosophy: 'Nature always operates by necessity, and according to the laws of pure mechanics, such as often remain unknown to us.'[16]

---

[13]   M. Foucault, *The Birth of the Clinic: An Archaeology of Medical Perception*, trans. A.M. Sheridan Smith, London, 1973, pp. xii–xv.

[14]   SM, p. 138.

[15]   See above, Chapter 3. Positions, however, varied greatly. The physician of the Apostolic palaces, Gaspare Reali, for instance (one of those who attended the autopsies at La Sapienza in 1706), in his *Exercitationes binae de convulsione, de motibus convulsivis cum succedaneo hydrope, de lacte, ac de pleuritide*, Rome, 1702, p. 128, posited the instability of somatic fluids but he used the argument to refute chemical medicine, rather than post-mortem evidence. Whether cardiac polyps were post-mortem coagulated blood or pathological concretions was much debated in seventeenth-century medicine; see, among others, M. Malpighi, *De polypo cordis* (1666), now in *Opere scelte di Marcello Malpighi*, ed. L. Belloni, Turin, 1969, pp. 191–216; T. Kerckring, *Spicilegium anatomicum, continens observationum anatomicarum rariorum centuriam unam*, Amsterdam, 1670; R.G. Mazzolini, 'Polyp', in *The Oxford Companion to the History of Modern Science*, Oxford, 2003, pp. 666–7.

[16]   Lancisi's quote, echoing polemical arguments by Malpighi, is in A.M. Borromeo, *Istoria dell'epidemia de' buoj accaduta nel Padovano l'anno MDCCXI ... aggiuntovi un altro ragionamento di Monsig. Lancisi, intorno all'epidemia de' cavalli*, Naples, 1712, p. 158, and continues: 'I confess meanwhile, that in the things of Nature which our senses do not penetrate, it is daring, and rather difficult, to venture our mind into the true properties of the effects. Therefore, considering the impossibility of seeing, or ... detecting by means of our senses the minimal parts of these exhalations, and much less of following them in the motion and actions they perform when they mix with liquors inside the cavities of the viscera and

Within the pre-eminence accorded to fluids, corpuscularianism was the other basic assumption of Lancisi's doctrine. Aneurysms (to which he later devoted a specific work, *De motu cordis et aneurysmatibus*, published posthumously), polyps, bone lamellae and atherosclerotic plaques are the kind of visible localised pathological formations whose interpretation ultimately rested on the assumption of the (invisible) corpuscular composition of bodily fluids. They are deemed to be formed through the action of imperceptible particles of air, blood or neural fluid, and in turn constitute further mechanical impediment to the motion of liquids and solids.[17]

Notwithstanding his additions to empirical knowledge, Lancisi's attempt at reconciling mechanism and chemistry eventually entailed an essential tension between visible and invisible, presumed and ascertained, perceived by the senses and established by reasoning. If all tissues and fluids are subject to the laws of physics, a number of pathological conditions can be deduced from physical concepts such as pressure, compression, weight (and from the work of physicists like Galileo's disciple Benedetto Castelli).[18] These eventually contradict localisation, since the hydrometric principles at times forestall any actual inspection of the impediments to circulation.

The tension between visible and invisible made medical knowledge reach different degrees of 'empirical denseness'. Lancisi's descriptions are especially detailed as regards cardiovascular ailments, as in this passage from Book Two:

> The heart, even though on the outside there was nothing that was evident apart from rather dry fibres that were furrowed lengthwise with some kinds of grooves, presented to us, however, a rare sight in its interior (in spite of the fact that it was completely empty of blood and polyps), indeed, it was one which a man would never forget: to wit: At the entryway of the large artery there were present in the

---

in other ducts, I am not embarrassed to consider this to be among the many things I ignore. [Nevertheless] I can see in the light of philosophical reasoning that these exhalations do adapt and accommodate in so as to impregnate the fibrous weave of the membranes and the small vessels of the oxes.' On different paradigms of visibility in seventeenth- and eighteenth-century science, see W. Bernardi, *Le metafisiche dell'embrione: scienze della vita e filosofia da Malpighi a Spallanzani (1672–1793)*, Florence, 1986; G. Giglioni, 'The Machines of the Body and the Operations of the Soul in Marcello Malpighi's Anatomy', in *Marcello Malpighi: Anatomist and Physician*, ed. D. Bertoloni Meli, Florence, 1997, pp. 149–74.

[17]   In the *historia* of the cobbler Stefano Ascieri, SM, p. 164, for instance, in the aneurysm of the aorta there was, according to Lancisi, 'a polyplike substance ... incrusted with great neatness into an arch' and, he adds, 'it is clear that a powerful obstruction against the pulsation of the blood toward the external part had thus been erected'. See also the description of a case of *cor bovis*, SM, pp. 185–96.

[18]   Explicit reference to Benedetto Castelli's *Delle misure dell'acque correnti* (1628) is in SM, p. 145.

individual semilunar cusps certain uneven and thin sarcomata, which, lengthened similar to a condyloma into fringes and flaps, projected into the aorta. ... there was no doubt whatever, but that those bodies were hanging there because they had their origin in the elongated fibres and vessels of the cusps, and indeed not because they had been compacted through similar adhesion. Finally there was found within the descending aorta a substance, uneven and round and of a truly polypous nature, which filled up almost the entire cavity.[19]

And indeed, in the pages devoted to the heart, mechanical philosophy and post-mortem experience reinforce each other in enabling Lancisi to reassess most available knowledge on the cardiovascular system and on the pathologies affecting cardiac valves, myocardium and coronary arteries.[20] On the other hand, when he deals with the brain and nervous system (the alterations of which are not easily detected by the naked eye), Lancisi's descriptions tend to become more vague and generic and to engender a sort of 'illusory localisation' of brain affections.

On closer inspection, Lancisi's work reveals several epistemic short circuits. In the first place, when narrating successful treatments, his explanations of the expulsion of noxious substances – variably described as viscous fluid, mucus or viscid lymphs – are strongly reminiscent of the ancients' evacuation of peccant matter.[21] After the patient's death and dissection, greater emphasis is put on the visible ailments; in describing these, however, the visible is never disentangled from what is only assumed by analogy. Fluids are especially revealing in this respect, as Lancisi supposedly infers their 'vices' from the kind of lesion detected but actually always postulates a few basic operations – fermentation, erosion, ooze. The notion of fibres as endowed with intrinsic properties and the focus on microstructures (small glands, fine vessels) provides useful assistance in refining his theory, but does not entirely solve the tensions that are inherent to a view of the body as a mere hydrostatic machine. Excerpts such as the following imply an analogy in scale (from small to infinitely small) and in category (from normal to morbid) from what is visible/known to what is invisible/unknown.

An excessive amount of these spirits ... can at some time, by too great a pressure and distension of the cortical glands of the brain, compress the passages of the

---

[19]   SM, p. 162.

[20]   E. Hamroui, 'L'invéntion de la pathologie cardiaque entre philosophie et expérience (1628–1749)', *Micrologus*, 11, 2003, pp. 555–75, esp. pp. 564–8.

[21]   Discussing the apoplexy of a prelate, for instance, Lancisi writes that the canonical sublingual phlebotomy freed the 'blood [intercepted] in the vessels chiefly at the base of the brain and at the root of the tongue with the mucus adhering to it', SM, p. 141; SM, p. 143, phlebotomy '[removed] the obstructions of the lower abdomen'; again pp. 147–54, he mentions the 'fattier lymph that adhered particularly to the base of the brain'.

nerves to such a degree that there is no room left for the animal liquid that is about to flow through.[22]

These conceptual shifts are enhanced by physical concepts such as strength, pressure and speed, postulated by Lancisi as universally valid in the physical world.

Admittedly, analogy was a basic tenet of modern physiology, the main epistemic premise of post-Harveyan normal, morbid and comparative anatomy. Moreover, Lancisi's especially recurrent application of analogy partly depended on his aspiration to deliver a *doctrina absoluta* of sudden death encompassing its ultimate theoretical and empirical demonstration. A noticeable hiatus separates the descriptive and the theoretical sections of *De subitaneis mortibus*, even within the *historiae* in Book Two. Whereas post-mortem reports follow a dry descriptive register meant to provide the empirical knowledge of facts, the *scholia* are instances of causal reasoning. In the latter, all pathological findings as well as any symptom ever recorded during the course of the deceased's illness must be provided with an explanation. This all-embracing approach, however, makes it extremely difficult to select and prioritise visible post-mortem ailments when it comes to framing the actual morbid process and, ultimately, the death of one particular patient. Accordingly, case histories are in fact plausible stories. The way in which Lancisi reconstructs the story of Cardinal Sacripanti's unfortunate manservant, whose demise in January 1706 had terrified the people of Rome, is indeed revealing in this respect.

Antonio M. Brilli, a stout, 'intemperate' 50-year-old man, had long suffered pain in his chest and diaphragm, swelling of his limbs and hydrops. One night, he woke up seized by an attack of urticaria. He soon felt relieved thanks to the cool night air, but while walking back to work the next day, all of a sudden he was struck dead in the street. Autopsy revealed a great quantity of fat in the viscera (the gall bladder, Lancisi notes, seemingly contained 'real pus'), around the pericardium, in the pulmonary artery and aorta; the heart was enlarged, especially in the right auricle and vena cava; a seemingly congenital hole pierced the skull, while the cerebral vessels and sinuses were filled with blood and the brain ventricles with 'turbid serum'. Lancisi's interpretation underscores the 'corrosive corpuscles and sulphurous lymph' that stemmed from the gall bladder and mixed with other fluids, progressively irritating the fibres and seeping into the brain and spinal marrow. In order to devise a rational, coherent picture, the papal archiater brings forth the physiological principles and the mechanic laws enunciated in the first part of his treatise to assist him in conjecturing the entire pathological process from its very onset. It thus becomes easy for him

---

[22]   SM, pp. 21–2.

to conjecture, that the cause of this sudden death was that mass of thickening blood and serous matter, since fluids, deprived of their oleo-volatile parts, and redundant with fixed salts, because of their lack of proper fluidity, started to adhere within the tiny arteries of the meninges, within the sinuses and within the remaining vessels of the brain. There ... with the muscular fibres of the dura mater, and all the villi that intertwine in the cortex of the cerebrum and with the cerebellum impaired, and because of the delayed movement of the blood, with pressure exerted upon the fibres and glands of that very cortex to such a degree as to bring about the obstruction of the secretory oscula of the nerve fluid, a sudden stroke of the fluids and solids within the brain occurred, which we can designate as a most powerful apoplexy accompanied by a deadly syncope ... because of the concurrent resistance to the movement of the thick and resinous blood which poured down at that time through the cavities of the heart.[23]

In other words, tracing the history of disease backwards from the dissecting table mostly produced a plausible, likely account.

Therefore, it can safely be argued that the modern 'pathological paradigm' – that is, the assumption that dissection represents one main key to access both the healthy and the pathological functioning of the human body – was already fully outlined in Lancisi's 1707 *De subinaeis mortibus*. Lancisi set forth the basic theoretical, ideological and methodological coordinates of a modern anatomo-localistic medicine; this, however, brought with it its own peculiar, constitutive ambiguities, inconsistencies and shortcomings, which must not be overlooked at risk of writing a selectively linear history of medicine.

Autopsy vs 'Heteropsy'? Social Networks and Credibility and the Use of Post-mortem Evidence

Admittedly, one major difficulty in assessing an early eighteenth-century pathology like Lancisi's depends on the traditions of medical historiography. Traditionally, historians of medicine have tended to study the evolution of the modern 'pathological paradigm' following two main lines of enquiry. One follows the development of morbid anatomy as an autonomous discipline, paying more attention to the first descriptions of pathological conditions as can still be identified today and less to the underlying medical theory; the other focuses on the genesis of modern anatomo-clinical medicine, intended as a system of knowledge elaborated through the systematic use of post-mortems and the observation of large numbers of patients in hospitals, and tends to consider

---

[23]   SM, pp. 181–2. In G.B. Avanzi's case, SM, pp. 197–206, Lancisi conjectures how pungent particles of the blood penetrated in the fibrous tissue of the vessels.

eighteenth-century medicine against this sole background. Also, the debate is still open among historians who see discontinuities between seventeenth- and eighteenth-century morbid anatomy and proper nineteenth-century anatomo-clinical medicine,[24] and those who posit an institutional and theoretical continuity in a long eighteenth century.[25]

In order to move a step forward in this debate and highlight the originality of *De subitaneis mortibus* in the context of eighteenth-century medical culture, it might be useful to reconsider the practice of dissection in terms of intellectual and material resources and of social configurations. By focusing on access to the living and the dead body, we will be able to shed light on the coexistence of various styles of thought and various ways of dealing with post-mortem evidence without concealing them in a linear narration. The practice of dissection and the trust placed in morbid anatomy, which at first glance might seem universal, rapidly proves to have been rather more fragmented.

In their tracts on sudden death, two early eighteenth-century university-trained physicians, da Sylva and Evangelista, whose work I introduced in the first chapter, resorted to the same circulatory and fermentative theories as Lancisi; moreover, both briefly mentioned the autopsies carried out at La Sapienza under the papal archiater's supervision. But what da Sylva knew of the outcomes of the autopsies he had only heard from his colleagues. He described post-mortem lesions in generic terms like 'lacerated vessels',[26] in very much the same way as a laymen like Valesio did in his diary. Manifestly, the Portuguese physician had not inspected the corpses with his own eyes, and autopsy reports appear as bookish as the classical and medieval texts he quoted in his writings. As for Evangelista, here is his account of what could be found in the corpses:

> Dirt in the blood therein produced by a fondant ferment which, enervating it little by little, dissipated its spirits and made it inert, and by stagnating in the head

---

24   Foucault, *Birth of the Clinic*; E.H. Ackerknecht, *Medicine at the Paris Hospital, 1794–1848*, Baltimore, 1967; Long, *A History of Pathology*; R.C. Maulitz, *Morbid Appearances: The Anatomy of Pathology in the Early Nineteenth Century*, Cambridge, 1987; Cosmacini, *Storia della medicina*, pp. 221–30. New insight in seventeenth- and eighteenth-century medical anatomy is now offered by Cunningham, *The Anatomist Anatomis'd*.

25   L. Premuda, 'Die anatomisch-klinische Methode: Padua-Paris-Wien-Padua', *Gesnerus*, 44, 1987, pp. 15–32; O. Keel, *L'avénément de la médecine clinique moderne en Europe, 1750–1815: politiques, institutions et savoirs*, Montreal, 2001; G.B. Risse 'Methodological Perspectives in Hospital History', in *Institutions of Confinement: Hospitals, Asylums, and Prisons in Western Europe and North America, 1500–1950*, ed. N. Finzsch and R. Jütte, Cambridge, 2003, pp. 75–97. See also C. Hannaway and A. La Berge, eds, *Constructing Paris Medicine*, Amsterdam, 1999.

26   M. da Sylva, *Romanorum lachrymae subitaneis mortibus effusae exsiccantur*, Rome, 1706, p. 8.

and in the chest, caused the said oppressions all of a sudden, and ... symptoms ... compressing and irritating the nerves.

In short, he gave his readers an explanation rather than empirical information.[27] Although both da Sylva and Evangelista could have easily attended the autopsies in the university anatomical theatre, they made unproblematic use of 'heteropsies' – that is, dissections recounted by others.[28] Port-mortem findings were for them but an element among others, and not the foremost. Admittedly, their choice had a stringent social rationale. Since they had not practised the autopsies first hand, they could not claim them to sustain their medical opinion and assert their professional authority. In their books, they were keener to narrate their own successful treatments, following a well-tested style of polemic which they deployed in order to stand out in the professional marketplace. Da Sylva and Evangelista's medical style is one of reasoning and learning, in which experience is still interchangeable with textual traditions of medical and non-medical origin, and the notion of medical evidence is indistinguishable from deductive logic.

Conversely, Lancisi wrote about bodies he had examined and corpses he had inspected. His prominent position in the Roman medical system is one of the elements we need to take into account in order to understand *De subitaneis mortibus*. Lancisi's career encompassed important positions which made him familiar with different social and medical worlds. A renowned physician and a leading figure in the professional elite in the capital, he customarily treated prelates and members of the aristocracy, thus gathering their long, detailed medical histories and first-hand clinical observations.[29] Frequently solicited as a consultant to other physicians, he gained access to further case histories. And when death took away one of his patients, he could proceed unhindered with their post-mortem (most often in the home of the deceased, sometimes in the church where the funeral would take place) with all the gravity and dignity that his institutional role bestowed upon him.[30]

---

[27]   A. Evangelista, *Lettera informativa intorno le cause delle morti improvise*, Rome, 1706, unpaginated; he adds in another passage: 'whosoever will want to reflect incidentally over those cadavers that were open in public [in Rome], will certainly gather from the dilated vessels in the ventricles of the heart ... the vice of the blood that lacked in fluidity'.

[28]   I owe this definition to I. Maclean, *Logic, Signs and Nature in the Renaissance: The Case of Learned Medicine*, Cambridge, 2002, p. 207.

[29]   On the physical examination of patients by early eighteenth-century Italian physicians and its relevance to pathological anatomy, see M. Nicolson, 'Giovan Battista Morgagni and Eighteenth-Century Physical Examination', in *Medical Theory, Surgical Practice: Studies in the History of Surgery*, ed. C. Lawrence, London, 1992, pp. 101–34.

[30]   D. Harley, 'Political Post-Mortems and Morbid Anatomy in Seventeenth-Century England', *Social History of Medicine*, 7, 1994, pp. 1–28.

As *archiatra*, or physician to the pope, Lancisi also personally supervised those public autopsies which had been ordered by the pope and, as such, implicitly endowed with a greater value. True, the unfortunate servants and craftsmen, whose mortal remains were shown in public by virtue of their humble origins only, met the *sector* without any accurate clinical history. Nevertheless, Lancisi was at the centre of a network that brought him information which, both in quantity and quality, was not available to others; hence, he was able to garner from doctors and family members 'the history of their normal and abnormal condition' albeit with some gaps 'especially in relation to the irregularity of the pulse'.[31]

Notwithstanding Lancisi's downplaying of differences, the social context in which post-mortem dissections took place and the background of the deceased did in reality have an impact on his clinical practice. The long and thorough medical history of Monsignor Spada in Book Two of *De subitaneis mortibus* shows how highly post-mortem examinations were regarded in society, and hints at the fact that they allowed for the creation of collective ideas about disease and death. Social expectations, however, paradoxically put the anatomo-pathological method under greater stress. The higher the social status of patients, the more information was available to the physician, but at the same time, the greater also the need to provide an explanation for each recorded symptom. It is no coincidence that this is the only case Lancisi supplied with an extra section entitled *aetiology* – that is, a preliminary explanation of the prelate's infirmity after his clinical history and before the autopsy report and the *scholium*. Readers can clearly perceive how difficult it was for the papal archiater to fit each symptom within a credible reconstruction of the evolution of the disease up to the patient's death, and to arrange the pathological findings in order of relevance and importance.[32]

In truth, the social context in which medical knowledge was acquired with regard to post-mortem evidence did not only stem from the relationship between doctor and patient,[33] but also came into play with respect to the physician's relationship to his professional community. In the early eighteenth century, access to corpses often worked as a sign of professional distinction and as a manifestation of modernity, rather than as an epistemic tool, as clearly demonstrated by yet another tract on sudden death published in Rome, Antonio Bernabei's *Dissertazione delle morti improvvise nella quale si ragiona*

---

[31]   SM, p. 131.

[32]   SM, pp. 115–30.

[33]   Cultural conditionings deriving from the uneven social position of doctors and patients are especially underscored by N.D. Jewson, 'Medical Knowledge and the Patronage System in Eighteenth-Century England', *Sociology*, 8, 1974, pp. 369–85; D. Porter and R. Porter, *Patient's Progress: Doctors and Doctoring in Eighteenth-Century England*, Oxford, 1989.

delle perucche e degli acidi (*Dissertation on the sudden deaths in which it is word of wigs and acids*).[34]

Bernabei came from Cossignano in the Marche, as did a considerable number of prelates, curial officers and medical practitioners.[35] Compared to da Sylva and Evangelista, he was better integrated into influential circles, had illustrious patients and good connections. This is probably the reason why in 1706 Bernabei personally attended at least one of the autopsies at La Sapienza, which he later described in his book with a wealth of details.[36] Despite the fact that Bernabei boasted about having taken part in the dissections, he still declared himself to be sceptical about their meaning, writing words that would have well suited the conservatives and empiricists who opposed Malpighi and his followers. According to Bernabei, in fact, autopsies were invalidated by the time that had elapsed from the death of the person until the opening of his or her corpse. Hence, lesions and haemorrhages deemed to be the cause of sudden demise were actually the result of the convulsions of the dying person, and were the effect rather than the cause of death. Short of reviving vivisection, he states provocatively that corpses

> do not shed much light which enables us to see the true causes of deaths clearly, since in the last days and the last hours of life the whole machine of man is upset, overturned and transformed.[37]

Trust in morbid anatomy is not the only thing setting Bernabei apart from Lancisi, whom he nevertheless quoted, praised and openly copied in his own

---

[34] A. Bernabei, *Dissertazione delle morti improvvise nella quale si ragiona delle perucche e degli acidi*, Rome, 1708.

[35] On the curial recruitment from the Marche, see B.G. Zenobi, *Ceti e potere nella Marca pontificia: formazione e organizzazione della piccola nobiltà fra '500 e '700*, Bologna, 1976; C. Weber, ed., *Legati e governatori dello Stato della Chiesa (1550–1809)*, Rome, 1994. In *De subitaneis mortibus* Lancisi refers to Bernabei once, who in turn claims to have been treated by the papal archiater and other important doctors when he was ill.

[36] Bernabei, *Dissertazione delle morti*, p. 2: 'In one of them of about 60 years of age, of a sanguine complexion, we observed the rupture of the vessels, since in the first cavity [that is, the head] there was blood between the two meninges, and in the ventricles of the brain a big quantity of serum that distended their diameter: however, the cerebellum was not damaged. In the second cavity [that is, the thorax], the pericardium was very much dilated by a large blood clot, poured from the vena cava, which was lacerated near the right auricle of the heart. Likewise, the diameter of the aorta artery appeared very large, and its orifice encrusted with a soft callous matter of an ashy colour; the right side of the lungs was found adhering to the ribs. In the lower cavity [that is, the belly] we found no morbid condition but the bile in the gall bladder of a yellowish colour.'

[37] Ibid., p. 4.

work. Indeed, it followed much the same structure as *De subitaneis mortibus*, moving from a section on sudden death in general to one devoted to the unfortunate events that had occurred in Rome. Like Lancisi, Bernabei intended to classify the various kinds of unexpected death into three categories. But he distinguishes workers and servants who collapsed 'while they were walking, or eating, or in church'; those who 'felt themselves drowning, and were anxiously toing and froing through the house gasping for breath and begging for prompt assistance'; and those killed by the 'mortal stroke' of apoplexy.[38] Hence, unlike Lancisi's, Bernabei's classification is not based on post-mortem evidence but on syndromes of signs related to the three traditional cavities of the body – abdomen, chest and head respectively – the 'three cavities whence this sort of death might be suspected to ensue'. Like Lancisi, Bernabei professes modern tenets and repeatedly cites Descartes, Bellini, Borelli, Sylvius, Redi, Malpighi and Cole. Unlike Lancisi, however, Bernabei sees diseases as chemical, not mechanical, ailments, which are related solely to the physiology of the bodily fluids. His analysis is also based on Willis's chemical-circulatory pathology, into which he integrated the theories of fibres put forward by his Roman colleagues such as Baglivi and the selfsame Lancisi, but the whole verges towards a generically modernised humoralism. In other words, post-mortem dissections did not offer Bernabei any insight into pathology. Discussion of post-mortems seems to be for him just a rhetorical device which signals to his readers that he had access to the most prestigious circles of the Roman medical world.

In Bernabei's view, sudden death is the outcome either of a 'stomach syncope' or a 'suffocating catarrh, produced by a superabundance of serums, or lymphs or serous blood tending to stagnation'; it can also ensue from humoral plethora that makes fibres 'distracted and nearly semi-convulsed', unable to ensure blood circulation, or even from blood and nerve fluid 'by reason of an acid substance or coagulating salt'.[39] Human blood, with its very tiny 'reddish little globules' as described by Christiaan Huygens,[40] is considered particularly liable to contamination by noxious particles which render it too dense or too watery thereby preventing circulation. The fluids in the nervous system also turn bad and are unable to flow. This process thus alters the balance between vital and animal spirits as postulated by the ancients, who are eventually brought back into play in Bernabei's argument. On these eclectic premises, Bernabei sets out to search for the primary cause of each form of ailment.

---

[38]   Ibid., pp. 5–6. The stomach syncope had already been mentioned by Galen; see C.R.S. Harris, *The Heart and the Vascular System in Ancient Greek Medicine, from Alcmaeon to Galen*, Oxford, 1973, p. 441.

[39]   Bernabei, *Dissertazione delle morti improvise*, p. 10.

[40]   Ibid., p. 19.

Historians have emphasised that the category of cause in early modern learned medicine was an open field, in which all data (including autopsies) could and should be included.[41] This is true in Bernabei's work. Since according to the canonical definition, apoplexy is 'a rapid deprivation of sense and motion' due to a shortage of 'animal spirits flowing [in the nerves] together with nerve fluid', then

> All that can impede this motion [of animal spirits]... shall cause apoplexy. And since these effects depend on the natural perfection of fluids and of solids, anything that harms their natural composition is either the immediate or the pre-disposing cause of sudden deaths.[42]

The external origin of the imbalance of blood and nervous fluids can be found in bad food, alcohol, and in the toxic mercury ointments provided by quacks against the French pox. These account for the many dead among the populace. Bernabei recalls the case of a worker who died after having drunk brandy on an October morning in 1706, and adds confidently that

> If we had opened the body of this man, we would have found the real cause for such sudden death in his last cavity [that is, the abdomen], just as in other corpses [the cause] has been detected either in the stomach or in the spleen, in the liver or the gall bladder from whence bilious liquor [serves] to increase fluidity to the other humours of the body.[43]

During the dissections at La Sapienza, he continues, he heard 'from professors there that in other corpses either the pancreas, or the stomach, either the spleen or the liver were found variously contaminated and bruised'.[44] These observations

---

[41]   Maclean, *Logic, Signs and Nature*.

[42]   Therefore – I need not underscore Bernabei's eclectism – 'such [causes] will be the vitiated ferments of the stomach, the exceedingly acid pancreatic juice, the enlarged or inert bile and the reflux of the lymphs from the hypochondria and from the two superior ventricles, [when they] mix in the vena cava with blood that is made nearly cadaveric for the repeated circulations and that cannot ferment properly; and even more so if they contain more austere acid tending to coagulate than balsamic volatile acid necessary to fermentation, they will cause this mixture of acids and vitriolic particles and other thousands of various type and potency, composed by corpuscles which according to Pierre Gassendi are hook-shaped or coppery, to produce through its motion through the [bodily] canals painful sensations ... in those small nerve fibres; moreover, it will let the more serous as well as the fibrous parts of the blood amass, so that they will become like a jelly; hence, because the circulation of fluids and spirits is hindered, the loss of motion and sense [of apoplexy] will ensue'. Ibid., p. 18.

[43]   Ibid., p. 7.

[44]   Ibid.

corroborate Bernabei's modern humoralism, in spite of the fact that in the previous pages of his tracts he had described unmistakable cardiac laceration.

Bernabei maintains that lead pipelines might be an additional source of noxious acids, and this enables him to praise Clement XI for repairing the Roman aqueducts. According to Bernabei, imbalances in the blood and nervous fluids could mostly be attributed to external agents such as those found in corrupt air (even though he does not exclude the possibility of miasmas and astral influence). Air is 'that spirit that penetrates all, moves all, pushes all', and there is no 'disease that has not its small seed' in air, for it can carry an excess of noxious, irritating and acrid particles. Once again, despite the rather old-fashioned physiology on which he draws now and then, he is keen to show off his up-to-date scientific knowledge and refers to Gassendi, Borelli and Lionardo di Capua to demonstrate the corpuscular nature of air. Accordingly, he makes modern physics agree with Hippocrates, suggesting that each locality abounds in peculiar salts, which would explain the discrepancies in the mortality rates of different towns. In Rome, 'bituminous, sulphurous, arsenic, vitriolic corpuscles and others filling the air' predispose bodies to 'sudden, deadly diseases'. After the earthquake 'many began to suffer vertigo, palpitations or hypocondriac and melancholy affliction; not a few precipitated in acute, deadly fevers'; the situation was worsened by the lack of snow, whose round flakes would have captured the 'arch shaped' acid molecules.[45] The unhealthiness of the air and climate of Rome had, after all, been known 'since Galen's times'.[46]

Bernabei rejects the idea of an epidemic of sudden deaths. Environmental conditions, however bad, do not harm the body unless the individual disposition is unhealthy – that is, unless there is a previous abnormal accumulation of acrid corpuscles (which are otherwise necessary and useful). So, with some inventiveness, he suggests that the new fad for wigs, which had spread among all sorts of people in Rome, was the real origin of unexpected deaths. Hair is in fact like so many small 'fistulas' that help the body purge itself of 'excremental matter' which, if trapped within by a wig, may produce acidity and even minute worms 'if we are to believe father Athanasius Kircher's microscope'.[47] Malpighi provided the anatomical rationale for the idea that wigs suppress natural evacuations, while the low mortality rate in female monasteries – where no wigs were worn – provided an alternative form of evidence to support his argument.[48]

---

45   Ibid., pp. 27–8, 31.

46   Ibid., pp. 24, 36, 38–9.

47   Ibid., p. 48. The allusion here is to the work of the renowned Jesuit polymath A. Kircher, *Scrutinium physico-medicum contagiosae luis, quae pestis dicitur*, Rome, 1658, which offered an experimental demonstration of Aristotelian generation *ex putri*.

48   Bernabei, *Dissertazione delle morti improvvise*, p. 51. A similar argument can be found in earlier medical writing on various topics, especially plague; see, for example, G. Roscio, *De postrema pestilentia urbis Romae*, Rome, 1665.

At that time, wigs were a popular though hotly debated accessory. Quinto Settano (Ludovico Sergardi), a renowned poet, had censured this new French fashion in his *Satyrae* of 1704. In December 1707, Cardinal Vicar Carpegna had to reiterate the prohibition against the wearing of hairpieces by ecclesiastics. Bernabei thus translated the moral disapproval for wigs which was currently being voiced by ecclesiastics and moralists into medical condemnation. His book is full of literary references and satirical interludes (like one *Ragguaglio contro le perucche in Parnaso*, News-sheet against wigs from Parnassus, in the style of Traiano Boccalini's notorious political satire *Ragguagli dal Parnaso*) and was clearly intended for a fashionable, sophisticated readership. For many readers, wigs seemingly represented a more obvious, visible evidence than autopsies, while for a medical practitioner like Bernabei, though well connected and aware of the contemporary developments in pathological dissections, post-mortem results were still very close to literary heteropsies.

The Body Ambiguous: Domenico Mistichelli, an Anatomist who was not a Pathologist

It has been argued that the origin of anatomo-localistic medicine is to be found not in the holistic, qualitative approach of learned medicine, but in the surgical approach to the sick body, given the extent to which surgeons focused on the solid parts and on localised lesions such as wounds.[49] Early modern Italy arguably offered a favourable context to the intellectual genesis and social acceptance of this kind of anatomo-localistic medicine since the social separation between physicians and surgeons was relatively weak and hospitals had been medicalised at a relatively early time.[50]

This interpretation could certainly be applied to Rome. The Roman College of Physicians granted academic qualifications both in medicine and surgery and in surgery, degrees that differed widely from the barber-surgeons' patents *in levibus* (for minor operations). Doctors in medicine and philosophy commonly taught and practised major surgery. At the university of Rome, as I have indicated, professors of anatomy also taught a three-year course in surgery based

---

[49]   O. Temkin, 'The Role of Surgery in the Rise of Modern Medical Thought', *Bulletin of the History of Medicine*, 25, 1951, pp. 248–59; G.B. Risse, 'La sintesi fra anatomia e clinica', in *Storia del pensiero medico*, ed. Grmek, pp. 291–335.

[50]   On the medicalisation of Italian hospitals, see A. Pastore, 'Gli ospedali in Italia fra Cinque e Seicento: evoluzione, caratteri, problemi', *Sanità, scienza e storia*, 1–2, 1990–91, pp. 71–8; A. Scotti, 'Malati e strutture ospedaliere dall'età dei Lumi all'Unità', in *Storia d'Italia, Annali 7, Malattia e medicina*, ed. F. Della Peruta, Turin, 1984, pp. 235–96. On the social status of surgeons, see S. Cavallo, *Artisans of the Body in Early Modern Italy: Identities, Families and Masculinities*, Manchester, 2007.

on the Hippocratic treatises *De Vulneribus Capitis, de Fracturis* and *de Ulceribus*. Moreover, hospitals (where the post of head surgeon was customarily held by a physician or at least a university-trained surgeon) created opportunities for scientific and professional exchanges between doctors and surgeons. Hospitals also were the place where medical dissections took place with the assistance of both physicians and surgeons.

This interpretation could also explain Lancisi's approach to pathology. As we have seen, at first he familiarised himself with both normal and morbid anatomy dissections in the hospital of Santo Spirito. He was then granted a university chair in anatomy and surgery. In his lessons on tumours, for instance, he clearly strove to interpret lesions in histological terms.[51] Later in his life, he created a library at Santo Spirito for medical students and apprentice surgeons and fostered a tighter connection between medicine and surgery.[52]

However, the mere performance of autopsies on deceased patients was not in itself sufficient for the practice to acquire the status that would enable it to be used as a clinical tool. The *Trattato dell'apoplessia* (*Treatise on apoplexy*), by the physician Domenico Mistichelli, another Roman contemporary of Lancisi's, is a case in point.[53]

Mistichelli was a hospital practitioner. Born in Fermo in 1675, he graduated from Rome and after a stint as assistant at the hospital of S. Maria della Consolazione, he was appointed physician at the hospital of Fatebenefratelli on Tiberina Island. He would later accept the post of town physician in the city of Ancona, where he died in 1717. At the time when the sudden deaths were frightening Rome, he was already established as a valid Cartesian anatomist.[54] And in his 1709 treatise on apoplexy he still wore the anatomist's hat.

Mistichelli's book was clearly inspired by *De subitaneis mortibus* and was likewise divided into a general section on apoplexy and a more specific part on the particular events in Rome, appended with clinical and post-mortem reports. It begins with a comprehensive, up-to-date introduction to the anatomy of the brain and heart, where the author presents his own research, as well as that of others, on many disputed topics.

---

[51]   See especially Ms BLR, Lancisi 153, *Prolusio ad praelectiones de tumoribus anni 1695*, fols 154–72.

[52]   G.M. Lancisi, *Dissertatio de recta medicorum studiorum ratione instituenda*, Rome, 1715. The raising of standards in the teaching of anatomy and surgery in religious institutions included barber-surgeons, as demonstrated by the new rules for apprenticeship inserted in the *Statuti, ordini, e costitutioni dell'Università, e Collegio de' Barbieri di Roma*, Rome, 1713.

[53]   D. Mistichelli, *Trattato dell'apoplessia in cui con nuove osservazioni anatomiche e riflessioni fisiche si ricercano tutte le cagioni e spezie di quel male e vi si palesa fragli altri un nuovo et efficace rimedio*, Rome, 1709.

[54]   *Lettres de G. Desnoues ... et de mr. Guglielmini ... sur différentes nouvelles découvertes*, Rome, 1706, pp. 205–11.

Mistichelli was a devoted anatomist. Using various techniques (maceration in liquids, ink injections, microscopy and so forth), he was able to describe the crossing of the medulla oblungata fibres and to explain the phenomena of inverted paralysis and cross-lateral control which had been known since antiquity (and recently observed by Lancisi with regard to brain tumours).[55] In his tract he was aware of the risk of artefacts when dealing with histological preparations, and he was prepared to contradict Malpighi and Willis on the micro-anatomy of the brain's grey matter, the glandular nature of which he firmly denied. In contrast, and relying on the ideas of his prominent Roman colleagues, Antonio Pacchioni, Giorgio Baglivi and Lancisi – if only to demonstrate his proximity to the city's medical elite – he turned his attention to the central role of the meninges in the functions of the nervous system.

Mistichelli argued that meninges are the 'expansion of the tunics of the carotid and cervical arteries and of jugular veins'; animal spirits are produced in their 'fibrous interstices' and then propelled by their contraction and dilation in the nerves, or more precisely in the membranes that envelop nerves and muscles, including the heart (in this he was drawing on Baglivi, but citing Aristotle and Andrea Cesalpino instead). Meninges also communicate *partem per partem* the material impressions sent by sensorial organs to the brain, where the immaterial soul interprets them.[56] Mistichelli thus intended to have his say in the great debate of the century over 'how animal motion is made'.

Firm in his (Cartesian) anatomical and philosophical premises, Mistichelli undertook the study of apoplexy 'or sudden death'. If apoplexy is what Galen described as a sudden deprivation of sense and motion in the whole body,

> since sense and movement are brought about by the animal spirits and the nerves, it must be deduced that in apoplexy, by which those functions are halted, the affected parts are the animal spirits or the nerves, or both; even better, since this ailment renders the whole body senseless, one has to conclude that the lesion is impressed at the origin of all the nerves, that is to say, at the meninges that cover the brain, or the medulla oblongata, which are the root of the nerves.[57]

---

[55] Mistichelli, *Trattato dell'apoplessia*, p. 58 and plate 1; P. Capparoni, 'Domenico Mistichelli e la sua scoperta della decussatio pyramidum', *Atti dell'Accademia di storia dell'arte sanitaria*, 5, 1939, pp. 261–75; M. Neuburger, *The Historical Development of Experimental Brain and Spinal Cord Physiology before Flourens*, ed. and trans. E. Clarke, Baltimore, 1981, pp. 57–8. Cross-lateral control – that is, the appearance of symptoms in the part of the body opposite to that in the head that suffered injury – had been a known phenomenon since antiquity, mentioned by Hippocrates and studied by Areteus; see E. Clarke and C.D. O'Malley, *The Human Brain and Spinal Cord: A Historical Study Illustrated by Writings from Antiquity to the Twentieth Century*, Berkeley, CA, 1968, pp. 280–83.

[56] Mistichelli, *Trattato dell'apoplessia*, pp. 19–21; see also p. 60.

[57] Ibid., p. 45.

And further,

> If the origin of the nerves is twofold, that is [there is] a proximate one, which are
> the meninges, medulla oblongata and spinal medulla, and a remote one, that is
> the heart, the carotid and cervical arteries, *which constitute the meninges*, one can
> reasonably recognise the affected parts in apoplexy, and not only the parts inside
> the skull, but also those enshrined in the thorax. Indeed, if the heart is seized by
> syncope, or any other ailment, and ceases to propel blood into the meninges, then
> apoplexy necessarily ensues.[58]

This comprehensive explanation of apoplexy was based on reason and authority.
It was part of Mistichelli's conventional nosography. In contrast to Lancisi's
(whose endeavour was to find the appropriate definition for unstructured
medical events such as 'sudden deaths'), Mistichelli's is an analysis of causes.
Mistichelli was therefore hesitating between a pathological approach reminiscent
of Lancisi's and a scholastic classification. According to the 'inclusive causality'
of early modern medicine, a cause is whatever precedes and stirs up a certain
illness, hence there can be remote or external causes such as the abuse of non-
natural things, traumas, suppressed or excessive evacuations, narcotic vapours,
excessive study, asthma, aneurysms, constitution of the body, age, time of the
year and so on. There are also internal or 'near' causes which, according to Galen,
pertain to the body itself: lymph, 'serous, viscous catarrhs', blood, polyps in the
heart, 'swelling in the skull', convulsion of the brain membranes, obstruction of
the veins.

> Each and every one of these causes, both internal and external, can contribute to
> bringing about a single effect such as sudden death; therefore, it is not surprising
> that [medical] authors have always disagreed in their works on its true origin,
> since the dissections of corpses have revealed different causes [of death].[59]

Mistichelli tries to classify the various types of apoplexy according to their
'origin', a term which is partly the equivalent and partly the opposite of 'cause'.
His imitation of Lancisi is apparent in his classification of the different types:
apoplexy from wounds, from the constriction or relaxation of solids,[60] and
from the coagulation or dissolving of liquids (plus a special kind of 'narcotic'

---

[58]   Ibid., pp. 45–6, my italics.

[59]   Ibid., p. 52.

[60]   This notion, although reminiscent of Hippocrates and the ancient Methodists, was
clearly inspired by Baglivi's *De fibra motrice et morbosa*. It should be recalled that in the same
year, 1709, Herman Boerhaave published his hugely influential *Aphorismi de cognoscendis et
curandis morbis*, through which the pathology of constricted and relaxed fibres was made
canonical.

apoplexy). Still, Mistichelli argues that only dissection can ultimately reveal the manifold causes of apoplexy, as the recent 'frequent Roman apoplexies' showed when

> In each a varying and different first origin was found, since in some serum in the brain cavities was observed; in others excessively fluid blood almost like a red serum; in others overabundance of blood; in others extravasated blood; in others iatids; in others soft and flaccid meninges; in others polyps in the sinus of the dura mater; in others, polyps in the ventricles of the heart; in others, aneurysms, or dilated arteries that [were] disrupted near the heart; in others *vomicae* in the lungs; and in others further ailments that had been generated long ago which suddenly, either because of laceration or pressures, or because of overflow, came to be the immediate causes of sudden death.[61]

Mistichelli therefore rooted his theory in post-mortem evidence; autopsies, however, rather than establishing the cause of death, are used to show how the same disease can be defined in terms of various dysfunctions and that apoplexy (that is, loss of sense and motion) is underlain by several causes. They also show how 'the beginnings of this evil varies, and in like manner the various ways in which the disease operates'.[62] To him, signs and symptoms were not a key for deciphering different morbid processes, but an element already provided by doctrine; therefore, the physician's task was to elaborate a comprehensive theory that accounted for all 'the phenomena that accompany apoplexy'.[63]

Mistichelli's 'inclusive causality' and the scholastic framework behind his modern mechanical and chemical explanations become more evident when he discusses 'the various reasons that may have produced the frequent apoplexies in Rome in the years 1705 and 1706'. Mistichelli is mainly interested in proving the rationality of his theory by establishing a causal chain reaching back to universals – and what is more universal than air?

As a modern natural philosopher, Mistichelli considers air both as a physical agent (which by virtue of its elasticity and its 'innumerable little arches or springs' rarefies and condenses the humours in the body) and as a chemical agent (its nitrous part, indispensable for the motion of the blood and the distillation of animal spirits, can coagulate with 'urinary spirits, or ammoniac vapours').[64]

---

[61] Mistichelli, *Trattato dell'apoplessia*, pp. 52–3.

[62] Ibid., p. 52. Hence there are apoplexies originating from 'blows to the head or to the stomach', wounds in the pericranium or 'cracking of the skull', 'by defects of the convulsed solid parts', 'by defects of the relaxed and soft solid parts' or by the 'density of fluid parts'.

[63] Ibid., p. 103.

[64] Ibid. p. 82.

As shown by John Mayow and others,[65] in the lungs, blood is combined with a number of active chemical substances, which mix and react with those already in the body and affect the blood and nervous fluid; therefore, it can be asserted that the universal cause of apoplexy is air.

Why then, 'if the causes of apoplexy were universal in Rome, was the illness not universal and common to all'?[66] The answer is commonplace – the sick person had 'in himself some particular principles condensing the spirits' – and so, too, is the general conclusion: the apoplexies in 1705 and 1706 began in bodies which were already susceptible

> by reason of some volatile ammoniac principles or some fixed and oily ones, as the nearest and concomitant cause; or on account of the impure constitution of the Roman air, which too readily compresses and dilates, as the universal cause; or due to the bad weather, namely, the southern and northern winds, as an occasional and predisposing cause; and, lastly, because of the consumption of certain foods and unripe fruits, which were full of fixed and rigid salts, as a remote and external cause.[67]

Once again, the author's objective is to link individual cases with universal theory through open, flexible categories of causes. The argumentation as a whole is quite revealing of the tenacity of old-fashioned causal reasoning, according to which each different factor contributes equally to producing a diseased condition.

The second part of Mistichelli's book is concerned with the 'practice' of treating apoplexy. Following the traditional conventions found in any good handbook, he organises remedies into three categories: surgical operations,[68] medical remedies (pharmaceutics) and preventive measures (hygiene). In the appendix Mistichelli also presents 'several notable cases by reason of the event or of the opening of the cadavers' that are meant to corroborate his theory. Upon examination, the dead at the hospitals of Consolazione and Fatebenefratelli all

---

[65]   Mayow is quoted repeatedly; on his chemical theory, see R.G. Frank, *Harvey and the Oxford Physiologists: A Study of Scientific Ideas*, Berkeley, CA, 1980, pp. 224–32; A. Clericuzio, *Elements, Principles and Corpuscles: A Study of Atomism in the Seventeenth Century*, Dordrecht, 2000, pp. 149–51. Mistichelli tried to integrate Mayow's chemical stance with the more mechanical approach of Boyle and Borelli to respiratory physiology, treating nitre as the 'elastic' component responsible for air compression and dilation.

[66]   Mistichelli, *Trattato dell'apoplessia*, p. 98.

[67]   Ibid., pp. 99–100.

[68]   In his view, there is no disease for which 'manual operation ... is more ideally suited' than apoplexy; ibid., p. 111.

showed some kind of alteration in the meninges.[69] Thus post-mortems conform to the medical doctrine of both the ancients and modern physiologists.

Mistichelli's work can be seen as mirroring his position in the Roman medical system. As a hospital physician, he was part of a dense network connecting the major city hospitals (and was therefore aware of current research); but as an unprivileged practitioner, he was excluded from, and in competition with, the medical elite.[70] So, he criticises celebrities like Malpighi, though implicitly relying on their authority to justify his anatomical endeavours, and he refers instead to Aristotle and Galen, using the traditional scholastic presentation of arguments. He introduces new observations – his book is yet another source showing that dissections were routinely practised in Roman hospitals – but makes little use of them while searching for universal explanatory principles encompassing all clinical manifestations of apoplexy. Lastly, he does not try to correlate clinical and post-mortem observations, even though he has direct access to sick people in hospital beds.

One of the reasons for this lies in the social status of the hospital patients whom Mistichelli treated, and occasionally dissected. Unlike Lancisi, who was physician to courtiers and prelates, Mistichelli could not rely on detailed medical histories, especially since patients were often unconscious when admitted to the hospitals he worked for, as both 'specialised' in traumas. It was therefore more difficult for him to correlate symptoms and post-mortem findings. His descriptions of the autopsies are rather cursory. Even more notably, during dissection Mistichelli often only inspected the head of the deceased patient, since according to the canonical definition of apoplexy the head was the seat of disease.[71]

---

[69] Ibid. pp. 164–6: in some cases, Mistichelli found during autopsy 'pus on the dura mater whence the latter appeared of a livid yellow colour, and its cavities were full of partly clotted and partly dissolved blood', in others 'a quantity of pus between the dura mater and the pia mater, the meninges livid and the substance of the brain soft', and the vessels of the meninges 'turgid with black, murky blood' and the pia mater covered with hydatids.

[70] Some of Mistichelli's clinical observations are included in Lancisi's SM, p. 102. Mistichelli claimed that he did not publish his book earlier because he was aware that Lancisi, who as papal archiater and a member of the College of Physicians was a much more prominent figure, was writing his own treatise.

[71] The following description is among the longest and exemplifies Mistichelli's style as a pathologist: 'Pietro, 30 years of age, arrived ill with a malignant fever from the Pontine marshes and was admitted to the hospital of Benefratelli after four days illness on the day of 9 November 1705. He was placed in bed no. 11; he was purged and his fever augmented with delirium; he was refrigerated with emulsions and the appropriated distilled water called alexiphamarkon; diaphoresis was also administered, but to his detriment, since delirium turned into lethargy, and lethargy in a strong apoplexy, and on the 19 of the same month he died. *The skull was opened*: the sanguineous vessels of the meninges were turgid with black, cloudy blood especially in the cavities; the pia mater had many hydatids; the medulla of the

Dissection, in any case, was not (any longer) innovative in itself, and normal anatomy was not the same thing as morbid anatomy. The wealthy and well-organised hospitals of Rome could provide many observations on the sick and the dead, but these did not necessarily produce innovation either in normal or pathological anatomy unless they were related to a new notion of medical truth.

Cause of Disease or Cause of Death?

Mistichelli was an anatomist, not a pathologist. Lancisi, in contrast, endeavoured to correlate the sick patient's symptoms with post-mortem findings. His practice of anatomy lies behind a few important clinical remarks, such as the warning that 'many symptoms, which according to appearances appertain to respiration, have their diseased root entirely in the heart itself and in the vessels appended'.[72] As I have indicated, the content of Book One of *De subitaneis mortibus* is designed to give precedence to the organs or fluids that are the ultimate cause of death, on the grounds that a good clinician must seek to anticipate whether and where the lesion is forming in order to intervene.

Historians of medicine have passed diverging judgements on Lancisi's achievement with respect to real advancements in pathological localisation. Some have regarded Lancisi's notations as 'intellectual short-cuts' that he was able to reach because of his bedside intuition rather than his medical theory.[73] On the whole, however, it can be argued that by emphasising the value of post-mortems, the papal archiater added to the traditional descriptions of suffocation (asphyxia), syncope and apoplexy. These syndromes are renamed on the basis of

brain was pale, covered with innumerable blood dots, whence blood poured that seemed putrid, and serous for the most part'; Mistichelli, *Trattato dell'apoplessia*, p. 166, my italics.

72   SM, p. 54.

73   See Cosmacini, *Storia della medicina*, p. 186. Lancisi is listed among the founders of scientific cardiology in most nineteenth-century handbooks and histories of cardiology such as J.O. Leibowitz, *The History of Coronary Heart Disease*, Berkeley, CA, 1970, pp. 3–4; J.I. McDougall and L. Michaels, 'Cardiovascular Causes of Sudden Death in "De Subitaneis mortibus" by Giovanni Maria Lancisi', *Bulletin of the History of Medicine*, 46, 1972, pp. 486–94; H.A. Snellen, *History of Cardiology: A Brief Outline*, Rotterdam, 1984, pp. 37–8, who particularly praises the description of excrescences in cardiac valves and aneurysms; L.J. Acierno, *A History of Cardiology*, London, 1994, p. 56; P.R. Fleming, *A Short History of Cardiology*, Amsterdam, 1997, pp. 3–4 and 135, who points to Lancisi's understanding of the link between pathology of the heart and respiratory symptoms, and to his description of excrescences from infective endocarditis, as does G. Weber, *Aspetti poco noti della storia dell'anatomia patologica tra '600 e '700: William Harvey, Marcello Malpighi, Antonio Cocchi, Giovanni Maria Lancisi: verso Morgagni*, Florence, 1997, p. 62.

the obstructions in the flow of air, blood and nervous fluid revealed by autopsy rather than on the basis of symptoms which, in scholastic medicine, defined their essence. There is a shift in the *locus affectus* theme: it is no longer sufficient to locate the affected cavity (the head, the chest or the belly) or the organ that has suffered the most damage; it is necessary to understand how deadly lesions are produced in the delicate structure of the body-machine.

It has been noted elsewhere that Lancisi did not consider visible lesions on a corpse to be the disease or its cause.[74] They are merely the localised outcome of a morbid process and the manifest facts from which a physician who knows normal anatomy and physiology may conjecture on causes. Scholars who emphasise the discontinuity in the history of modern medicine such as Foucault and Ackerknecht consider the quest for causes as the fixed perimeter within which early eighteenth-century anatomo-localistic medicine in its early stage (that is, in the period from Malpighi to Morgagni roughly speaking) first tackled the problem of pathological localisation. Indeed, early eighteenth-century medicine still read symptoms as an effect of systemic unbalances, and sought the ultimate origin of disease distinguishing it from organic damage. In contrast, in the nineteenth-century anatomo-clinical medicine illness and the morbid process on tissues are one and the same.[75]

This interpretation seizes on a peculiar aspect of modern 'rational' medicine: the obsession with cause. The *scholia* in Book Two of *De subitaneis mortibus* bear witness to the papal archiater's obstinate search for the very first cause that triggered the morbid process, tracing back to the natural, organic cause of disease and death from an autopsy.

Among the consequences of such modern rational empiricism – or empirical rationalism – is an understanding of causality that proceeds a step further in the wake of the collapse of Aristotelianism and Galenism, which still confusingly provided the organisation for practical medicine. In scholastic medicine, the six Aristotelian causes adapted for medical learning by Galen and Avicenna were logically deduced by medical experts from particular to general and in reverse. As we have seen with medical authors such as da Sylva, Evangelista, Bernabei and Mistichelli, causes were not assigned any hierarchical order in relation to

---

[74] E. Hamraoui, 'L'oeuvre d'Hippocrate revisitée par la pensée médicale des Lumières: l'exemple des traités médicaux de G.M. Lancisi (1654–1720)', in *Hellénisme et hippocratisme dans l'Europe méditerranéenne: autour de D. Coray*, ed. E. Andréani, H. Michel and E. Pélaquier, Montpellier, 1996, pp. 101–9.

[75] Foucault, *Birth of the Clinic*, p. 142; V. Hess, 'The Foundation of Morphological Pathology in Cultural Context', in *Traditions of Pathology in Western Europe: Theories, Institutions and their Cultural Setting*, ed. C.-R. Prüll, Herbolzheim, 2003, pp. 21–40; Risse, *La sintesi fra anatomia e clinica*, pp. 307–8. In the interpretation favouring 'discontinuity' an important role is played by the patients' depersonalisation, assumedly brought about by the nationalisation of hospitals during the French Revolution.

individual patients. On the contrary, according to Lancisi, all too frequently 'the blame for being the real causes of sudden deaths is placed on certain factors which should instead be looked on as precipitating'. However, even he admits that 'the causes which are able to bring about sudden death are innumerable and are usually, in their various ways, so intermingled among themselves that you will rarely find one that is simple'.[76] As I have already pointed out, his main tenet is that, once the time of dissection has come, the proper cause of any single death can be traced back or conjectured from the visible lesions. The chain of causality is modified accordingly, since the diverse factors causing disease and, eventually, death are reorganised and prioritised: the roots of disease remain multiple and vary in each sick person, but some consist of the circumstances and an individual's constitution and habits which may produce a defect if they combine in the wrong way, while others are concrete ailments which ultimately bring about death.[77] In other words, there is a necessary cause for each syndrome and each death, rather than many possible causes for all clinical manifestations of a given disease.

It must be borne in mind that, unlike works on general pathology such as Bonet's *Sepulchretum* or Morgagni's *De sedibus et causis morborum per anatome indagatis*, Lancisi's *De subitaneis mortibus* is a treatise on death. The section in Book Two devoted to the events of 1705 and 1706 in Rome, in particular, does not deal with any specific illness, but instead with the conditions that have ultimately caused those particular deaths. Since Lancisi's investigation moved across the borders of forensic medicine, medical theory and practical medicine, it inherently implied searching for causes. It is also important to recall that the first task assigned to physicians during the Roman medical investigation on sudden death under Clement XI was the discovery of plausible causes for each 'accident'. Moreover, physicians were able to assert their authority precisely because they met social expectations in this regard. Again, one can but note how specific historical circumstances shape scientific facts.

The interplay between medico-legal and medical concerns underlies several aspects of Lancisi's work. Because he investigates unrelated cases of sudden death, Lancisi can use pathology reports as *ex post* indications for clinical purposes,

---

[76]   SM, pp. 11–12.

[77]   The classification of proximate and remote causes was a much debated issue in medieval and Renaissance medicine; nevertheless, in practice the sophisticated Aristotelian distinctions were blurred when applied to concrete cases. See P.F. Ottosson, *Scholastic Medicine and Philosophy: A Study of Commentaries on Galen's Tegni (ca. 1300–1450)*, Naples, 1984; D. Jacquart, 'Medical Scholasticism', in *Western Medical Thought*, ed. Grmek, pp. 197–40; on the eighteenth century, with special reference to Boerhaave's work, see L.S. King, 'Some Problems of Causality in Eighteenth Century Medicine', *Bulletin of the History of Medicine*, 37, 1963, pp. 15–24.

and he needs not venture into the subtleties of nosology and definitions. Lancisi attempts to establish post-mortem diagnosis using lesions as diagnostic tools. Shifting the emphasis from prognosis to diagnosis, albeit *a posteriori*, he moves a step towards an anatomo-clinical approach to disease.[78] Since Lancisi's book is not about diseases but about death, his demonstration pivots around functional somatic systems rather than the head to toe scheme of practical anatomy (including Morgagni's *De sedibus*). In fact, Lancisi puts forward an understanding of vital functions as essentially interdependent. Heart, lungs and brain with their respective appendages are functional systems and principles of physiological organisation, autonomous and interconnected at the same time, from each of which (and not only from the heart-centre) life and death can be understood. This was arguably the beginning, in terms of organs at least, of that 'decentralisation of life' which would continue throughout the eighteenth and nineteenth centuries up to cellular pathology.[79]

In brief, the combination of mechanical philosophy and the anatomo-pathological method enabled Lancisi to revive the traditional issue of the hierarchy of vital functions. Eighteenth-century medical literature on death, from Morgagni to Bichat, would basically build on his interpretive grid.[80] More specifically, Lancisi's classification of the causes of sudden death laid the foundation of subsequent medical scholarship. The French pathologist and an authority in forensic medicine Paul Brouardel still referred to it in the late

---

[78]   P. Lain Entralgo, *La historia clínica: historia y teoría del relato patográfico*, Madrid, 1950, pp. 203–9; F. Cid, 'La nosologia morgagniana en la historia de la patografia', in *De sedibus et causis: Morgagni nel centenario*, ed. V. Cappelletti and F. Di Trocchio, Rome, 1986, pp. 109–18.

[79]   Hamroui, 'L'invéntion de la pathologie cardiaque'; B. Kisch, 'What Keeps Men Alive? A Survey of the History of Thoughts About Life and Death', in *The Historical Development of Physiological Thought*, ed. C. McC. Brooks and P.F. Cranefield, New York, 1959, pp. 309–34.

[80]   P. Astruc, *Essai sur Jean–Baptiste Morgagni*, Paris, 1950, pp. 37–9; C.A. Defanti, *Soglie: medicina e fine della vita*, Turin, 2007, pp. 57–63. According to Foucault, *Birth of the Clinic*, pp. 143–8, Bichat's *Recherches physiologiques sur la vie et la mort* (1802) was the first medical tract in which the relationship between life and death was subverted epistemologically and death was fully incorporated in the notion of life, rather than conceived as antithetic. It should be added, however, that the second part of Bichat's *Recherches* was devoted to sudden death; sudden death is treated according to a functional approach reminiscent of Lancisi, although Bichat's tissular pathology differed from Lancisi's mechanical organic pathology.

nineteenth century,[81] and the present classification of causes of sudden death is not too distant from Lancisi's.[82]

I am not arguing that searching for the cause of death was ever an epistemically unproblematic operation. Quite the opposite. It bore its specific complications. Indeed, *De subitaneis mortibus* set a number of constitutive aporia that would shape further medical research on the causes of death. In the first place, autopsy inevitably gives certain lesions priority over others, given the different degrees of 'descriptibility' of ailments, especially those affecting the heart and those affecting the brain. In the former, description and explanation, lesion and illness tend to coincide and thus become an immediate cause of death. Even today, heart diseases (particularly coronary heart disease) are used in medico-legal documents as obvious causal explanations.[83]

Secondly, the notion of cause of death is altogether ambiguous. Overall, in the course of the eighteenth century, cause of death came to be more and more closely identified with lesions found during autopsy. This would continue in the late nineteenth and twentieth century, even though, in the framework of cellular pathology and experimental physiology, death ceased to be viewed in terms of organic interdependence and came to be understood as the cessation of intracellular biochemical communication in the brain and in the heart; in other words, death became truly *invisible* on the dissecting table.[84] The 'pathological paradigm' implied the continuous superimposition of causes of disease and causes of death for Lancisi as well as for his heirs. It should also be noted that the notion and terminology of causality was still fairly unstable in eighteenth- and nineteenth-century medicine, and causes and circumstances were still used interchangeably.[85]

There was then a certain ambiguity in the social role that doctors had conquered through their dealings with death, especially when death was

---

[81]   P. Brouardel, *La mort et la mort subite*, Paris, 1895, and, before him, N.M. Sormani, *Monografia sulle morti repentine*, Milan, 1834. In the influent *Dictionnaire encyclopédique des sciences médicales*, ed. A. Dechambre, vol. 9, Paris, 1875, pp. 517–79, E. Bertin's entry 'Mort, physiologie' argues the uselessness of isolating a specific notion of sudden death from death in general, but a few pages later, G. Tourdes in 'Mort, médecine légale', pp. 690–708, deals with sudden death following Lancisi's arguments, and attributes to Lancisi the idea of the 'tripod of life' (lungs, heart, brain) that was later made canonical by Bichat.

[82]   L. Soimero, M.T. Tasini and M. Faggioli, *Morte improvvisa: storia del concetto, cause e meccanismi*, Rome, 1992, pp. 70–86.

[83]   S. Timmermans, *Postmortem: How Medical Examiners Explain Suspicious Deaths*, Chicago, 2006, pp. 35–62.

[84]   B. Fantini and M.D. Grmek, 'Le definizioni di vita e di morte nella biologia e nella medicina contemporanee', in *Bioetica*, ed. A. Di Meo and C. Mancina, Rome and Bari, 1989, pp. 163–200.

[85]   A. Fagot-Largeault, *Les causes de la mort: histoire naturelle et facteurs de risque*, Paris, 1989, pp. 261–84.

unexpected, sudden or suspicious. In their aspiration to always provide an explanation for legal, sanitary or simply diagnostic purposes, medical experts tended – and still tend – to 'reduce a necessary event to an accidental event … designating as cause a circumstance that cannot happen if it does not happen',[86] and thus retained a loose, nuanced notion of causality. They 'pathologised' the causes of death, while at the same time climbing back (more or less deliberately) from causes to predisposing or triggering factors of death. By the late eighteenth and early nineteenth century, it therefore became clear that pathological investigations on the cause of death needed to be compounded by much more information of various kinds. Scientific statistics – and not only Hippocratic-style observations or Enlightenment 'natural histories' of disease – would only enable medicine to reformulate the whole issue of causes, incidence and prevention of sudden death.[87] And it should be added parenthetically that such an evolution required the reform and secularisation of demographic control, which never took place in Papal Rome.

All of this, however, did not exhaust the problem of sudden death in the eyes of early modern physicians. Thorny ethical and professional issues surrounded the end of life, and to these we will now turn our attention.

---

[86]   Ibid., p. 1.

[87]   C.A Wunderlich, *Handbuch der Pathologie und Therapie*, vol. 1, Stuttgart 1852, pp. 53–6. One of the first attempts to correlate autopsy reports and epidemiological data in Italy was G. Ferrario, *Statistica delle morti improvvise e particolarmente delle morti per apoplessia nella città e nel circondario esterno di Milano dall'anno 1750 al 1834*, Milan, 1834, whereas Sormani, *Monografia sulle morti*, and Freschi, *Sulle cause della morte improvvisa e sulla loro maniera di agire*, Florence, 1850, kept a clinical stance. On the slow evolution of the conceptualisation of the causes of death in nineteenth-century mortality statistics, see G.B. Risse, 'Cause of Death as a Historical Problem', and K. Coddell Carter, 'Causes of Diseases and Causes of Death', *Continuity and Change*, 12, 1997, pp. 175–88 and 189–98 respectively.

PART III
The Lost and the Saved: Sudden Death as an Ethical and Religious Issue

Chapter 6
Death and the Doctors: Scientific Queries and Ethical Dilemmas

At the Confines of Life: Sudden Death, Apparent Death, Gradual Death

The alarm caused by the sudden deaths was slowly subsiding, when in February 1707 another horrifying story of death circulated in Rome. A young woman married to a draper 'was believed dead' after a miscarriage and taken to the church of San Giacomo in Scossacavalli for the funeral. Although, as it was later reported, 'in burying her, the undertaker found her warm and ... told the parish priest and her husband', nobody believed him, so that 'she was buried in a coffin', and after a while the horrific discovery was made of 'the said coffin, [which had been] sealed with nails, all scratched; [this was] the manifest sign ... that when she was buried, she was not dead as everybody claimed'.[1] Soon, the phobia of overhasty interment, of apparent death and of being buried alive, would spread throughout Europe.[2]

In truth, fear of premature burial had already had a very long tradition indeed. Tales of apparent deaths and untimely funerals had inhabited popular culture and literature for centuries and could be read in Pliny, Apuleius, Boccaccio and Matteo Bandello. They were not wanting in medical texts either. Although the diagnosis of death was a marginal problem in Graeco-Roman medicine,[3] the topic was explored by some medical authors, more or less indulging in terrifying details. The problem of apparent death was closely associated with sudden death and particularly with apoplexy, as this could impair involuntary motions such

---

[1] *Diario di Clemente XI*, 22 February 1707. On fears aroused by the introduction of sealed coffins, see M. Vovelle, *La mort et l'Occident de 1300 à nos jours*, Paris, 1983, p. 453.

[2] M. Patak, *Die Angst vor dem Scheintod in der 2. Hälfte des 18. Jahrhunderts*, Zurich, 1967; I. Stoessel, *Scheintod und Todesangst: Äusserungsformen der Angst in ihren geschichtlichen Wandlungen (17.–20. Jahrhundert)*, Cologne, 1983; C. Milanesi, *Morte apparente e morte intermedia: medicina e mentalità nel dibattito sull'incertezza dei segni della morte (1740–1789)*, Rome, 1989; M. Schwegler, *Erschröckliches Wunderzeichen oder natürliches Phänomenon? Frühneuzeitliche Wunderzeichenberichte aus der Sicht der Wissenschaft*, Munich, 2002, pp. 157–81; J. Bodenson, *Buried Alive: The Terrifying History of Our Most Primal Fear*, New York, 2001.

[3] M.D. Grmek, 'Les indicia mortis dans la médecine gréco-romaine', in *La mort, les morts et l'au-de-là dans le monde romain*, ed. F. Hinard, Caen, 1987, pp. 129–44.

as respiration and, in its most severe manifestation, induce the appearance of death. The risk of apparent death in apoplectic patients, however remote, was commonly acknowledged by medical experts.[4]

Ascertaining death with the utmost thoroughness to prevent tragic mistakes or unmask deceit was an issue of particular interest to forensic medicine. It should be recalled, incidentally, that ascertaining death was not a customary task of physicians, who intervened in suspicious cases only. Medico-legal authors such as the Sicilian physician Fortunato Fideli admitted that ascertaining death beyond doubt was a difficult operation but also suggested simple empirical criteria to perform it.[5] The chief proponent of early modern medico-legal common sense, the papal Protomedicus Paolo Zacchia, considered that putrefaction was the only infallible sign of death, yet in practice he did not advocate postponing funerals any longer than the customary 24 or 48 hours.[6]

In the second half of the seventeenth century, medical interest in the issue of apparent death was rekindled by mechanical philosophy and corpuscular chemistry. In his *De miraculis mortuorum*, the German doctor Christian Friedrich Garmann set out to expose tales of live burials and moving dead, attributing any sign of apparent survival of the corpse to the mere effect of residual chemical components and circulation of fluids.[7] And yet, as denunciation of myths and legends went on, so did, seemingly, the fear of apparent death. Already at the beginning of the eighteenth century the city of Weimar seemingly planned to build a morgue – that is, a specific place where corpses would be deposited for a period of time long enough to ascertain their actual death.[8] In 1714 in Rome, Clement XI tellingly issued a decree prohibiting

---

4   As did Arnold of Villanova, *Practica medicinae*, book I, chap. 23, and later D. Terilli, *De causis mortis repentinae tractatio*, Venice, 1615, p. 102; F. Ranchin, *De morbis subitaneis*, in his *Opuscula medica*, Lyon 1627, p. 595. 'Hysterical suffocation' (that is, suffocation by the uterus) was another illness to which apparent death was commonly attributed. Book VII of Pliny's *Natural History* was among the most cited sources on this topic, together with Celsus, *De medicina*, II, 6. On apparent death of drowned persons, see T. Bonet, *Medicina septentrionalis collatitia*, Geneva, 1686, vol. 1, pp. 431–44.

5   F. Fideli, *De relationibus medicorum libri quatuor*, Palermo, 1602, pp. 196–9.

6   I refer to the 1661 Lyon edition of P. Zacchia, *Quaestiones medico-legales*, pp. 161–72. See M.P. Donato, 'La morte repentina, tra dubbi diagnostici e speranze di rianimazione (secc. XVII-XVIII), in *Storia della definizione di morte*, ed. F.P. de Ceglia, Milan, 2014, pp. 199–214.

7   Originally printed in Leipzig in 1670, and republished by B. Herrmann and S. Benetello, *Über die Wunder (Dinge) der Toten*, Göttingen, 2003, who incidentally correct the interpretation of Garmann's work by P. Ariès, *The Hour of Our Death*, trans. H. Weaver, London, 1981, pp. 354–8.

8   Reference to this early German project is given only by P. Brouardel, *La mort et la mort subite*, Paris, 1895, p. 21. The *Leichenhaus* was actually built at the end of the eighteenth century in Weimer and elsewhere in Germany; see A. Josat, *De la mort et de ses caractères*,

burial of dead hospital patients 'before the due space of time of at least twenty hours, or even longer, *in accordance with the prudent judgement of experts*, so as not to have any doubt over their death, as prescribed in the Roman ritual'.[9] In fact, the official Roman ritual of 1614 prescribed a generic *debitum temporis intervallum* (due lapse of time) before burial, though it explicitly advised extra caution in the cases of sudden death.[10] The contradiction between the scientific stance and popular fears surrounding apparent death is only superficial. The breakdown of Aristotelianism undermined the traditional perception of death, and thus modern natural philosophy charged dying with new implications and concerns. The question of the confines of life and death began to be invested with unprecedented urgency.

As I have indicated, life – or rather the living being – was the object of inexhaustible speculations and interminable disputes in medieval and early modern medicine, whereas death received relatively little attention. If the ceasing of breathing and heartbeat were enough to define death in practice, in theory it was conceived essentially as deprivation, the loss of the material essence and immaterial principle of life. This was further complicated by the fact that scholastic medicine acknowledged the existence of Aristotle's and Galen's three souls and faculties, and that the animal immortal soul was at once an organic principle and the individual's essence.[11] Hence, death was most commonly

Paris, 1854, pp. 167–209. On France, see B. Bertherat, 'La mort en vitrine à la morgue à Paris au XIXe siècle (1804–1907)', in *Les narrations de la mort*, ed. R. Bertrand, A. Carol and J.-N. Pelen, Aix-en-Provence, 2005, pp. 181–95.

[9]   *Ordini e decreti per li spedali di Roma*, Rome, 1714, later reprinted in *Bullarium Clementis XI pont. max.*, Rome, 1723, pp. 599–600, my italics. Another symptom of the spreading fear of premature burial can be found in last wills and testaments. In 1694, for instance, Malpighi donated his body to his disciples to dissect but asked that they wait for two days before dissection. Analogous requests became frequent in the 1730s according to P. Chaunu, *La mort à Paris: 16e, 17e, et 18e siècles*, Paris, 1978, pp. 39–41; M.A. Visceglia, 'Corpo e sepoltura nei testamenti della nobiltà napoletana (XVI–XVIII secolo)', *Quaderni storici*, 17, 1982, pp. 583–614.

[10]   G. Catalani, *Rituale romanum Benedicti papae XIV jussu editum et auctum, perpetuis commentariis exornatum*, Padua, 1760, vol. 1, p. 384, did in fact admit that the custom was to bury the dead right after funerals within 24 hours, and even immediately if the corpse was visibly decaying.

[11]   Grmek, 'Les indicia mortis'; M.S. Pernick, 'Back from the Grave: Recurring Controversies over Defining and Diagnosing Death', in *Death: Beyond Whole-Brain Criteria*, ed. R.M. Zaner, Dordrecht, 1988, pp. 17–74. It is not by chance that the entry 'death' is missing in most sixteenth- and seventeenth-century medical dictionaries, for instance in the popular B. Castelli, *Lexicon medicum Graecolatinum ... ex Hippocrate, et Galeno desumptum*, Venice, 1607. Obviously, in the Christian West, the Aristotelian notion of soul was compounded with more or less pronounced Platonic elements that also fostered a conception of death as separation and passage.

described as the extinction of innate heat and radical moisture, up to the final moment in which the last breath was exhaled, and at the same time the immortal soul departed from the body. The popular metaphor of the lamp, comparing life to a lamp whose flame burns out the oil, was still commonly used throughout the seventeenth century.[12]

Although any natural philosopher and medical author from Aristotle onwards acknowledged death as a basic component of life (only living beings can die),[13] death did not constitute an explanatory principle, nor was it the autonomous object of scientific discourse. As we have seen in the previous chapters, sixteenth- and seventeenth-century medical writers who addressed sudden death could not solve the ambiguity of Christianised Aristotelian biology. Accordingly, they considered death at once as the departing of the rational, immortal soul from the body and a process of deprivation of innate heat, but they did not attempt to clarify the connection between these two events. In his *Mortis repentinae examen*, for instance, Paolo Grassi gave a succinct, broad definition of death in opposition to life,[14] and then endeavoured to establish whether death can ever be described as natural (a topic of much debate among ancient *auctoritates*) and how it is possible that the body is corrupted after it is deprived of heat. Grassi ruled out the question by drawing a distinction between heat, spirit and natural

---

[12]   T.S. Hall, 'Life, Death and the Radical Moisture: A Study of Thematic Patterns in Medical Theory', *Clio Medica*, 6, 1971, pp. 3–23; C. Crisciani, 'Aspetti del dibattito sull'umido radicale nella cultura del tardo medioevo (secoli XIII–XV)', *Arxiu de textos catalans antics*, 23–4, 2005, pp. 333–80. On death as privation, see R.W. Albury, 'Ideas of Life and Death', in *Companion Encyclopedia of the History of Medicine*, ed. W.F. Bynum and R. Porter, London, 1993, vol. 1, pp. 249–80.

[13]   A. Pichot, *Histoire de la notion de vie*, Paris, 1993, pp. 35–127. In Aristotelian biology the soul is the founding principle in the definition of living beings. Death, in the strict sense of the word, is a minor topic in comparison with corruption. A strong ambiguity persisted in Aristotle's distinction between natural and violent death; see D. Ross' commentary to his edition and translation of *Parva Naturalia*, Oxford, 1955; R.G. Harris, *The Heart and the Vascular System in Ancient Greek Medicine, from Alcmaeon to Galen*, Oxford, 1973, pp. 170–72; R.A.H. King, *Aristotle on Life and Death*, London, 2001, pp. 130–38. Avicenna drew a distinction between natural and accidental end of life in his *Canon*, Book I, fen 1, doc. 3, chap. 3, while addressing the *complexio* of different ages; see O. Cameron Gruner, *A Treatise on the Canon of Medicine of Avicenna Incorporating a Translation of the First Book*, London, 1930, p. 72. On later re-elaborations of Avicenna's doctrine, see N.G. Siraisi, *Avicenna in Renaissance Italy: The Canon and Medical Teaching in Italian Universities after 1500*, Princeton, 1987, pp. 315–24; C. Crisciani, L. Repici and P.B. Rossi, eds, *Vita longa. Vecchiaia e durata della vita nella tradizione medica e aristotelica ancita e medievale*, Florence, 2009.

[14]   P. Grassi, *Mortis repentinae examen ... cum brevi methodo praesagendi et praecavendi*, Modena, 1612, p. 6: 'all philosophers and physicians define natural death as the corruption of innate heat by deprivation of radical moisture. As a matter of fact, the longer that heat remains in the moisture, the longer we live.'

soul on the one side, and animal soul, which 'comes from outside and is immortal', on the other. Whereas the separation of the immortal soul amounts to death, natural heat still lingers in the corpse and corrupts it. As for Terilli, he drew on Aristotle's *Parva Naturalia* in asserting that death is 'the dissolution of the soul that was inherent to innate heat' – that is, it is the moment when the vegetative soul is deprived of heat, its prime mover. Nonetheless, he rapidly reverted to the more comfortable metaphor of the lamp and endorsed the ceasing of heartbeat as the best practical criterion for defining death.[15]

Altogether, the hylomorphism underpinning Christian scholastic philosophy and theology promoted a notion of death as passage or transit.[16] It was the transition from one condition to another, from the living to the dead body, each with its own metaphysical principle, while the immortal soul passed from this to the other world,[17] regardless of the contiguity of the two realms and the contacts that the living and the dead might still have.[18] Things changed dramatically in mechanical physiology. Although it was still necessary to accept the scholastic doctrine of the immortal soul as *forma corporis* (which was after all an article of faith since the Council of Vienne of 1311–12, and again reaffirmed in the Lateran Council of 1513), the expulsion of Galenic and scholastic inferior souls and faculties from animal economy entailed a new articulation between life and death too. Instead, ancient atomistic and other non-Aristotelian theories

---

[15] Terilli, *De causis mortis repentinae*, pp. 3–12.

[16] This was regardless of how early modern philosophers viewed the relationship of soul (or souls) and body, on which see E. Michael, 'Renaissance Theories of Body, Soul and Mind', in *Psyche and Soma: Physicians and Metaphysicians on the Mind–Body Problem from Antiquity to Enlightenment*, ed. J.P. Wright and P. Potter, Oxford, 2000, pp. 147–72.

[17] This raised serious questions on the resurrection of the flesh and individual identity at the time of Judgement, because of the difficulty in clarifying the connection between the substantial form of the living body and that of the dead body; the status of the corpse and of the separated soul remained problematic even after Benedict XII condemned the thesis on the purging souls' insensitivity in 1336, on which see C. Walker Bynum, *The Resurrection of the Body in Western Christianity, 200–1336*, New York, 1995. A particularly thorny subject in this respect was the corpse of Jesus in the sepulchre; see T. Gregory, 'Per una fenomenologia del cadavere: dai mondi dell'immaginario ai paradisi della metafisica', *Micrologus*, 7, 1999, pp. 11–42; A. Boureau, *Théologie, science et censure au XIIIe siècle: le cas de Jean Peckham*, Paris, 1999, pp. 87–136. The issue of individual identity after death in view of resurrection was made no less problematic by modern atomist and corpuscular natural philosophy; see L. Dacome, 'Resurrecting by Numbers in Eighteenth-Century England', *Past and Present*, 193, 2006, pp. 73–110.

[18] J.-C. Schimitt, *Les revenants: les vivants et les morts dans la société mediévale*, Paris, 1994; G. Zarri, 'Purgatorio "particolare" e ritorno dei morti tra Riforma e Controriforma: l'area italiana', *Quaderni Storici*, 17, 1982, pp. 466–97.

regarding death and dying were revived.[19] If life was nothing else than animal economy and motion, then death was also to be 'somatised' in the mechanisms of the body alone, and it no longer coincided with the extinction of the physical and metaphysical principles of life. Moreover, if life was but the organisation of organic aggregates in motion, death was not merely the passing from one reality to another, but rather a process of disintegration.

Lancisi's contribution to the philosophical and medical debate on death must be set in such a context. In *De subitaneis mortibus* he briefly examined the *indicia mortis* with a few considerations pertaining to forensic medicine. Although he acknowledges the difficulty of ascertaining death, he disregards it. Detecting death is only a matter of careful examination of the circulation of air and blood, as these are always necessary to life, however diminished and barely perceptible.[20] For the papal archiater, apparent death is just a false problem when set against the background of a sound knowledge of the interdependence of vital functions such as his. His doctrine, he claims, also enables the explanation of some common phenomena that may wrongly suggest residual vital activity of the corpse (like intestinal gas or male erection). In his opinion, cases of premature interment – a tragic eventuality in times of plague – are to be imputed to the negligence and ignorance of undertakers and church attendants, and doctors should raise awareness of such risks both in the government and among the population.[21]

Lancisi's speculations, however, transcended practical concerns. Drawing together ideas that were scattered throughout contemporary life sciences, he advances a definition of death as the

> true and in every way complete cessation of the movement of air, blood, and nerve fluid within and through the organs of major function, which have truly and completely lost their natural movements. And this cessation *has to be indeed so stable and constant, that there is no longer any possibility of reviving it by means of any natural power.*[22]

---

[19]   On conceptions of the relationship of soul and body in non-Aristotelian ancient philosophies, see H. von Staden, 'Body, Soul and Nerves: Epicurus, Herophilus, Erasistratus, and Galen', in *Psyche and Soma*, ed. Wright and Potter, pp. 79–118; on Lucretius's notion of death as disaggregation, see C. Segal, *Lucretius on Death and Anxiety: Poetry and Philosophy in De Rerum Natura*, Princeton, 1990.

[20]   Following Galen, sixteenth- and seventeenth-century medical writers explained apparent death by maintaining that air intake was made through perspiration instead of respiration. Lancisi rejected this idea.

[21]   SM, p. 42.

[22]   SM, p. 7, my italics. See above, Chapter 4, on the equation of life with motion, be it the motions of blood according to Harvey's doctrine re-elaborated by Willis and Hoffman within a chemical-mechanical framework, or of air, as for Mayow and Borelli.

Two distinct time frames are introduced to provide a novel account of sudden death. One encompasses the pathological process and distinguishes between the slow, underlying action of illness up until the breaking point; the other concerns death itself. Reasserting the Catholic notion of death as the moment in which the soul departs from the body, Lancisi nevertheless argues that it occurs in stages and is always preceded by symptoms, however slight. Of course, death is a precise 'point in time' but its course is a sufficiently long succession of stages to allow understanding, slowing down, and sometimes even stopping or reversing the process altogether.

Consequently, death is defined as the natural outcome of 'natural senescence and gradual disintegration' of the bodily mechanisms that are responsible for the motion of life, and the final halt of motion coincides with the soul departing and becoming a separate entity.[23] Referring to the authority of Aretaeus, Lancisi thus offers a mechanistic interpretation of death as the 'dissolution of the links of nature' between the parts, and specifically between the fibres. As I have indicated in Chapter 4, fibres had a great relevance in mechanical physiology in order to overcome the strongest aporias of Cartesian dualism and consistently materialise life and, consequently, death. The intrinsic dilatability and contractibility of fibres accounted for all those involuntary motions of organs and tissues that constitute life itself. This conceptual innovation paved the way to a new perception of partial life phenomena, like the classic problem of the excised heart still beating.

The 'decentralisation of life' would continue throughout the eighteenth and nineteenth centuries, when modern vitalist biology would reframe the whole issue of the duration of death and of the time span necessary for the destruction of an organism. Therefore, what Claudio Milanesi aptly termed 'intermediate death' and 'imperfect death'[24] would become crucial themes by the end of the eighteenth century, and undergo a more precise conceptualisation in the fields of experimental physiology and cellular biology in the following century. It then became possible to posit a substantial 'space-temporal structuration of death,

---

[23] The rational soul is described by Lancisi as 'departing' in the extreme instant, which implies that the separation of the soul coincides with death rather than causing it. The same was also true for Descartes, as underscored by Pichot, *Histoire de la notion*, pp. 348–9; M.D. Grmek, 'Les idées de Descartes sur le prolongement de la vie et le mécanisme du vieillissement', *Revue d'histoire des sciences*, 21, 1968, pp. 285–302. The causal link between the separation of the soul from the body and death was already blurred in scholastic medicine, due to the inconsistency between Aristotelian and Galenic biology and religious dogma.

[24] Milanesi, *Morte apparente*, rightly points out that in the eighteenth century medical discourse confusion between apparent and partial death subsisted. See further F. Duchesneau, *La physiologie des Lumières: empirisme, modèles et théories*, The Hague, 1982; R. Rey, 'L'anima, il corpo, il vivente', in *Storia del pensiero medico, Dal Rinascimento all'inizio dell'Ottocento*, ed. M.D. Grmek, Rome and Bari, 1996, pp. 195–257.

postulating different hierarchic levels and determining various "stages" of death';[25] this in turn led to the distinction between organic (that is, cardiac-circulatory and cerebral) death, potentially reversible, and irreversible cellular death.

In contrast, late seventeenth- and early eighteenth-century medical writers mostly spoke of *apparent* death, instead of partial death, meaning a state in which vital motions persisted in a slow or imperceptible manner. This idea maintained the distinction between reanimation and resurrection which was fundamental in view of the religious acceptance of the new medical discourse on life and death.[26] We shall return to this point. Yet, it was mechanical physicians, and particularly Lancisi, grappling with sudden death in Clement XI's Rome, who began the re-interpretation of death. Notwithstanding religious dogmas, by explaining the living being as a structured organism, mechanical medicine voided the notion of death as separation; instead, the ancient Democritean vision of death as disaggregation and complete and irreversible stasis was recovered. Accordingly, irreversibility came to be a major criterion for the definition of death in medical and lay literature.[27]

In a nutshell, a notion of death as a process was now put forward, at least in regard to functional, organic interdependence, and this was enough to alter the stance on death from a clinical standpoint. Indeed, in *De subitaneis mortibus* Lancisi argues that although death technically occurs at a precise moment, it is invariably preceded by a succession of stages during which physicians can intervene. One purpose of medical research is to learn how to predict the risk of death and delay its process with experimentally tested remedies. Since 'there is neither any cause nor any illness capable of killing with extreme swiftness, which does not bring about its effects through divisible moments in time', improved medical knowledge means that even seemingly unexpected deaths might, in future,

> be foreseen through some hidden and extraordinary symptom, and then delayed for some little while through the administration of a medicine, at least for the benefit of the soul.[28]

---

[25]   B. Fantini and M.D. Grmek, 'Le definizioni di vita e di morte nella biologia e nella medicina contemporanee', in *Bioetica*, ed. A. Di Meo and C. Mancina, Rome and Bari, 1989, p. 184.

[26]   This aspect is underscored by S. Timmermans, *Sudden Death and the Myth of CPR*, Philadelphia, 1999, pp. 31–8.

[27]   As in the entry 'Mort (médécine)' of Diderot's *Encyclopédie*, Neuchâtel edn, vol. 10, 1765, pp. 718–19, and even more clearly in the entry 'Oeconomie animale', ibid., vol. 11, 1765, pp. 360–66. Among medical authors, see F. Hoffmann, *De certo et rationali mortis in morbis praesagio* and *De generatione mortis in morbis*, in his *Opera*, Geneva, 1761, vol. 6, pp. 181–7 and 244–50.

[28]   SM, pp. 6, 13.

Since death implies the *permanent* and *final* cessation of motion, there exists a time when some kind of action can be exerted to preserve this motion or reactivate the circulatory systems before their stasis becomes irreversible. Thus, the concept of death as a process provided not only the foundation of medical knowledge of death and dying, but also a new power for physicians to act upon it.

First, Do No Harm?

The question is, to all appearances, as simple as this: if death happens in time, how far and to what extent can physicians intervene?

As is well known, an expectant attitude had been predominant in Western medicine since antiquity. In the 'Hippocratic triangle' – the sick person, the disease and the doctor – medical art was conceived as support for the sick in their fight against illness. Hence, medicine must imitate the healing powers of Nature and accompany the various stages of disease with a full awareness of its own limitations. Nothing resembling emergency medicine existed. Swift action was recommended in some circumstances and for a number of afflictions, at least in performing procedures such as purging and bleeding which could predispose the body either to a natural reaction or to further treatment. However, far more numerous were the cases (including surgical ones) for which a maximum of caution was prescribed, following Hippocrates, since a rash or ill-timed intervention might worsen the patient's conditions and even have lethal consequences.[29]

Of course, within the general tendency outlined above, there were instances of a more energetic attitude, and even testimonies of emergency medicine *avant-la-lettre*, both in texts of learned medicine and in 'popular' medicine aimed at a lay readership.[30] But even when a swift intervention might be deemed advisable, what course should be taken? Could or should any medicinal or surgical remedy

---

[29] H. von Staden, 'Incurability and Hopelessness: The "Hippocratic corpus"', in *La maladie et les malades dans la Collection hippocratique: actes du VIe Colloque international Hippocratique*, Québec, 1990, pp. 75–112. On the notion of 'due time' in Hippocratic medicine, see E. Garcia Novo, 'L'urgence de l'intervention théraupetique', in *Aspetti della terapia nel Corpus Hippocraticum: atti del IX Colloque intérnational Hippocratique*, ed. I. Garofalo et al., Florence, 1999, pp. 75–88.

[30] Ranchin, *De morbis*; R. Hawes, *The Poore-Mans Plaster-Box: Furnished with Diverse Excellent Remedies for Sudden Mischances ... Directions, Whereby a Man May Know by What Means a Person, Being Found Dead, came by his Death*, London, 1634; J. Pechey, *A Plain and Short Treatise of an Apoplexy, Convulsions ... and Several Other Violent Diseases that Come of a Sudden ... Shewing the Sick or By-Standers What Ought Presently to be Done*, London, 1698; J. Pechey, *Of Sudden Diseases*, London, 1714; see also G. Norman, '"Helps for Suddain Accidents": Stephen Bradwell and the Origin of the First Aid Guide', *Bulletin of the History of Medicine*, 67, 1993, pp. 51–73.

be applied, even those unheard of in previous practice? Should an all-out attempt be made in desperate cases?

Answers to these questions tended to be overwhelmingly negative. Still following Hippocrates, there was general agreement on the inappropriateness of undertaking treatment for cases that were considered incurable, although it was generally accepted that doctors should not deny patients what we would now call palliative care.[31] While religious literature strove to promote acceptance of sickness and death (though at the same time health and life were considered a gift of God to preserve),[32] medical deontology was nearly unanimous in underscoring the limits of the healing art. Following the great ancient masters, medical authors subscribed to the restricted scope of their action and rejected the possibility of subjecting the incurable or terminal patient to therapeutic experiments indefinitely.

In fact, the Hippocratic Oath forbade doctors from administering poisonous drugs to accelerate the patient's death, a practice that was probably commonplace in antiquity.[33] In addition to the Oath (which at any rate did not have the prescriptive character it would acquire in the nineteenth century)[34] and other deontological texts (like *Decorum* and *The Law*), many other *loci*

---

[31]   D.W. Amundsen, 'The Physician's Obligation to Prolong Life: A Medical Duty without Classical Roots', *Hastings Center Report*, 8, 1978, 4, pp. 23–30; J. Jouanna, *Hippocrate*, Paris, 1992, pp. 153–9. In the Hippocratic Corpus there are several passages in favour of treating the incurable, as discussed in R. Wittern, *Grenzen der Helkunst: eine historische Betrachtung*, Stuttgart, 1982; von Staden, 'Incurability and Hopelessness'. Treating incurable patients was a professional dilemma for early modern physicians, on which see M. Stolberg, *Die Geschichte der Palliativmedizin: medizinische Sterbebegleitung von 1500 bis heute*, Frankfurt, 2011, pp. 57–72.

[32]   Inducing acceptance of sickness and death was the priest's duty, according to the *Rituale romanun Pauli V P.M. iussu editum*, Rome, 1614, p. 84, and yet refusing medical care was sinful according to the canon law expert T. Azzio, *Tractatus novus legalis de infirmitate, eiusque priuilegijs, et effectibus*, Venice, 1603, pp. 92–3, and the theologian O. de Bonis, *Arte teorica e pratica per aiutare nello spirito gl'infermi*, 2nd edn, Rome, 1686, p. 17. It must be made clear that awareness of the limits of the medical art did not mean that dying patients were not given any cure, although this was obviously in proportion to the families' financial situation, as shown for seventeenth-century England by I. Mortimer, *The Dying and the Doctors: The Medical Revolution in Seventeenth-Century England*, Woodbridge, 2009.

[33]   L. Edelstein, 'The Professional Ethics of the Greek Physician', *Bulletin of the History of Medicine*, 30, 1956, pp. 391–419; D. Gourevitch, 'Suicide Among the Sick in Classical Antiquity', *Bulletin of the History of Medicine*, 43, 1969, pp. 501–18; P. Carrick, *Medical Ethics in Antiquity: Philosophical Perspectives on Abortion and Euthanasia*, Dordrecht, 1985.

[34]   V. Nutton, 'Beyond the Hippocratic Oath', in *Doctors and Ethics: The Earlier Historical Setting of Professional Ethics*, ed. A. Wear, J. Geyer-Kordesch and R. French, Amsterdam, 1993, pp. 10–37; V. Nutton, 'Hippocratic Morality and Modern Medicine', in *Médecine et morale dans l'Antiquité*, ed. H. Flashar and J. Jouanna, Geneva, 1997, pp. 31–56.

in the Hippocratic Corpus reiterated the basic precept of the doctor–patient relationship, namely avoiding harm to the patient, as stated in the celebrated passage in *Epidemics* I,11: 'The physician must ... have two special objects in view with regard to disease, namely, to do good and to do no harm.'

In practice, the 'no harm' principle was translated into a refusal of violent treatment, futile care and experimental therapies, even in the most hopeless cases. The vast majority of medical authors were in agreement over these points, however wide their theoretical and confessional differences might be. A Catholic physician attending a Counter-Reformation cardinal like Vincenzo Carrari, for instance, exhorted his readers never to be *audax vel temerarius* in applying treatment; only if light drugs proved ineffectual might energetic and painful remedies be used, but without ever resorting to experimentation.[35] In pretty much the same vein, the celebrated Sephardic physician in Hamburg Rodrigo da Castro emphasised that the art of medicine must merely help Nature, and that a practitioner should never stray from traditional therapeutics dictated by the established medical canon.[36]

Medical authors were corroborated in their prudent orientation by jurists. Failure to conform to the customary rules of the medical art could have legal consequences for practitioners. Several distinguished commentators on medical legal matters substantiated this interpretation. In the chapters *de medicorum erroribus* of his *Quaestiones medico-legales*, Paolo Zacchia not only reasserted the prohibition of precipitating death with poisonous drugs or excessive bloodletting, but also recommended extreme caution in any other treatment. Zacchia equally forbade the use of all experimental or violent remedies, as well as life-endangering surgeries even for incurable or lethal diseases; in such cases, physicians must only treat the most severe symptoms. He drew even more stringent restrictions, within their respective fields, for surgeons and apothecaries.[37]

Obviously, all of the foregoing does not mean that an expectant attitude would be adopted by doctors with all patients and at all times. But it undoubtedly discouraged therapeutic audacity and hazardous attempts, even in cases with a

---

[35]   V. Carrari, *De medico et illius erga aegros officio opusculum*, Ravenna, 1581, pp. 155–78. In truth, ordinary cures were painful and violent *per se*, the reason why Galenic medicine was criticised by non-academic practitioners; see A. Wear, 'Medical Ethics in Early Modern England', in *Doctors and Ethics*, ed. Wear, Geyer-Kordesch and French, pp. 98–130.

[36]   R. da Castro, *Medicus politicus, sive de officiis medico-politicis tractatus*, Hamburg, 1614, pp. 97–100.

[37]   Zacchia, *Quaestiones*, pp. 408–26, on whom see H. Karplus, 'Medical Ethics in Paolo Zacchia's "Quaestiones Medico-Legales"', in *International Symposium on Society, Medicine and Law*, ed. H. Karplus, Amsterdam, 1973, pp. 125–34; A. Marchisello, '"Culpa habet sociam peonam": la responsabilità del medico nelle Quaestiones medico-legales di Paolo Zacchia', in *Paolo Zacchia: alle origini della medicina legale, 1584–1659*, ed. A. Pastore and P. Rossi, Milan, 2008, pp. 221–48.

foregone conclusion. A patient and his relatives could take a doctor to court with the accusation of having administered unorthodox treatment. The toxicity of some 'violent' drugs such as antimony[38] was a recurrent theme in early modern medical controversies throughout Europe, and one that gave rise to trials, indictments and prohibitions. To put it in the crude words of polemical writing, the good 'Roman Catholic physician' should seek first and foremost to avoid inflicting death at his hands, and those who did not observe this principle were but 'empirics and charlatans'.[39]

Because of the obvious danger of surgery, such an obligation was spelled out with greater clarity in surgical texts. Here advisable caution became a categorical precept, if only because a mistake during surgery would be immediately visible to everyone and impossible to attribute to the hidden morbid operations of the body. Not by chance, concerns of reputation – that is, how to avoid putting one's reputation at risk by engaging in desperate cures – were already thoroughly examined in Hippocratic surgical texts such as *De fracturis*, which almost invariably urged circumspection and renunciation. It could be added, incidentally, that medical reticence about precarious treatment was possibly increased by the Counter-Reformation condemnation of magic. Medieval medicine had been fascinated by the possibility of prolonging life.[40] Late sixteenth-century Catholic doctors, in contrast, were compelled to declare explicitly that the end could not be delayed in any possible way. The doctor's duty merely consisted in procrastinating and watchfully monitoring his patients' senescence until they reached their natural demise in such a way as to match the Christian ideal of the good death.[41]

Early modern physicians' fundamental attitude towards the sick and the dying also applied to those swift, unexpected maladies that led to rapid death. Following Hippocrates and Galen, apoplexy was universally considered one such desperate condition, and commonly ranked among those not to be treated, since chances for recovery were extremely slim.[42] As Hippocrates recommended,

---

[38]   R.I. McCallum, *Antimony in Medical History: An Account of the Medical Uses of Antimony and Its Compounds since Early Times to the Present*, Edinburgh, 1999. On the contracts passed between treating physicians and patients, see G. Pomata, *Contracting a Cure: Patients, Healers, and the Law in Early Modern Bologna*, Baltimore, 1998.

[39]   *Risposta apologetica per sincerare la verità di tutto quello, che si ritrovò nell'apertura del cadavere di un gran personaggio in Roma*, Venice [but Rome], 1684, p. 14.

[40]   G.J. Gruman, *A History of Ideas About the Prolongation of Life: The Evolution of Prolongevity Hypotheses to 1800*, Philadelphia, 1966; Crisciani, 'Aspetti del dibattito sull'umido radicale', pp. 357–76; C. Crisciani, ed., *Alchimia e medicina nel Medioevo*, Florence, 2003.

[41]   Grassi, *Mortis repentinae examen*, p. 18; Azzio, *Tractatus novus legalis*, p. 96.

[42]   Incurable disease included innate affections such as blindness, deafness, congenital humpback and elephantiasis, and acquired pathologies such as cancer; see Castro, *Medicus*

incurable patients should not be subjected to useless efforts, and many experts believed that this was the case with both apoplexy and syncope, and that even traditional Graeco-Roman and Arabic surgical methods were to be avoided, for instance the application of cauteries, meant to reactivate vital and animal spirits, to different parts of the body. In the seventeenth century the application of red-hot irons was indeed commonly criticised and rejected. Fierce debates were also sparked by another fashionable burning remedy, the scarifying cupping glasses which several medical authors considered appropriate to drain humours and revive animal spirits in apoplexy or at least to inflict enough acute pain on the patient to prevent him or her from slipping into a coma.[43]

In other words, right up to the early eighteenth century Christian physicians (regardless of whether they belonged to the Roman Catholic Church or Reformed confessions) did not attempt to prolong life or precipitate death, did not interfere with death and always abstained from any drug *mortem vel retardantibus, vel accelerantibus* (accelerating or retarding death), any drug which, like opium, 'can open the door from which life escapes'.[44]

The 'epidemics' of sudden deaths in the Rome of Clement XI appears to be a turning point also with regard to medical treatment for the dying. At the very least it fostered the emergence of a significantly more interventionist approach, to the extent that action was now always urged in an attempt to resuscitate those unfortunate persons struck by violent, sudden ailments, including extremely serious ones.

In fact, a reaction against hasty and defeatist diagnosis of foetal death and death of premature infants had already emerged in Catholic theology and medicine at the end of the seventeenth century.[45] We shall go back to this significant topic in the next chapters, as it is partly related to the resuscitation

---

politicus, pp. 175–6.

[43] Ranchin, *De morbis*, p. 599; D. Panaroli, *Iatrologismorum, seu medicinalium observationum Pentecostae quinque*, Rome, 1652, pp. 265–6; G. Piccini, *Antipyrapoplepathia siue de cauteriorum abusu in apoplexia*, Spoleto, 1668. Cauteries were in contrast recommended for apoplectics in F. Bacon, *Historia vitae et mortis*, London, 1623, p. 162.

[44] E.G. Struve, *Dissertatione solenni mortis theoriam medicam ... sub praesidio D.N. Georgii Ernesti Stahlii*, Halle, 1702, pp. 37–40. On the means commonly used by laypersons to end agony, see M. Stolberg, 'Active Euthanasia in Pre-Modern Society, 1500–1800: Learned Debates and Popular Practices', *Social History of Medicine*, 20, 2007, pp. 205–21.

[45] A few theologians and obstetricians had in fact already suggested drastic remedies like caesarean section in difficult childbirths in order to administer baptism to the endangered infant and save his or her soul, such as the Jesuit T. Raynaud, *De ortu infantium contra naturam per sectionem caesaream, tractatio qua reliqui item conscientiae nodi ad matrem alvo gerentem*, Lyon, 1637, and the surgeon P. Peu, *La pratique des accouchemens*, Paris, 1694, p. 334. See N. Filippini, *La nascita straordinaria: tra madre e figlio la rivoluzione del taglio cesareo*, Milan, 1995.

of the dying. As for interventionism in relation to the dying, once again Lancisi was among the earliest and most explicit voices in this debate.

In Chapters XII and XIII of *De subitaneis mortibus*, the pope's physician addressed the problem of sudden death from a prognostic standpoint, classifying diseases as curable and incurable. The latter included sudden rupture of large vessels or aneurysms, and severe haemorrhage or apoplexy affecting the elderly, whose tissues were no longer able to recover sufficient elasticity. Yet Lancisi urged physicians never to underestimate chances for survival and to intervene in any case. Sometimes, he argues, asphyxiated, strangulated or apoplectic persons deemed lost, and even those pronounced dead, can return to life spontaneously or with the assistance of the medical art. Especially in cases of apoplexy and hysteria, 'a wise physician ... should rarely be so abjectly helpless that he is without hope'.[46]

Lancisi praised the ancient philosophers' ideal of the good death, painting an idyllic picture of the perfectly serene demise of Socrates, who had waited patiently for his end surrounded by friends and disciples. In this respect, he prefigured a new Enlightenment sensibility towards death. But he soon re-assumed the mantle of the Catholic physician. Christians cannot abstract the moment of death from the destiny of afterlife, and no consideration whatsoever regarding a dignified departure should prevail over salvation. This is why the faithful should beg God to spare them from unexpected death, and at the same time physicians must do anything in their power to gain time.[47] The main reason for such interventionism is expressly linked to the temporal duration of death. For no condition, however serious, be it syncope or the most violent apoplexy,

> no matter how fast they are usually wont to kill, has there ever been found an instance where some moments of time do not elapse before we come to that particular moment in which that *absolute fixedness* of fluids and solids sets in, which, after the departure of the soul, we call death.[48]

In Lancisi's view, this should encourage physicians to try out any available means. They must quickly decide on a course of action, and play their cards without fearing for their professional reputation.

Admittedly, the Hippocratic-Galenic medical tradition had already acknowledged the eventuality of apparent death and spoken of corpses with residual signs of life. Life, however, could never be recovered, since according to Aristotle it was possible to pass from possession to privation, but not the opposite. Instead, with the mechanisation of life and the circulatory physiology

---

[46]   SM, p. 37.

[47]   SM, p. 68.

[48]   SM, p. 11, my italics.

of modern mechanical medicine, the stress was laid on the resumption of motion and the reanimation of 'suspended' life. Since sudden death is induced only by that which

> most quickly, persistently, and severely harms the fluids or solids already mentioned, or deprives them of their alternate movements so that these movements cannot be restored by any means of art or nature[49]

then, sooner or later, medicine will find a way to avert, procrastinate and slow down death. Accordingly, the use of drastic methods, such as applying hot irons to the skull or feet of the agonising person, was recommended as a means of inducing 'maximum stimulation' to the nerves.[50] When they succeeded in snatching a patient from the clutches of death, especially those who had been given up as dead, physicians were acting almost like gods.[51]

From the notion of death as a process, therefore, Lancisi inferred an obligation for physicians to always intervene and try to impede that process. Other medical writers in the Roman debate on sudden death insisted on this point. Domenico Mistichelli, in particular, claimed to have written his *Trattato dell'apoplessia* in Italian 'so that anyone who is not a doctor can learn to be one, in order to help his fellow men in such circumstances'.[52] Mistichelli was the most confident advocate of resuscitation by means of red-hot irons applied to the soles of patients' feet, and explained the rationale of this treatment on the basis of his general neurological theory. If motion is communicated *partem per partem* through the nerves, to and from their peripheral terminations – that is, from the feet up to the meninges and vice versa – then cauteries do have a beneficial stimulating effect on the brain and the heart. When compared with the chance of resuscitating patients seized by apoplexy, burns on the feet are an insignificant secondary effect, and it is

> a mistake born of imprudent fearfulness, deserving of condemnation on the part of Hippocrates, that the majority of men care more to see people dying in desperation without remedy than to see an operation administered that in spite of all its apparent atrociousness is extremely beneficial.[53]

---

[49] SM p. 12.

[50] SM, p. 109. In one case, an old woman struck with apoplexy in 1705, Lancisi described the 'immediate application' of scarifying cups, cauteries, blistering remedies and spirits of ammonia, which allowed her to regain consciousness and undergo further treatment the next day.

[51] SM p. 37.

[52] D. Mistichelli, *Trattato dell'apoplessia*, Rome, 1709, 'Proemio'.

[53] Ibid., p. 171.

To prove the benefits of cauteries, in the appendix of his treatise Mistichelli reports the case of a man received in desperate condition in the hospital of Fatebenefratelli. Although the cure eventually proved ineffectual, the patient was at least momentarily awakened through cauterisation, which 'liberated [his] capacities and made this sick man capable of receiving Holy Sacraments, and able to put his temporal and spiritual affairs in order'.[54]

Hence, mechanical philosophy offered not only an explanatory key for sudden death but a therapeutic strategy as well. Moreover, the unprecedented emphasis on the duration of death recast the issue of medical intervention. The clarification of the process of sudden death in time and the mechanistic understanding of the body provided the rationale for a rapid and energetic treatment. Although these were eventually limited to red-hot irons or the evergreen phlebotomy, and no clear indication of when it was best to intervene was given, the change in attitude paved the way for subsequent, more sophisticated resuscitation techniques. Moreover, the same arguments also induced moderate optimism. If it was true that unexpected deaths were always preceded by hidden morbid conditions, efforts could reasonably be made to slow these down, even though they eventually proved incurable and lethal.

Some historians and historians of medicine divide eighteenth-century doctors into 'fence-sitters' and interventionists with respect to illness and death. It is a distinction that correctly applies only to the famous debate initiated in the mid-eighteenth century, and which continued for over a century, about the uncertainty of the signs of death. With regard to the end of life, by contrast, Enlightenment physicians were on the whole more interventionist than their predecessors, and this included the prime advocate of an expectant attitude in the *querelle* over death diagnosis, the French physician Jacques-Jean Bruhier. In his extremely popular *Dissertation sur l'incertitude des signes de la mort*, Bruhier analysed the available resuscitation techniques and concluded his overview, plagiarising Lancisi, by writing that when resuscitation is successful 'one may say in truth that doctors raise the dead'.[55] Jean-Jacques Menuret de Chambaud concluded the entry 'Mort (médécine)' in volume X of Diderot and d'Alembert's

---

[54]   Ibid., p. 169.

[55]   [J.J. Bruhier], *Dissertation sur l'incertitude des signes de la mort, et l'abus des enterremens, et embaumemens precipités*, vol. 2, Paris, 1745, p. 466. The first volume of Bruhier's work was but the translation of Danish-born anatomist J.-B. Winslow's *Quaestio medico-chirurgica ... An mortis incertae signa minus incerta a chirurgicis, quam ab aliis experimentis?*, Paris, 1740, which was in fact nothing other than a synthesis of the medico-legal section of Lancisis's *De subitaneis mortibus*. It is worth noting that Winslow had previously addressed the very 'Roman' topic of the brain meninges' role in animal economy in his early *An cordis motus a dura meninge?*, Paris, 1703. See also P. Dionis, *Dissertation sur la mort subite et sur la catalepsie*, Paris, 1710; J.S. Möller, *Dissertatio ... in qua mortis subitaneae non vulgaris causas et remedia*, Wittenberg, 1723.

Encyclopédie (1765) with an identical sentence. Chambaud was indeed critical of ruthless, useless medical treatment, but nevertheless recommended trying all possible remedies (including violent ones) against sudden death, in the hope of reactivating vital motion.[56] In the course of the eighteenth century, several new techniques and tools appeared that were presumed to save drowned, asphyxiated persons and those seized by apoplexy, and assistance for resuscitation was organised in several European cities. However, the synergy of conceptual and institutional factors necessary for the birth of proper emergency medicine would not occur for another two centuries.[57]

With respect to medical resuscitation, some historians have argued that the eighteenth- and nineteenth-century widespread phobia of premature burial was the price that medicine paid for medicalising death, and that the fear was in proportion to the hope of reanimation that medicine now claimed to be able to offer.[58] Other scholars have played down the impact of early emergency medicine, arguing that the eighteenth-century medicalisation of dying was rather induced by a new, non-religious ideal of painless death, in which the dying person was to be relieved from suffering by virtue of the doctor's assistance and the use of opium.[59] Recent studies have also underscored the discrepancy between medical discourse on resuscitation, with its attendant social and technological organisation, and the actual rate of success of cardio-pulmonary resuscitation (CPR) – a discrepancy that they nonetheless consider an additional proof of the medical profession's primacy in the management of death.[60]

These three interpretations are more complementary than it would seem. True, it would be incorrect to assume that the new eighteenth-century medical interventionism became a generally shared approach. Although medicine had just begun to take into consideration the possibility of interrupting the destruction of a dying organism, the dominant orientation was still one of waiting and not intruding on death. Suggestions to refrain from futile care abounded in deontological literature up until the twentieth century. Nonetheless, in the

---

[56]   'Mort (médécine)', in *Encyclopédie*, Neuchâtel edn, vol. 10, 1765, pp. 718–19.

[57]   A. Larcan and P. Brullard, 'Remarques concernant la prévention, la notion d'urgence et l'organisation des secours au XVIIIe siècle', *Histoire des sciences medicales*, 13, 1979, pp. 271–8; M. Nurok, 'Elements of the Medical Emergency's Epistemological Alignment: Eighteenth–Twentieth-Century Perspectives', *Social Studies of Science*, 33, 2003, pp. 563–79; M. Goulon et al., *La réanimation: naissance et développement d'un concept*, Paris, 2004.

[58]   Pernick, 'Back from the Grave'; M. Alexander, 'The Rigid Embrace of the Narrow House: Premature Burial and the Signs of Death', *Hastings Center Report*, 10, 3, 1980, pp. 25–31. I. Illich, *Medical Nemesis: The Expropriation of Health*, London, 1975, includes this argument in his criticism of the modern medicalisation of life.

[59]   D. Porter and R. Porter, *Patient's Progress: Doctors and Doctoring in Eighteenth-Century England*, Oxford, 1989, pp. 47–8.

[60]   Timmermans, *Sudden Death and the Myth*.

event of an especially dreaded demise such as sudden death, medical approaches did begin to change. And such change can be traced back to early eighteenth-century Rome and to Lancisi's work. This is where the long history of (the hope of) resuscitation started.

Above all, I wish to emphasise the religious roots of this shift in sensibility towards death, which historiography has generally interpreted in terms of secularisation. The opposition between the assumedly traditional, Christian, resigned acceptance of death, and a novel Enlightenment activism, which supposedly was the symptom of a new secular passion for life, seems to me rather misleading. Lancisi and his Roman colleagues shared a clear objective indeed: to gain enough time to administer the sacraments or to allow for sincere contrition. As Mistichelli wrote,

> If ever these [red-hot irons] only brought us back to life for a few moments, if they made us return only to pronounce Domine miserere mei, if they awakened us to a simple act of inner contrition, then theirs would be a great fire, and a supreme remedy.[61]

They thus extended to death religious considerations that had originally emerged with regard to birth, in the first debates on caesarean delivery and the christening of foetuses.

It must be added that the religious connotation of medical interventionism in respect of the dying would become truly evident much later. In the nineteenth century, it actually marked the dividing line between Catholic and agnostic or atheistic doctors in their attitudes towards extraordinary lifesaving techniques. The latter would be accused of professional laxism by the former, bent on extolling the sanctifying value of pain and the virtues of medical resuscitation for the sake of the salvation of the soul. Catholic practitioners thus became the most fervent users of all kinds of chemical and surgical interventions at the end of life, and were supported in this by those theologians who regarded the scientific notion of imperfect death as a sacramental opportunity.[62] Lay physicians, in contrast,

---

[61]   Mistichelli, *Trattato dell'apoplessia*, p. 172.

[62]   The chief supporter of administering sacraments to manifestly deceased persons on grounds of the duration of death before definite cellular death was the Spanish Jesuit J.B. Ferreres, *La mort réelle et la mort apparente et leurs rapports avec l'administration des sacrements*, Paris, 1905; conversely, an orthodox Thomist like A. Michel, in his article 'Mort', in *Dictionnaire de théologie catholique*, vol. 10, 2, Paris, [1911] 1929, cols 2486–500, refuted the administration of sacraments to persons in a state of 'intermediate death', arguing that although the vegetative soul enabled residual bodily functions, after the departure of the rational soul they no longer enjoyed the status of individuals; he conceded sacraments only to cases of 'apparent death' following sudden attacks when vital functions could be presumably reactivated. See also C.A. Defanti, *Soglie: medicina e fine della vita*, Turin, 2007, pp. 77–9.

tended to favour a 'philosophical' acceptance of natural death and, following the Enlightenment ideal of the painless good death, did not spare sedation, sometimes leading to surreptitious forms of euthanasia.[63]

Salutary Truth or Merciful Lie? Ethics and Etiquette towards the Dying

Let us return to the early eighteenth century. The thorny issue of the physician's duties towards the dying was not limited to emergencies. And surely, in respect to ordinary practice, despite the emergence of an interventionist attitude aimed at averting unexpected death and similar accidents, the traditional expectant attitude towards the dying was an enduring one. A celebrated physician and outspoken proponent of mechanical medicine like Friedrich Hoffmann (who was a Lutheran, but who may be considered Lancisi's counterpart in respect of his institutional position, philosophical tenets and medical ideas) asserted in his *Medicus politicus* that a physician was not meant to treat everything, and when faced with 'the most serious afflictions, the physician must not despair nor desist from treatment, but nevertheless always act cautiously and heed the counsel of other colleagues'.[64] He furthermore suggested prescribing so-called 'heroic' medicines (heroic because of the pain they caused) with extreme caution, to avoid visiting sick patients during such strong treatments and finally, with a fair dose of realism, to 'always form a circumspect prognosis in malignant and acute diseases'.[65]

As pointed out in Hoffmann's dry compendium, death posed a number of extremely sensitive deontological questions: how should the doctor introduce the eventuality of a swift passing, when he deemed it probable because of the patient's underlying pathological conditions or lifestyle? When and to whom should a fatal prognosis be disclosed?

Caution was undeniably the key word in this respect too. Of course, no doctor would hesitate to warn in general terms of the risks arising from excessive indulgence in food, drink and sex. Dangerous from a medical viewpoint and sinful from a religious one, such vices could potentially lead to a departure so abrupt as to allow no time for a medic or a priest to be summoned. But announcing an actually impending death to a particular patient was a completely different story.

---

[63]   A. Carol, *Les médecins et la mort: XIXe–XXe siècles*, Paris, 2004.

[64]   F. Hoffmann, *Medicus politicus sive regulæ prudentiæ secundum quas medicus juvenis studia sua et vitæ rationem dirigere debet*, Leiden, 1738, pp. 181–4, discussed in J. Geyer-Kordesh, 'Ethics in the Eighteenth Century: Hoffmann in Halle', in *Doctors and Ethics*, ed. Wear, Geyer-Kordesch and French, pp. 153–80.

[65]   Hoffmann, *Medicus politicus*, pp. 220–34.

Since the Fourth Lateran Council of 1215, it was the precise duty of any Christian treating physician to ensure that the patient took confession, regardless of the kind and degree of his or her infirmity. Physicians should not worry that calling for a priest at the sickbed could be interpreted as an indication of imminent death. Moreover, they should not hesitate to reveal a negative prognosis. This was the opinion of several writers on medical ethics, especially during the heyday of the Counter-Reformation in the late sixteenth century. Probably the most pious and rigorous among Italian medical moralists, Giovan Battista Codronchi, a physician from Imola in Central Italy, was adamant on this point: the end does not justify the means. Hence, optimism might very well be beneficial to healing, and yet this was no excuse for not calling the priest, since the sick patient needed to be aware of the time he or she had left and put it to good use. Consequently,

> We must not heed Galen who, being a pagan, urges audacity and daring when he says that the physician must always promise recovery, though he be despairing as to the health of the sick.[66]

Thirty years later, this same precept was reiterated by a Portuguese physician practising in Rome, Gabriel Fonseca.[67] Severe ailments commonly reputed to have a rapid adverse course, like apoplexy, epilepsy and syncope, obviously commanded greater urgency. Scipione Mercurio (who had in fact been a monk before graduating in medicine) enumerated such circumstances and added that family members erred and sinned when they hastened to reassure their sick loved one, even when he or she was suffering from 'a most serious accident, or vehement fever, or dizziness, or sudden fatigue without previous cause, or unusual fainting' (that is, all the prodromal signs of an impending abrupt death).[68]

Yet, exceptions and limitations to this medical orthodoxy were commonplace. First, innumerable passages in the writings of the *auctoritates* could be relied upon to justify discretion. Neither Hippocratic nor Galenic writers questioned the physician's obligation to disclose prognosis as quickly as possible, in order not to create false expectations (which, moreover, could harm the physician's reputation), and yet listed many reasons for procrastinating. In his *Commentary on the Epidemics* of Hippocrates, for instance, Galen maintained that the treating physician had to be fully aware of the patient's personality before revealing anything, and always watch not to grieve the sick person with bad news,

---

[66]   G.B. Codronchi, *De christiana ac tuta medendi ratione*, Ferrara, 1591, pp. 57–9.

[67]   G. Fonseca, *Medici oeconomia: in quae ad perfecti medici munus attinent brevibus explanantur*, Rome, 1623, pp. 91–7.

[68]   S. Mercurio, *Degli errori popolari d'Italia*, Venice, 1603, fols 129r–v and 124r–126v.

thus aggravating his or her condition. Galen's injunction enjoyed enormous popularity in medieval and early modern medical literature.[69]

Second and most importantly, prognosticating death with any accuracy was inherently difficult. By common consensus, there were only a few reliable *signa mortifera*, such as the peculiar changes in the face described by Hippocrates' *The Book of Prognostics* (the so-called *facies hippocratica*). A physician was better able to recognise the signs of recovery than those of death – so the medieval experts claimed. A wrong prognosis of death was more shameful than failing to cure. In point of fact, some medical authors argued the opposite: it would be better to exhibit pessimism and then to take full credit in case of the patient's recovery. At any rate, it was in no one's interest to speak too much, too soon or too confidently.[70]

Even among the pious Counter-Reformation physicians, therefore, a call for moderation was not wanting. For instance, Vincenzo Carrari reminded physicians of their obligation to ensure confession for their sick patients and warned them not to play down the seriousness of illness just to delay calling the priest. But at the same time Carrari also recalled that, according to many canonists, doctors were required to treat any ill person, including the unrepentant.[71] The majority of authors in medical deontology proved even more reticent than Carrari, and variously motivated prudence in prognostication, if not actual ambiguity, on the basis of theoretical reasoning (that is, the difficulty of detecting any unmistakable sign of imminent death) and moral justification (that is, compassion towards the sufferer), along with more prosaic considerations pertaining to their professional status. Another early seventeenth-century Italian doctor, Giovanni Colle, perfectly summed up this detached approach when he advised his fellow physicians to always show an imperturbable face and offer hope to the sick and his or her friends and family, but 'from time to time, to defend oneself from slander, also declare that the illness is serious and in need of the utmost care'.[72] The Milanese physician Giovan Battista Selvatico even permitted some small lies if the treating doctor was not able to decipher the patient's malady right away.[73]

---

[69]   J. Jouanna, 'La lecture de l'éthique hippocratique chez Galien', in *Médecine et morale*, ed. Flashar and Jouanna, pp. 211–53, insists on the shift in meaning from Hippocrates' medical notion of prognostic caution (that is, avoiding wrong prognostics) to Galen's moral notion (not lying). See also A. D'Alessandro, 'La morte nella medicina greca e romana', in *Storia della definizione di morte*, ed. F.P. de Ceglia, Milan, 2014, pp. 97–122.

[70]   M.R. McVaugh, 'Bedside Manners in the Middle Ages', *Bulletin of the History of Medicine*, 71, 1997, pp. 201–23; D. Jacquart, 'Le difficile pronostic de mort (XIVe–XVe siècles)', *Médiévales*, 46, 2004, pp. 11–22.

[71]   Carrari, *De medico*, pp. 157–63.

[72]   G. Colle, *Cosmitor medicaeus triplex, in quo … consultationes medicinales et quaestiones practicae enucleatae proponuntur*, Venice, 1621, p. 29.

[73]   G.B. Silvatico, *Controversiae medicae numero centum*, Milan, 1601, pp. 132–5.

Generally, most authors sided with their fellow practitioners and verged on cynicism in advising caution. According to Rodrigo da Castro, patients are naturally suspicious and pusillanimous, and hence physicians must use utmost circumspection in making predictions. Indeed, in order to avoid the shame of error, they should be no less than 'ambiguous' in their prognosis unless there are unquestionable and infallible signs of death. Of course, it is always good practice to discreetly suggest that the patient make his or her last will and put temporal affairs in order.[74]

A few Catholic writers attacked da Castro, as did the Genoese and former Jesuit Girolamo Bardi in his *Medicus politico-catholicus* summarising canonical law enforcements,[75] but others substantially agreed with him. A Roman Catholic physician teaching and practising in Rome, like Pietro Castelli for instance, taught his students that the surest way to take full credit for patients' recovery and avoid the stigma of failure was to always claim that the affection was critical and difficult to treat. If the patient's condition deteriorated, the wise doctor was to send only an assistant to ask for news; and should the patient be already dead, the assistant should be instructed to say that he merely wished to ascertain the precise time of death. Arnold of Villanova had made the same suggestion four centuries earlier.[76]

Writing from the heart of Roman Catholicism, with the authority that his position as papal protomedicus bestowed upon him, Paolo Zacchia advocated detachment too with his usual equitable predisposition. On the one hand, physicians must abide by their obligation to persuade patients to confess and receive the last communion, but, on the other hand, they should refrain from issuing an overly pessimistic prognosis except in response to explicit and insistent requests, or when it was not otherwise possible to 'avoid a great scandal', namely with notorious sinners to whom the Church could later refuse burial in consecrated land. Of course, the good doctor must avoid excessive optimism too, lest he distract a patient from seeking spiritual health. Yet, it was not up to him, but to relatives, friends and priest, to give the sick any bad news. Ultimately, however, doctors could not abandon their patients if they refused confession.[77]

At the beginning of the eighteenth century, therefore, the medical profession was still divided in regard to deathbed ethics and etiquette, but

---

[74]   Castro, *Medicus politicus*, pp. 126–33.

[75]   G. Bardi, *Medicus politico catholicus seu Medicinae sacrae tum cognoscendae, tum faciundae idea*, Genoa, 1643, pp. 238–40 and 340.

[76]   P. Castelli, *De visitatione aegrotantium: pro suis auditoribus et discipulis ad praxim instrunedis* (1630), which I am quoting from W. Schleiner, *Medical Ethics in the Renaissance*, Washington, DC, 1995, pp. 47–8. Castelli drew on Arnold of Villanova's *De cautelis medicorum*, discussed in J. Ziegler, *Medicine and Religion c. 1300: The Case of Arnau de Vilanova*, Oxford, 1998, pp. 250–58.

[77]   Zacchia, *Quaestiones*, p. 403.

generally inclined to silence. As for Lancisi, while advocating intervention at all costs for the salvation of the soul if not of the body, he was far less prompt in regard to telling the truth to patients. Prognostication was indeed a complex matter. Following Hippocrates and Galen rather than Counter-Reformation theologians, Lancisi maintained that patients should be left in the dark about most things, and the 'disgrace' of erroneous prognostics be avoided.[78] A few years later, his successor at the Roman Protomedicate, Domenico Gagliardi, wrote in his *Idea del vero medico* (*Ideal of the true physician*) that although lying was bad, it was nevertheless advisable to remain vague.[79] On one thing Gagliardi was adamant, though: treating doctors must never wait for the supposedly right planetary conjunctions before administering treatment. Otherwise, the patient 'will go to heaven to look more closely at his unlucky stars'.[80] In the course of the eighteenth century, the doctor's role would progressively become that of a trusted friend and adviser to his patient. Accordingly, compassionate silence would finally prevail over religious preoccupations in spite of the repeated opposite recommendations of some more rigorous authors.[81] Proponents of silence would then become the absolute majority, albeit with some nuances, in nineteenth-century medical deontology.[82] It was, after all, yet another subtle form of the increasing medicalisation of death, and an expression of the physicians' power over the dying.

Whether zealous or reticent, in any case, early eighteenth-century physicians did not linger around the dying person when the end was truly near. Hoffmann crudely warned his students how unpleasant it was to be close to agonising patients and their smell of putrefaction, and had no qualms about suggesting that they interrupt their visits.[83] It would take a few more decades until doctors considered it their duty (and their prerogative) to assist the dying up to the very last moment. At the beginning of the eighteenth century, in contrast, they still willingly surrendered this office to priests, who at any rate claimed it vigorously.

---

[78] SM, pp. 37, 55, 62 and 65.

[79] D. Gagliardi, *Idea del vero medico fisico, e morale, formata secondo li documenti, ed operazioni d'Ippocrate*, Rome, 1718, pp. 207–9 and 177–80.

[80] Ibid., p. 63.

[81] P. Vecchi, 'La mort dans l'Encyclopédie', in *Transactions of the Fifth International Congress on the Enlightenment*, Oxford, 1980, vol. 2, pp. 986–94; Porter and Porter, *Patient's Progress*, pp. 144–52.

[82] Carol, *Les médecins et la mort*, ch. 1; M.L. Betri, 'Il medico e il paziente: i mutamenti di un rapporto e le premesse di un'ascesa professionale (1815–1859)', in *Storia d'Italia, Annali 7, Malattia e medicina*, ed. F. Della Perruta, Turin, 1984, pp. 209–32.

[83] Zacchia, *Quaestiones*, pp. 405–9; Hoffmann, *Medicus politicus*, p. 219. On the attitude of late eighteenth-century medical authors, see R. Porter, 'Thomas Gisborne: Physicians, Christians and Gentlemen', in *Doctors and Ethics*, ed. Wear, Geyer-Kordesch and French, pp. 252–73.

Chapter 7

In the Hour of Death

Physicians' Duties and Clerics' Prerogatives at the Deathbed

In theory, the subordination of doctors to the clergy with regard to curing the sick and dying had been established for a long time. The Fourth Lateran Council of 1215 had decreed that the soul was a much more valuable asset than the body, and that physicians should not induce sufferers to do anything that might endanger their spiritual health.[1] No one should be allowed to die without confession and viaticum. The 1215 canons thus put an unprecedented pressure on all actors on the stage of death – the sick, their families, the priests and the doctors – to make passing and bereavement truly Christian events as well as salutary moments.[2]

The Counter-Reformation Church reasserted and clarified the obligations of treating physicians. In 1566, the bull *Super gregem* by Pius V enjoined doctors – under penalty of infamy, the paying of a fine and the stripping of their university degree – to urge patients to go to confession before embarking on treatment. It also forbade them to provide assistance to those who still refused sacraments after three visits.[3] This rule was revived in the *Rituale Romanum* of 1614. In the chapter *de visitatione et cura infirmorum*, the Roman official liturgical book reiterated the prohibition on doctors taking actions aimed at preserving physical health that might be in any way detrimental to the patients' spiritual health, and entrusted control over physicians caring for the sick and dying to parish priests. Indeed, priests had to admonish patients not to give in to doctors' illicit orders, the devil's cunning or the blandishments of friends; instead, they must refrain

---

[1]   *Conciliorum oecumenicorum decreta*, ed. G Alberigo et al., Basel, 1962, p. 222: 'cum anima sit multo pretiosior corpore, sub interminatione anathemais prohibemus, ne quis medicorum pro corporali salute aliquid aegroto suadet, quod in periculum animae convertatur'.

[2]   J. Avril, 'La pastorale des malades et des mourants aux XIIe et XIIIe siècles', in *Death in the Middles Ages*, ed. H. Braet and W. Verbeke, Leuven, 1983, pp. 88–106; C. Treffort, *L'Église carolingienne et la mort: christianisme, rites funéraires et pratiques commémoratives*, Lyon, 1996, p. 55, points out the early diffusion of viaticum despite resistance from the clergy. See further F.S. Paxton, *Christianizing Death: The Creation of a Ritual Process in Early Medieval Europe*, Ithaca and London, 1990.

[3]   The norm was included in the 1595 statutes of the Roman College of Physicians and reasserted in those of 1636.

from 'fallacious and dangerous procrastination' and receive the sacraments while they were still unimpaired 'in their mind and their senses'.[4]

In fact, as I have indicated in Chapter 6, medical doctors willingly yielded to priests in the hour of death. Nevertheless they disclaimed the obligation to summon the priest. Medical ethical literature went no further than stating that it was doctors' duty to warn patients to confess. Therefore, clergy frequently rebuked treating physicians for their lax piety in this regard. Clerical insistence on this point would suggest that, in spite of canon laws, medical practitioners must have been rather lenient towards recalcitrant patients.[5] Physicians' obedience to papal decrees must be total and without 'glossing the canons' to find exceptions, warned the Dominican friar Bartolomeo D'Angelo at the height of the Counter-Reformation.[6] A doctor would commit sin if 'he recommended to the infirm anything that resulted in a prejudice to the soul', passed over calling his patients to repentance, did not conform to established medical practice, was not sufficiently diligent or failed to warn the patient of the risk of death.[7] Whoever prevented the patient from receiving the viaticum before succumbing to the disease would commit mortal sin, and even more at fault was a patient refusing it out of 'human respect, negligence or impiety'.[8] Jurists agreed with theologians. Physicians must necessarily announce the impending death, or at least have someone announce it in their place; prizing physical recovery before spiritual redemption or failing to remind patients of their obligation to confess their sins would definitely put them in the wrong.[9]

The risk of sudden death of patients whose conditions were seemingly not overly serious was precisely one of those instances when, according to theologians, the case for faith outweighed any medical consideration. At the cost of suffering a diminished professional reputation, treating physicians must not

---

[4]   *Rituale romanum Pauli V P.M. iussu editum*, Rome, 1614, pp. 74–6. It must be remembered that extreme unction could also be administered with a conditional formula when the person was in danger of death (for example, to soldiers or people undergoing surgery), see ibid., pp. 56–62; L. Godefroy, 'Extrême Onction', in *Dictionnaire de théologie catholique*, vol. 5, 1, Paris, 1924, cols 1818–2022.

[5]   As admitted by Catalani in the mid-eighteenth century in *Rituale Romanum Benedicti papae XIV jussu editum et auctum, perpetuis commentariis exornatum*, vol. 1, Padua, 1760, p. 278.

[6]   B. D'Angelo, *Ricordo del ben morire dove s'insegna a ben vivere e ben morire*, Venice, 1609, p. 178. The work was first published in 1576 and reissued in 20 subsequent editions.

[7]   O. De Bonis, *Arte teorica e pratica per aiutare nello spirito gl'infermi divisa in cinque parti*, 2nd edition, Rome, 1686, p. 24.

[8]   J. Crasset, *La douce et sainte mort* (1681), I have used the modern edition of Lyon-Paris, 1853, p. 164.

[9]   T. Azzio, *Tractatus novus legalis de infirmitate, eiusque privilegijs, et effectibus*, Venice, 1603, pp. 98–9.

delay advising patients to seek divine grace. In his very popular devotional tract on the preparation for death *L'huomo al punto* (*The man on the point*), the Jesuit Daniello Bartoli devoted no less than two chapters to the danger and ugliness of sudden death in sin. In a further chapter he expatiated on the sins of physicians and relatives who did not disclose to a sick person the ever-impending risk of an unforeseen demise.[10] At the beginning of the eighteenth century another Jesuit, Giuseppe M. Prola, had even stronger words in store for the 'fatal complacency' of doctors who put spurious therapeutic reasons before salvation merely to avoid speaking frankly to their patients, and then called the priest too late to comfort them in their agony.[11] It should be added that, whereas medical treatises strove to demonstrate that anyone had the religious and civil obligation to follow doctors' orders, canonists unsurprisingly never conceded medicine an equal authority to religion.[12] In the religious representation of the hour of death, at any rate, the presence of a physician just before and immediately after the fatal moment was not really contemplated.[13]

Whether collaborating or competing, with unity of purpose or in mutual suspicion, physicians and clergy did have at least one area in which they had to work together. Doctors of philosophy and medicine were called on to contribute to the revision of sacramental theology undertaken by the post-Tridentine Church. Through their science and experience, they must help specify the physical and mental states in which sacraments could be legitimately administered. Apoplexy, syncope and apparent death were common morbid conditions that raised delicate theological issues on which physicians had to provide clarification in order to settle the doubts of theologians: in which conditions could the risk of death be predicted and extraordinary measures resorted to? Did an individual need to be conscious to receive the sacraments? If not, which sacraments could the semi-conscious receive? Who determined such a state and how? What ailments irreversibly damaged sensory and intellectual capabilities? How were natural, preternatural and supernatural states of unconsciousness to be defined? Approximately how much time elapses between the prodromal signs of a sudden

---

[10] D. Bartoli, *L'huomo al punto cioè l'huomo in punto di morte*, Rome, 1667, pp. 197–222 and 316–24.

[11] G.M. Prola, *Giorno di vera vita consecrato all'apparecchio d'una santa morte ... terza impressione*, Rome, 1708, pp. 24, 58.

[12] G. Pomata, *Contracting a Cure: Patients, Healers and the Law in Early Modern Bologna*, Baltimore, 1998, p. 138.

[13] *Rituale romanum*, pp. 101–29; M. Cappuccino, *Dichiaratione dell'offitio de' morti, e delle cerimonie nell'essequie per le anime delli defonti. Secondo li riti cattolici di Santa Chiesa, e del rituale Romano riformato*, Rome, 1626. One of the salient aspects of the Catholic reform with regard to dying was that the priest was now requested to comfort the agonising person until the very last instant and not only administer the sacraments and then leave.

affection, the real crisis and death? When was it best to call a priest and should the laity be allowed to replace him in extraordinary circumstances?

Sixteenth- and seventeenth-century moral theologians borrowed heavily from medical writers, who in turn looked to theologians and commentators of Aristotelian-Scholastic philosophy for enlightenment when they wrote about life and death, sickness and health. Rome, of course, was one of the main centres where theological and medical scholarship on these topics was elaborated. Such expertise was indeed necessary to the activity of congregations and courts with universal jurisdiction, such as the Rota, the Holy Office and the Congregation of Rites. Not surprisingly, Paolo Zacchia devoted many of his *Quaestiones medico-legales* to the states of consciousness required for receiving a sacrament or sealing a notary deed. He also addressed the question of whether a dying man struck with a syncope was able to receive the sacraments and to make a testament, in what pathological conditions the priest and notary were to act *in articulo mortis* – that is, with special express procedures – and whether apoplectics could ever regain their full mental faculties.[14] These same questions also engaged several other canonists and moralists.[15] In addition, according to his early biographers, Zacchia devoted a specific treatise to the thorny subject of *De subitis et mortis insperatis eventibus, cumque praecognitione* (*On the cases of sudden and unexpected death, and how to foresee them*), now apparently lost.[16]

Sudden Death and Pastoral Dilemmas

There is no need to repeat it: sudden death had always been one of the central concerns of Christian pastoral care. A dangerous ugly death that did not allow time for repentance and salvation, *mors repentina* (abrupt death) upset the order of things. It was 'the absurd instrument of chance, which was sometimes disguised as the wrath of God',[17] an ignominious end that was opposite to the ideal of good death as an anticipated moment awaited in the company of family and community. It was so abhorrent as God's punishment that, during

---

[14]   P. Zacchia, *Quaestiones medico-legales*, Lyon, 1661, pp. 130–60, 236–40.

[15]   P. Riva, *De actis in mortis articulo commentarii*, Ticino, 1599, pp. 4, 89, 155 and 194 on extreme unction. Azzio, *Tractatus novus legalis*, pp. 32–5, lists the cases when it is possible to proceed *in articulo mortis*; pp. 134, 181 and 277 examine the sacraments with regard to various pathological conditions and states of unconsciousness; p. 30 discusses the ability to test. Among theologians, I only mention Z. Pasqualigo, *Theoria, et praxis in qua iura, obligationes, et privilegia eorum, qui in periculo aut articulo mortis constituuntur*, Rome, 1672, pp. 233–5, 451–5 and 335, where he treats the question whether it is possible to absolve someone who is struck with apoplexy while kneeling before the priest to give confession.

[16]   G. Marini, *Degli Archiatri pontifici*, Rome, 1784, vol. 2, p. 121.

[17]   P. Ariès, *In the Hour of Our Death*, trans. H. Weaver, London, 1981, p. 10.

what has been described as the first 'clericalisation of death' in the thirteenth century, ecclesiastics tried to alleviate the suspicion and aversion it aroused.[18] Consequently, abandoned corpses that were theoretically destined to be buried in unconsecrated ground because it was not possible to ascertain the deceased's state of grace were admitted into cemeteries, and their burial came to form one of the charitable deeds of religious confraternities. Without much success, though: well into the early modern age, sudden death, except on the battlefield, was still considered an infamous end.[19] Even as late as in the popular culture of the nineteenth century, the dangerous revenants and most terrifying ghosts were those of persons who had died suddenly (not necessarily from a violent death), as they were assumed to have subverted the times and rites of dying and mourning.[20]

As is well known, the Tridentine Church had recourse to the fear of death, and especially of sudden death, to discipline life. The hour of death was no longer the moment that could compensate for a sinful earthly existence as it had been in the Middle Ages. It was no longer the last chance to cast a fleeting thought to Jesus and the Holy Mother and shed a late yet salvific 'measly tear' (*lagrimetta*), as Bonconte of Montefeltro had done in Dante's *Purgatory* (V, 101–5): 'God's angel took me up, and Hell's fiend cried:/"O you from Heaven, why steal what's mine?/You may be getting his immortal part–/and won it for a measly tear, at that,/but for his body I have other plans!"'.[21] Instead, it was now the final act of a long preparation through penance, prayer and meditation. The entire time on earth had to be lived with the awareness of death. The *ars moriendi* literature changed accordingly, shifting from the moment of death to the experience of death throughout life. It also acquired a novel clerical connotation. It thus progressively diverged from

---

[18]   A. Bernard, *La sépulture en droit canonique du décret de Gratien au Concile de Trente*, Paris, 1933, pp. 113–30.

[19]   H. German-Romann, *Du bel mourir au bien mourir: le sentiment de la mort chez les gentilshommes français, 1515–1643*, Geneva, 2001, p. 200. Such an attitude persisted for a longer time in England, according to C. Gittings, 'Sacred and Secular: 1558–1660', in *Death in England*, ed. P. Jupp and C. Gittings, Manchester, 2000, pp. 147–74; and in Switzerland and Low Germany, according to S. Lauter, *Geschichten vom Tod: Tod und Sterben in Deutschschweizer und oberdeutschen Selbstzeugnissen des 16. und 17. Jahrhunderts*, Basel, 2007, pp. 132–5.

[20]   J. Delumeau, *La peur en Occident, XIVe–XVIIIe siècles: une cité assiégée*, Paris, 1978, pp. 75–96; V. Petrarca, 'Tecniche rituali per il controllo della paura: la festa dei morti in Sicilia tra XIX e XX secolo', in *Storia e paure: immaginario collettivo, riti e rappresentazioni della paura in età moderna*, ed. L. Guidi, M.R. Pelizzari and L. Valenzi, Milan, 1992, pp. 319–31.

[21]   'L'angel di Dio mi prese, e quel d'inferno/gridava: "O tu del ciel, perché mi privi?/Tu te ne porti di costui l'etterno/per una lagrimetta ch' l mi toglie"', *Dante Alighieri's Divine Comedy: Purgatory. Italian Text and Verse Translation*, trans. M. Musa, Bloomington, IN, 2000, p. 49.

the humanistic meditation on the experience of dying that had persisted in the early sixteenth century, gaining instead a straightforward catechetical intent in the framework of the Tridentine Catholic doctrine.[22] Spiritual assistance to the dying and prayer for the dead became fundamental missions for Counter-Reformation confraternities. These also devoted themselves with renewed vigour to the charitable burial of those poor souls struck by sudden death and left lying in the streets and fields or pulled out of water.[23]

Thus, sudden death was an omnipresent theme in a Catholic piety grounded in fear which, in the words of Robert Favre, often reduced faith to the fear of God, and fear of God to fear of death.[24] Pastoral literature focused on the terrors that had coalesced over centuries: dying unconscious, dying alone, dying suddenly.[25] In his classic book on the history of early modern attitudes towards death, Michel Vovelle estimates that, in the seventeenth century, six books out of ten on preparation for death explicitly addressed the topic of sudden death.[26] Moral and ascetic literature – those collections of good deeds, 'gardens of examples' and 'mirrors of virtue' warning Christians to flee distractions and maintain a way of life dominated by the thought of the afterlife – sifted through history and hagiography looking for instructive examples. The *memento mori* pervaded early modern figurative culture; more specifically, the theme of sudden death appeared prominently both in allegorical learned paintings and in popular prints, which mostly circulated the representation of the sinner's bad unanticipated demise. Indeed, according to many preachers, a sinner's death was always sudden, fatal and unprepared for, and doomed to damnation.[27]

---

[22]   A. Tenenti, *Il senso della morte e l'amore nella vita del Rinascimento* (1957), Turin, 1989, pp. 62–120, 311–52; A. Tenenti, ed., *Humana fragilitas: i temi della morte in Europa tra Duecento e Settecento*, Clusone, 2000, especially P. Scaramella, 'L'Italia dei trionfi e dei contrasti', pp. 25–98.

[23]   V. Paglia, 'Le confraternite e i problemi della morte a Roma nel Sei-Settecento', *Ricerche per la storia religiosa di Roma*, 5, 1984, pp. 197–220. Drowning was considered a form of sudden death but persons drowned in rivers were more easily suspected of having committed suicide than those lost at sea, whose disappearance was always considered accidental; see C. Treffort, 'Le corps du noyé et le salut de son âme dans la tradition chrétienne occidentale', in *Corps submergés, corps engloutis: une histoire des noyés et de la noyade de l'Antiquité à nos jours*, ed. F. Chauvaud, Paris, 2007, pp. 113–21.

[24]   R. Favre, *La mort dans la littérature et la pensée française au siècle des Lumières*, Lyon, 1978, p. 69, and on sudden death, pp. 85–92.

[25]   R. Chartier, 'Les arts de mourir, 1450–1600', *Annales ESC*, 31, 1976, pp. 51–76.

[26]   M. Vovelle, *La mort et l'Occident de 1300 à nos jours*, Paris, 1983, pp. 295–7. On England, where analogies with Catholic discourse on good or bad death prevailed, see R. Houlbrooke, *Death, Religion, and the Family in England, 1480–1750*, Oxford, 1998, pp. 183–213.

[27]   J. Delumeau, *Le péché et la peur: la cupabilisation en Occident (XIIIe–XVIIIe siècles)*, Paris, 1983, pp. 407–11.

It is quite obvious that Post-Tridentine Catholicism sparked the onset of a specific medical literature on sudden death at the end of the sixteenth century. Grassi, for instance, admitted his religious motives unreservedly: it was a matter of anticipating an event that endangered both the patients' soul and the general social order. He even concluded his scientific dissertation with some prayers against unexpected death that any reader who so desired could address to God and the Holy Mother.[28] For their part, ecclesiastical authors drew on medicine when they pointed to the difficulty of maintaining one's reason and willpower intact during physical suffering, and especially in pathological conditions such as apoplexy and syncope. Daniel Roche estimates that a quarter of the seventeenth-century religious discourse on dying revolved around disease and pain, and on the uncertainties and dangers they brought with them. Whether 'comforters' or 'terrorists', all ecclesiastics agreed on how difficult it was to turn to God in one's final moments on one's deathbed, when the mind and the body were weakened by infirmity.[29] The sick, wrote the French Jesuit Jean Crasset in his highly successful *La douce et sainte mort*, must not hesitate to put their worldly affairs in order at the very onset of their affliction, since, as their conditions worsened, they would be 'deprived of the use of the senses and destitute of forces: the former [condition] prevents one from receiving the [priest's] instructions, the latter from putting them into practice'. Also, if the final moment had not been well prepared, it aroused so much fear as to become a disease in itself that 'freezes the blood, grips the heart, stops the flux of spirits and hinders the use of all faculties'.[30]

Many Catholic writers used the theme of the loss of consciousness associated with sudden ailments to induce fear of unprepared death, since unconsciousness hampered confessional absolution and communion, leaving the dying to receive the last ointment only, at best. 'It is very difficult, at the extreme confines of life, to prepare well [for death]', wrote the Oratorian priest Francesco Marchese. When physical pain increases, he continued, then it is indeed hard to 'conceive that more intense pain for one's evildoings, to the degree that is appropriate at the end of a life spent in sin'. Without the grace of God, the soul 'by itself will not be capable, despite all efforts and the assistance lent by others, to fully repent of and grieve for its misdeeds'; moreover,

> There may be cases when, struck by sudden death, one is taken from this world, as happens daily to many persons who die of sudden death, or struck by apoplexy, are

---

28   P. Grassi, *Mortis repentinae examen ... cum brevi methodo praesagendi et praecavendi*, Modena, 1612, pp. 4, 96–8.

29   D. Roche, 'La Mémoire de la mort', *Annales ESC*, 31, 1976, pp. 76–119.

30   Crasset, *La douce et sainte mort*, pp. 164, 191, 86.

> instantly deprived of the use of their senses and speech ... thence ending their days like
> brute animals, without any consciousness of dying.[31]

'One thinks oneself in good health and yet carries death in one's chest ... Who can be sure of even one single moment of life, as one is continuously in danger of dying from many accidents?', the Lazarist priests admonished their flock wherever they preached.[32] The limits of the medical art and the superiority of spiritual healing over physical care were a leitmotif of all *ars moriendi* literature, and yet, medical explanations and terms were mobilised to increase the fear of death. Clinically realistic descriptions were sometimes introduced by ecclesiastics in their tracts, such as the following, written by the Spaniard Jaime Montanes at the end of the sixteenth century:

> The feet get cold ... the teeth almost black, the nose sharp, the eyes are blind and moist,
> the forehead becomes hard ... the ears livid and deaf, the tongue big, rough and black,
> the chest swells and the throat tightens, and one loses consciousness. [33]

The circularity of arguments between medicine and religion is well exemplified in the *Prattica per aiutare a ben morire* (*Handbook for those helping to die well*) by the Jesuit Juan Baptista Poza.[34] Poza's text, however, is also revelatory of the dilemmas besetting Catholic pastoral discourse, constantly hesitating between hope and fear, between the temptation to obsessively reiterate the risks of unanticipated death and the need to combat the popular fears and 'superstitions' associated with it. Poza did in fact devote a long chapter to sudden death in order to warn inveterate sinners, but he also took pains to refute the 'common belief that every sudden death is a sign of the wrath of God'. To prove his point, he drew up a list of 'saintly and exemplary persons who died abruptly and without

---

31   F. Marchese, *Preparamento a ben morire*, Rome, 1697, pp. 34, 39, 154. On Marchese, see I. Lavin, 'Bernini's Death', *Art Bulletin*, 54, 1972, pp. 161–86 and 'Afterthoughts on "Bernini's Death"', *Art Bulletin*, 55, 1973, pp. 429–36.

32   Roche, 'La mémoire de la mort', p. 105.

33   J. Montanes, *Espejo de bien vivir y para ayudar a bien morir*, quoted in A. Milhou-Roudie, 'Un transito espantoso: la peur de l'agonie dans les preparations à la mort et sermons espagnols du XVIe et XVIIe siècles', in *La peur de la mort en Espagne au Siècle d'Or: littérature et iconographie*, ed. A. Redondo, Paris, 1993, pp. 9–16, quotation at p. 12 (it is an obvious reference to the *facies hippocratica*).

34   I have used the Italian translation of J.B. Poza, *Prattica per aiutare a ben morire anco per quelli, che solo sanno leggere, e per imparare a ben vivere da quello che occorre, e si deve fare nel tempo della morte*, Rome, 1631 (the original Spanish version was first published in 1619). On the Jesuit, see V. Lavenia, '"D'animal fante": teologia, medicina legale e identità umana. Secoli XVI–XVII', in *Salvezza delle anime, disciplina dei corpi: un seminario sulla storia del battesimo*, ed. A. Prosperi, Pisa, 2006, pp. 483–526.

sacraments', and dwelled on a medical digression concerning the 'many causes that can provoke the sudden death of the righteous'.[35] Page after page, the Jesuit explained the functioning of the human body and all the accidents that can affect its main organs. Death comes 'whenever a vein or an artery or a main nerve melts, splits or breaks, because the heart is then damaged by being deprived of motion and air'; or it happens because 'thick substances or humours [are generated] which impede the passage of the blood and the spirits, and ... at times create such reflux to the heart that they drown it'; last but not least, in the 'instruments of respiration there similarly hide legions [of ailments] that cause sudden death'.[36] Poza illustrated the assortment of life-threatening diseases looming over man, but at the same time he turned medical knowledge into derision of doctors and their frantic search for prognostic signs. In point of fact, 'these deaths are natural effects, and obligations of nature', medicine is powerless, and one must simply thank God for keeping one alive despite countless physical pitfalls. Leading a righteous life, the Jesuit adds in passing, also includes relinquishing superstition and avoiding passing 'impertinent judgement over whether whosoever died suddenly died an evil death'.[37]

Vigilate itaque, quia nescitis diem neque horam (Matthew 25.13). It should be added that the papal condemnation of divination, issued by Sixtus V (bull *Coeli et terrae Creator*, 1586) and reasserted by Urban VIII (bull *Inscrutabilis*, 1631, which was issued after a disreputable affair regarding prophecies of the pope's death), dismissed as heresy all those death forecasts and horoscopes of which the medieval and Renaissance public had been so fond.[38] Foreknowledge of death was to be deemed God's special grace and one of the hallmarks of holiness.[39]

Plague remained a particularly dreaded form of rapid death. Medical notions in fact aided preachers and every plague outbreak renewed the oratory power of homilies that evoked the ravages of contagion and called to repentance in apocalyptic tones. Some preachers paradoxically insisted on the spiritual benefits of epidemics, which affected the body but healed the heart, as did another Jesuit, Etienne Binet, in his *Remèdes souverains contre la peste*. Against

---

[35] Poza, *Prattica*, p. 148.

[36] Ibid., pp. 155–7.

[37] Ibid., pp. 158 and 160.

[38] Nonetheless, the practice of astrology remained widespread, including in seventeenth-century Rome; see L. Fiorani, 'Astrologi, superstiziosi e devoti nella società romana del Seicento', *Ricerche per la storia religiosa di Roma*, 2, 1978, pp. 97–162; G. Ernst, *Religione, ragione e natura: ricerche su Tommaso Campanella e il tardo Rinascimento*, Milan, 1991, pp. 255–79; U. Baldini, 'The Roman Inquisition's Condemnation of Astrology: Antecedents, Reasons and Consequences', in *Church, Censorship and Culture in Early Modern Italy*, ed. G. Fragnito, Cambridge, 2001, pp. 79–110.

[39] E. Rébillard, 'La Belle mort des saints', in *Qu'est-ce que mourir*, ed. J.-C. Ameisen, D. Hervieu-Léger and E. Hirsch, Paris, 2003, pp. 148–64.

the plague and all other accidents and illnesses that lead to sudden death, Binet offered a number of simple spiritual remedies in line with the moral teachings of the Society of Jesus: taking frequent communion, participating in collective general confessions, venerating the Holy Mother of Jesus, reciting the litanies of the saints and the 'act of true contrition, which is the only remedy against sudden death', since, according to the Jesuit, no one dies so quickly as not to be able to recite it.[40]

On this last point, however, the opinions of theologians, preachers and physicians were far from unanimous.

Rigorism and Contrition

It is precisely within the context of a significant shift in theological opinions and religious sensibility on the subject of *in extremis* contrition at the end of the seventeenth century that the new urgency of the issue of sudden death must be understood. This was combined with a more active attitude towards the dying on the part of both medical doctors and clergy. The reorientation of Catholic theology and morals in the neo-Tridentine Church affected the areas of contact between religion and medicine. The appearance of the theme of sudden death in late sixteenth-century medical literature was an outcome of the Council of Trent and the Counter-Reformation; its re-elaboration at the beginning of the eighteenth century was a product of neo-Tridentinism.

Studies by Tenenti, Ariès, Vovelle, Chartier and Roche have demonstrated how the Christian discourse on death reached its apex in the second half of the seventeenth century. The form and content of it were shaped to suit what was now deemed a largely Christianised and disciplined society. Indeed, there was no more room for instant conversions. Everybody ought to prepare their passing in the solitude of their individual conscience, away from the comforting and yet superficial collective rituals of medieval piety. Last minute repentance seemed doubtful to all churchmen and preachers, regardless of their theological inclinations. All now emphasised how difficult it was for the sick and the dying to gain a valid penitential absolution. 'Will it be enough, after a debauched life,

---

[40]   Published in Paris in 1628, Binet's tract was translated into Italian as *Sovrani et efficaci rimedi contro la peste e morte subitanea* and published at the outbreak of the plague in Rome in 1656. On the plague as spiritual medicine, see A.L. Martin, *Plague? Jesuit Accounts of Epidemic Disease in the Sixteenth Century*, Kirksville, MO, 1996; E. Hipp, 'Plague as Spiritual Medicine and Medicine as Spiritual Metaphor: Three Treatises by Etienne Binet, S.J. (1569–1639)', in *Piety and Plague: From Byzantium to the Baroque*, ed. F. Mormando and T. Worcester, Kirksville, MO, 2007, pp. 224–36.

no longer able to talk, to shake the hand of the priest in order to obtain God's grace? Oh uncertain penance!'[41]

The threat of sudden death was still the ultimate weapon to urge conversion and preparation, whether by laying the stress on the infinite mercy of God, as did the Jesuit Crasset,[42] or by laying it on the eternal punishment of hell, as did the Oratorian Marchese. According to Marchese, only a confession made in a pristine state of mind and body, after rigorous self-examination and sincere contrition, could be an instrument of salvation, and

> experience reveals day after day how vain and deceitful is the hope of many persons who believe they [still] have a long series of years to enjoy, trusting in their youth, the robustness of their body, the liveliness of their spirits; and yet suddenly, in the fullness of their youth, they are mowed from the soil of this world by the scythe of death.[43]

At the end of the seventeenth century, however, ecclesiastics preaching 'benign' moral theology such as Crasset progressively gave way to the growing number of proponents of a strict moral attitude – including towards the dying – like Marchese. The tone of penitential literature became more severe, calls for an evangelical conduct of life more insistent, moral teachings stricter.[44] The neo-Tridentine wish to impose a more diligent sacramental practice and a rigorist interpretation of Christian moral doctrine intertwined with the renewal of Augustinian theology. This shift impacted all relevant moments of an individual's life from conception to death. The issue of sudden death, in particular, acquired an unprecedented urgency with reference to the burning question of attrition and contrition.

In the fourteenth session on penitential confession, the Council of Trent had defined contrition as the 'sorrow of the soul and hatred of sins committed, with the firm purpose of not sinning again' (*dolor ac detestatio ... de peccato commisso, cum proposito non peccandi de caetero*); perfect contrition arises from the love of

---

[41]   J. Nouet, *Retraite pour se préparer à la mort* (1679), quoted in H. Bremond, *Histoire littéraire du sentiment religieux en France depuis la fin des guerres de religion jusqu'à nos jours*, vol. 9, *La vie chrétienne sous l'Ancien régime*, Paris, 1932, p. 334, my italics.

[42]   Crasset, *La douce et sainte mort*, pp. 113–17; with the right preparation at any rate, the Jesuit adds reassuringly, 'bien que sa mort soit subite, elle n'est jamais imprévue', an argument that he derived from the *Ars bene moriendi* of his more illustrious brethren Roberto Bellarmino (1620).

[43]   Marchese, *Preparamento a ben morire*, p. 28.

[44]   J. McManners, *Death and the Enlightenment: Changing Attitudes to Death among Christians and Unbelievers in Eighteenth-Century France*, Oxford, 1981, pp. 191–233. Also in Protestant countries, and especially in England, the topic of sudden death was revived in late seventeenth-century preaching, as part of a general rebuke of the new urban and secular way of life; see Houlbrooke, *Death, Religion, and the Family*, pp. 211–13.

God, whom sin has offended, and it leads to justification. But it was also affirmed that imperfect contrition, or attrition – that is, remorse for the sin committed for fear of punishment – prepared the soul of the repentant sinner to receive grace during confession. Although insufficient without the sacrament of penance, still, attrition was defined as God's gift and an impulse of the Holy Spirit. Hence, both conditions were contemplated in the canons of the Council of Trent. In the final formulation of session XIV, 4, however, the Council Fathers stated that attrition could be conceived 'either from the consideration of the turpitude of sin or from the fear of hell and punishment' (*vel ex turpitudinis peccati consideratione vel ex gehennae et poenarum metu*),[45] leaving in the conjunction *vel* a wide margin for interpretation. Hence, sixteenth- and seventeenth-century moral theologians eagerly engaged in the exposition of the meaning of attrition, the infinitely various motives of the sinner asking for pardon, the degrees and types of attrition required for the confessor to give it.

Notwithstanding the Tridentine canons, or actually because of them, the second half of the seventeenth century witnessed the consolidation of the theological position that considered contrition the necessary prerequisite for justification. The misinterpretation of the conciliar canons by Jesuits, Capuchins and other proponents of the benevolent 'large' doctrine of justification was the preferred argument for those who, appealing to Augustine, called for reform of baroque sacramental practice. Some theologians referred to no less than St Bernard and St Anselm and taught that perfect contrition was an absolute requirement even during confession. Although not entirely new, this argument was now enhanced by the crisis of the spiritual and doctrinal middle ground which the Tridentine Church had settled upon after much tribulation. The more baroque moral casuistry had increased the number of exceptions and the 'opportunities' to hold the sacraments valid,[46] the more the rigorists called for strict uniformity. They invoked scriptural and patristic authority, the 'venerable antiquity' of early Christianity, and they accused casuists of introducing 'abusive' novelty and laxity, spoiling the Church's *pristinus decor*.

Consequently, a sudden and unexpected demise seemed fatal for salvation. If justification required the confession of all sins after a thorough self-examination and with the full awareness of the sins committed, then eternal life could hardly be gained at the time of death, especially if this occurred quickly and unexpectedly. If a true and sincere contrition was essential, then time and lucidity were needed. But both were lacking during agony, especially in the case of a sudden ailment. Hopes of salvation were thus shaken to their very foundation, the fear of death

---

[45]   *Conciliorum oecumenicorum decreta*, pp. 679–89, 'Doctrina de sanctissimis poenitentiae et extremae unctionis sacramentis'.

[46]   A good example of sacramental extreme probabilism is Pasqualigo, *Theoria et praxis*, on attrition pp. 218–83.

instilled and the danger of damnation for those who had not led a consistently virtuous life magnified.[47]

Among other things, rigorist theologians and experts in sacred history argued that in the primitive Church those who would not atone for their sins through public penance, or dubious or relapsed penitents would never receive absolution, not even on the point of death. Furthermore, *in extremis* repentance was always only inspired by fear. Especially in France and Flanders, many stigmatised the notion of attrition as a pernicious scholastic invention and a Jesuit sophistication, and maintained that the confessor could not attest to its sincerity. Therefore, sacraments administered to the dying were not necessarily valid; even extreme unction had to be administered to alert persons only to have any value.[48]

Sparked between the Jesuits and the Jansenists in the frontier lands of Flanders, the controversy over the so-called 'servile attrition' (the attrition motivated by mere fear of hell and punishment) inflamed Catholic Europe for decades. And it reverberated in Rome, where renowned theologians of opposed factions tried to redraw the official doctrinal line in their favour. The controversy was not a mere academic dispute since it resounded in ordinary preaching on penitential absolution and affected the administration of the sacraments, raising doubts and fears among the faithful. The contest was so bitter that it spurred the Holy Office to issue a first condemnation of several propositions on attrition in 1667.[49] It served no purpose, though. For years, Rome continued to receive requests from Flanders and France for a formal pronouncement on attrition and penance that would act as a check against the moral degeneration of laxist and

---

[47]   J. Delumeau, *L'aveu et le pardon: les difficultés de la confession, XIIIe–XVIIIe siècle*, Paris, 1992, pp. 128–35.

[48]   I shall mention only two authors: J. Morin, *Commentarius historicus de disciplina in administratione sacramenti poenitentiae tredecim primis seculis in Ecclesia Occidentali et huc usque in Orientali observata* [1651], Antwerp, 1682, pp. 719–92 on penitential practice with the sick and the dying; pp. 740–44 on the faithful struck with sudden illness and left without sense and the ability to talk to whom absolution must be withheld; pp. 47 and 505–15 on attrition as a Scholastic invention; E. Marten, *De Antiquis Ecclesiae ritibus libri quatuor*, Rouen, 1700, vol. 2, pp. 105–20 on extreme unction and the abuses introduced in the thirteenth century in regard to its administration. For an overview of the dispute, see A. Beugnet, 'Attrition', in *Dictionnaire de théologie catholique*, vol. 1, Paris, [1898] 1937, cols 2235–62, who, however, follows the attritionist position that finally prevailed in the nineteenth century. On the archeolatria (the worship of antiquity) of Jansenists and Augustinians, see B. Neveu, *Érudition et religion aux XVIIe et XVIIIe siècles*, Paris, 1994.

[49]   L. Ceyssens, 'L'origine du décret du Saint-Office concernant l'attrition (5 mai 1667)', in his *Jansenistica minora*, vol. 1, Malines, 1950, ch. 3. Note that servile attrition could have different degrees (servile, slaverly servile and so on). Already in 1658 the Holy Office had declared audacious the proposition according to which a heretic who performed an act of contrition *in articulo mortis* but persisted in error could be saved (Ms ACDF, S. Offitii, Dubia Varia 1570–1688, fasc. 23).

probabilistic moral theology. Such requests found active support among the increasingly strong rigorist faction in the Roman curia and papal court.

Alexander VII's condemnation of a number of laxist propositions in 1665 and 1666, including several relating to the confession in *articulo mortis* and attrition, marked the first substantial success of the rigorist party. It was further enhanced in 1679 by Innocent XI's condemnation of the proposition 'it is probable that natural honest attrition only is sufficient [for justification]' (*probabile est sufficere attritionem naturalem modo honestam*) and a number of other laxist ideas, along with the prohibition to follow a merely probable opinion in matters pertaining to the administration of sacraments.[50] Several books containing laxist morals or defending extreme probabilism were placed on the Index of Prohibited Books. Although the pontificate of Alexander VIII Ottoboni marked a temporary reversal of the Roman doctrinal line,[51] rigorists consolidated their position in all of the Church institutions. The *laxus opinandi modus* progressively lost ground even among the Jesuits (who in truth had never been unanimous in moral theology), to whom the Order's general congregation of 1696 forbade the teaching of several bold probabilistic principles.[52]

The condemnation of probabilism and laxism in 1679 has attracted the attention of historians with regard to baptism. It has been considered the starting point of a new attitude towards pregnancy, childbirth and birth. The 1679 Roman decrees rejected, among other things, irregular or hasty baptism rites, especially of unborn foetuses still in their mothers' womb, as well as any moral justification of abortion. Consequently, they arguably fostered the eighteenth-century affirmation of caesarean section and, ultimately, the prevailing of the unborn child's rights over the mother's, which, for all its piety, Counter-Reformation medicine had not contested.[53] It is true that the Holy Office refused to take a

---

50   H. Denzinger, *Enchiridion symbolorum definitionum et declarationum de rebus fidei et morum*, XL, ed. P. Hünermann, Bologna, 1997, particularly n. 2031 (on omitting sins during confession *in articulo mortis*), n. 2101 (on permission to follow probable opinion 'in spite of the surer one'), n. 2129 (on the simulation of sacrament), n. 2157 (on the validity of attrition). On the 1679 condemnation of laxism, see J.-L. Quantin, 'Le Saint-Office et le probabilisme (1677–1679): contribution à l'histoire de la théologie morale à l'époque moderne', *Mélanges de l'Ecole française de Rome. Italie et Méditerranée*, 114, 2002, pp. 875–960.

51   During Alexander VIII's papacy, attrition out of mere fear of hell was thus rehabilitated by the Holy Office, whereas the systematic postponement of absolution by confessors was condemned (cf. Denzinger, *Enchiridion symbolorum*, nos 2314–21). The peculiar circumstances of missions also gave rise to several doctrinal doubts and queries about the end of life, which were generally settled from Rome in favour of the rigorist interpretation (ibid., nos 2380–82).

52   M. Petrocchi, *Il problema del lassismo nel secolo XVII*, Rome, 1953, pp. 55–6, 95–103.

53   N.M. Filippini, *La nascita straordinaria: tra madre e figlio la rivoluzione del taglio cesareo*, Milan, 1995, pp. 87–8; A. Prosperi, *Dare l'anima: storia di un infanticidio*, Turin,

firm position on the animation of foetuses for several decades to follow,[54] but from the standpoint of moral theology 1679 undeniably marked a turning point. I argue that an equivalent shift can be appreciated at the other extreme of human experience. In particular, sudden death was made an increasingly frightening and tragic possibility by the papal pronouncements on attrition, probabilism and confession in *articulo mortis*.

Rigorist doctrines also implied a different strategy in daily spiritual care. The rigorist offensive undermined all those expressions of baroque piety, firmly rooted in the substrate of medieval beliefs, which attenuated the terror of a death without sacraments. For instance, official inquiries and condemnations by Church authorities in the late seventeenth and eighteenth centuries hit the so-called sanctuaries *à répit*, where parents took the puny little bodies of their stillborn babies to implore their momentary resurrection, long enough to have them baptised, and thus save their souls and bury their bodies in consecrated ground.[55] Similarly rejected was the popular belief that the excommunicated dead could sometimes appear in churches (in spirit, if not in their corporeal bodies) begging for absolution.[56] Throughout the Catholic world, spiritual assistance to the dying was revived with the aim of establishing greater control over the end of life, and renewed attention was also turned to the plight of those who died suddenly and alone and were left unburied.[57]

2005, pp. 283–5.

[54] A. Prosperi, 'Battesimo e identità cristiana nella prima età moderna', in *Salvezza della anime*, pp. 1–66. Other relevant documents are in ms ACDF, S. Offitii, UV 51, fasc. 4 and 5.

[55] These rites were fiercely criticised especially by French ecclesiastics and experts of early Christianity such as J.B. Thiers, *Traité des superstitions* (1679) and N. Alexandre, *Theologia dogmatica* (1694), on whom see L. Cavazza, 'La doppia morte: resurrezione e battesimo in un rito del Seicento', *Quaderni Storici*, 17, 1982, pp. 551–82; S. Seidel Menchi, 'Les pèlerinages des enfants morts-nés: des rituels correctifs pour un dogme impopulaire?', in *Rendre ses voeux: les idéntités pèlerines dans l'Europe moderne (XVIe–XVIIIe siècles)*, ed. P. Boutry, P.-A. Fabre and D. Julia, Paris, 2000, pp. 139–53; J. Gélis, *Les enfants des limbes: mort-nés et parents dans l'Europe chrétienne*, Paris, 2005.

[56] A. Calmet, *Traité sur les apparitions des esprits et sur les vampires ou les revenans de Hongrie* (1746), Paris, 1751, vol. 2, pp. 116–22; J.-M. Goulemot, 'Démons, merveilles et philosophie à l'Âge classique', *Annales ESC*, 35, 1980, pp. 1223–50.

[57] F. Lebrun, *Les hommes et la mort en Anjou au XVIIe et XVIIIe siècles*, Paris and The Hague, 1971, pp. 457–8; F. Hernandez, 'Être confrère des agonisants ou de la bonne mort aux XVIIe et XVIIIe siècles', in *Confréries et dévotions dans la catholicité moderne, mi-XVe–début XIXe siècle*, ed. B. Dompnier and P. Vismara, Rome, 2008, pp. 311–18. On the frontier land of Québec, which caused the pronouncements of the Holy Office in 1703 mentioned above, see G. Plante, *Le rigorisme au XVIIe siècle: Mgr. de Saint-Vallier et le Sacrement de pénitence, 1685–1727*, Gembloux, 1971; Y. Landry and R. Lessard, 'Causes of Death in Seventeenth- and Eighteenth-Century Québec as Recorded in the Parish Registers', *Historical Methods*, 29, 1996, pp. 49–57.

In Rome, the holy city whose exemplary character the papacy sought to reaffirm, doctrinal reorientation and neo-Tridentine reform of the care of the dying went hand in hand. New impetus was given to the confraternities that prayed for the dying and buried the dead, which had been rather inactive following their foundation in the early sixteenth century.[58] The institute of the apostolic visit – that is, the periodical inspection of churches and other ecclesiastical institutions that was the Roman equivalent of the bishop's tour of his diocese – was also given new impulse, and hospitals were particularly targeted. Improvements in their economic, religious and medical management were made with the aim of making illness and agony a time of spiritual rebirth, if not of physical healing.[59] In line with the predominant rigorist stance and the contritionist interpretation of justification, greater accuracy in the administration of the sacraments and especially penance was recommended to everybody.[60]

In short, disease and death were certainly not overlooked in neo-Tridentine Church discipline, which put greater pressure on clergy and laypersons. It would be hard to misinterpret the aim of the Major Penitentiary Cardinal Nicolò Ludovisi when he commissioned a second edition of the *Arte teorica e pratica per aiutare a ben morire* (*Theoretical and practical art for helping to die well*) by the Somascan Omobono de Bonis. This was a slender yet intransigent compendium on how to help the sick and the dying avoid the 'errors and sins committed by

---

[58]   M. Maroni Lumbroso and A. Martini, *Le confraternite romane nelle loro chiese*, Rome, 1963, on the archconfraternity of the Natività di Gesù Cristo degli agonizzanti (Nativity of Jesus Christ of the dying), p. 256, of Gesù e Maria, p. 157, of the Crocifisso agonizzante (of the Agonizing Crucified [Christ]), p. 109. On the confraternity of the Orazione e Morte (Oration and Death) which assisted sick labourers and buried dead bodies found in the fields, see G. Rossi, *L'agro romano tra '500 e '800*, Rome, 1988, pp. 231–52, who sees a turning point in the revival of this confraternity in the year 1672.

[59]   Records of relevant apostolic visits to the main city hospitals are to be found in ms ASV, Visita Apostolica, Acta 12 and 13; Ms VL, Chigi G III 85, apostolic visit to San Salvatore ad Sancta Sanctorum hospital and church (1677); Ms ASV, Misc. Arm. VII 56, apostolic visit to Consolazione hospital (1675–77); Ms ASV, Misc. Arm. VII 59, fasc. 3, visit to San Giacomo hospital (1677); ASV, Misc. Arm. VII 64, visits to Santo Spirito hospital (1660, 1677–79, 1696).

[60]   Clement IX ordered the religious of all orders to serve in the city's hospitals in turn, and the rotation of the confessors from the regular clergy was further improved by Innocent XI. In addition, Pope Odescalchi issued a pastoral *Instruttione* to impose a uniform method to be held in assisting the sick and the dying; see ms ASV, Misc. Arm. IV–V, vol. 9, fols 25–8. Innocent XII also ordered a new edition of the *Avvertimenti di san Carlo per li confessor ... con l'aggiunta delle propositioni dannate, bolle e altri decreti*, Rome, 1700 (Instructions by St Charles [Borromeo] to the confessors ... with an Addition of Prohibited Propositions, Bulls and Other Decrees), reprinted again under Clement XI in 1702 and in 1703. Pope Albani issued new regulations for the distribution of viaticum too (*Regole ed istruzzioni che si devono asservare nell'accompagnamento del Santissimo Viatico*, Rome, 1701).

the sick in their affliction, the physicians in their cures and the priests in their guidance of the infirm'.[61] An edict issued in 1699 by Rome's cardinal vicar reminded doctors that they had taken the oath imposed by Pius V not to treat unrepentant patients. Even decisions surrounding burials in consecrated land seemingly became less lenient.[62]

Inevitably, the discourse on death changed too. Not only in the distant regions of Northern Europe, but also in the very centre of the Catholic world, Rome, the last decades of the seventeenth century witnessed a wave of writings on the preparation for death by rigorist authors. Whereas 'benign' moral theology – without necessarily degenerating into laxism – had recommended to priests a compassionate, benevolent approach in assisting the dying, a novel rigour now pervaded manuals for confessors, instructions of moral theology, homilies and orations. Preachers of all orders, including the Jesuits,[63] instilled the fear that only a true heartfelt contrition guaranteed divine forgiveness. Following the rigorist 'narrow morals', they insisted on a scrupulous preparation before receiving sacraments, thus increasing the anxiety of all good Catholics in the face of unanticipated death. In the presence of a God who is a 'just punisher' who sends earthquakes, wars and 'all the most bitter sufferings, the most incurable diseases, the most deadly plagues', as Francesco Marchese (who was promoted apostolic preacher by Innocent XI) described him, 'who amongst us will be able to boast assurance about the remission of their errors, even after [receiving] the priest's absolution?'[64]

---

[61]   O. De Bonis, *Arte teorica e pratica divisa in cinque parti...*, 2nd edn, Rome, 1686, p. 17.

[62]   It is difficult to ascertain from the incomplete documentation available in ms ACDF, S. Offitti, St. st. M 3, but it would appear that in pronouncements concerning burials in unconsecrated ground or exhumations the Holy Office, leaving its customary caution, tended now more often to delegate decisions to bishops after a thorough examination of the deceased's last actions (as indeed it was prescribed by the *Rituale Romanum*). Moreover, the rules reprinted at the behest of Cardinal Carpegna in 1707 (*Statuta antiqua de Officio camerarij cleri Romani, et iuribus funeralibus ecclesiarum, praesertim parochialium Almae Vrbis, una cum additionibus, seu declarationibus novissime*, Rome, 1707, p. 80) reaffirmed the prohibition to concede burial in consecrated ground to the excommunicated and to notoriously unrepentant sinners; they also enjoined that the cardinal vicar be consulted expressly *si aliquot ermerserit dubium, an in communione catholica, vel statu peonitentiae obierint* (if any doubt arose as to whether he died in communion with the Catholic Church or in a state of penitence).

[63]   L. Albicini, *Gesù nella sua Passione modello de' cristiani moribondi ... per benefizio de' fratelli delle Congregazioni della Buona Morte, erette nelle chiese de' padri della Compagnia di Gesù*, Bologna, 1719.

[64]   F. Marchese, *Massime di pietà e fruttuose instruzioni espresse in cento discorsi detti nelle adunanze solite di san Filippo Neri*, Rome, 1699, p. 121. The 'strict' doctrine on contrition and attrition is summarised by F.M. Campione, *Dissertatio theolgico scholastica de necessitate aliqualis saltem imperfecti amoris Dei*, Rome, 1698; F.M. Campione, *Instructio pro se*

This was the climate in Rome when the mysterious sudden deaths began in 1706. And if one places them against the backdrop of the rigorist offensive that had been waged in religious life for decades, it is easier to understand the emotion and alarm they aroused. Who could be assured of salvation any longer?

It must be noted that in conjunction with the series of 'accidents' that dismayed the citizens of Rome, there was a surge in controversies on the topic of attrition. Between 1703 and 1709, not in a remote province but in the very centre of Roman Catholicism, a bitter dispute over grace and attrition pitted the Jesuit Baldassarre Francolini, influential professor of moral theology at the Roman Seminary, against the staunchest defender of contritionism, Pierre Lambert Le Drou of the Hermits of St Augustine. Le Drou was every bit as eminent as Francolini, having been the former rector of the faculty of theology at Louvain, bishop of Porphyria and former member of the delegation of theologians from Louvain who had demanded the formal condemnation of laxism in Innocent XI's times.[65] The main congregations of cardinals in charge of doctrinal orthodoxy tried to silence the most virulent attacks. But if in 1703 the Holy Office foiled the attempt of the general of the Society of Jesus, Tirso Gonzales, to rekindle the debate on probabilism, acting on him *cum suavitate*, in 1706 the Congregation of the Index had to ban yet another caustic booklet against the 'laxist' Francolini.[66] On 4 June 1706, the Holy Office felt compelled to remind the opposing parties that the proposition 'natural attrition is sufficient for the validity of the sacrament of penance, and supernatural [intervention] is not needed to bear fruit' had been prohibited by Innocent XI. The Holy Office,

---

praeparantibus ad audiendas confessiones, Rome, 1704, in particular pp. 30–31, 64, 122. In his *Instruttione per gl'ordinandi, cavata dal Concilio di Trento, rituale e pontificale romani, e da' decreti per il clero di San Carl*, Rome 1702, pp. 414–18, however, Campione, while maintaining the contritionist doctrine, admitted several exceptions *in articulo mortis*.

[65]   B. Francolini, *Veteris ecclesiae rigor in administrando sacramento poenitentiae*, Rome, 1704; B. Francolini, *Praesentis ecclesiae benignitas in administrando sacramento poenitentiae*, Rome, 1705; B. Francolini, *De dolore ad sacrae poenitentiae rite suscipiendum necessario*, Rome, 1706; B. Francolini, *De disciplina poenitentiae libri tres*, Rome, 1708. On the opposite front, P.L. Le Drou, *De contritione et attritione dissertationes quatuor quibus ostenditur non requiri in reconciliationis sacramento prefectam et se solo justificantem contritionem*, Rome, 1708, on which see J.J.I. von Döllinger, *Geschichte der Moralstreitigkeiten in der römischkatholischen Kirche seit dem sechzehnten Jahrhundert*, Nördlingen 1889, pp. 282–96. Another champion of the attritionist camp in Rome was Giovanni Antonio da Palermo, *Scrutinium doctrinarum qualificandis assertionibus, thesibus, atque libris conducentium, exemplis propositionum a conciliis oecumenicis, vel ab Apostolica Sede ... refertum*, Rome, 1709.

[66]   Ms ACDF, S. Offitii, Censurae librorum 1703, fasc. 38; the pamphlet in contention was *Francolinus cleri romani paedagogus, laxioris in administrando poenitentiae sacramento disciplinae magister, commentitiae rigoristarum secta fictitiarmque in ecclesiam veterem ac recentem calumniarum impugnator observationibus historico-critico-moralibus exagitatus*, Cologne, 1706.

furthermore, bitterly deplored disputes continuing in defiance of the papal prohibition on further debating attrition.[67]

Clement XI too tried to remain equidistant from the theological and political parties embroiled in such controversies. He summoned theologians of all schools and inclinations in the special congregation appointed to draft the bull *Vineam Domini* against Jansenists, including advocates of strict Augustinianism like Le Drou. Mindful of keeping the balance between the factions in appointing cardinals, in need of counsel as he was, and desirous of support to overcome his uncertainties,[68] in 1706 the pope bestowed the cardinal's hat on the two champions of the opposing sides, Lorenzo Casoni and Carlo Agostino Fabbroni.

Hence, if the rigorist stance on death allows us to understand the fear aroused by the wave of sudden deaths at the beginning of the eighteenth century, the theological warfare that was tearing the Church and the Roman curia apart helps explain Clement XI's decision to resort to science and seek a medical answer to a mystery that created such acute fear and raised such difficult questions for the Church. Neo-Tridentine Catholicism had intensified the anxiety that abrupt death had always instilled in the collective imagination and sensibility, and made the need to decipher it more urgent than ever.

Theologians' disputes on attrition dragged on for decades. At any rate, whatever their theological and moral tenets were, all preachers and pastors found motivation in the Roman events of 1706 to revive penitential fervour. Sudden death enjoyed further popularity in public preaching. The spate of sudden deaths was not yet over when Abbot Agostino Taia – a churchman and a man of letters highly appreciated at court – took inspiration from the circumstances for his gloomy *Meditazioni ... da farsi in tempo di malattia* (*Meditations for the times of illness*).[69] The following year, the echo of the sudden deaths in Rome resounded in Paris. The archbishop of Paris, Cardinal de Noailles, emanated an *ordonnance* on the spiritual care of the sick, in which he stigmatised the sinful reticence of physicians who did not disclose the dangers of illness to their patients, disregarding 'the unfortunate experience of so many sufferers whom a sudden and unforeseen death takes away and dooms for eternity'.[70] In truth, a few physicians did actively consider the spiritual dangers of sudden death and contributed, in their own way, to the religious discussion about the end of life.[71]

---

[67] On this affair, see the vote by the theological consultant, the Conventual Franciscan Giovanni Damasceno in ms ACDF, S. Offitii, UV 51, fasc. 10.

[68] P. Stella, *Il giansenismo in Italia*, vol. 1, *I preludi tra Seicento e primo Settecento*, Rome, 2006, p. 97.

[69] A. Taia, *Meditazioni ... da farsi in tempo di malattia*, Rome, 1706.

[70] I am quoting from Bremond, *Histoire du sentiment*, p. 350.

[71] Lancisi was in line with the rigorist stance; see SM, pp. 68, 96. P. Dionis, *Dissertation sur la mort subite et sur la catalepsie*, Paris, 1710, p. 151, recommended choosing a good spiritual counsellor who was especially able to provide guidance in the art of dying.

Some ecclesiastics drew on the deadly events in Rome to rekindle the controversy between theological factions, as did the Jesuit Giuseppe M. Prola in reprinting his *Giorno di vera vita consecrato all'apparecchio d'una santa morte* (*A day of true life devoted to the preparation for a holy death*). The work is severe in tone, reflecting the Society of Jesus' reorientation in moral theology, and it makes explicit reference to the grim events of the time:

> How many amidst your acquaintances, or perhaps amidst relatives or neighbours were taken away by sudden death? How many were seized all of a sudden this year? Alas you know it. They were well informed that during the previous year many had perished unexpectedly. Do you think that any of them ever seriously said to themselves ... soon it might befall me?'

It is therefore necessary, wrote Prola, to prepare for death through constant meditation and frequent confession and communion, before disease (and the atrocious medical treatment) prevents the necessary rigorous scrutiny of conscience and repentance, for which 'certain infirmities do not allow either time or ease. Raging delirium, deep lethargy, violent pain ... obscure reason and make man no longer have mastery over himself.'[72] After such stern warnings, however, Prola did not miss the opportunity to open fire against the Jansenists, assuring his readers that 'contrition regardless of its degree is contrition' and can be 'so intense as to extinguish the sin deserving of punishment, so that if you died today you could immediately fly and reach the highest immortal happiness.'[73]

The first decades of the eighteenth century witnessed an increasing number of comments on sudden death in homiletics and devotional literature, which included discussions of the bad deaths of the wicked and the worldly. When in 1723 the French Regent Philippe d'Orléans passed away suddenly in the arms of his mistress, his end seemed to many a striking confirmation of the warnings from preachers and doctors alike about the risks of a life of vice and excess. Was there really no aid, no protection against such a *mala mors* as was sudden death?

---

[72]   Prola, *Giorno di vera vita*, p. 17.

[73]   Ibid., pp. 23, 57, 94.

Chapter 8
Looking for a Heavenly Protector: Saint Andrew Avellino, the 'Apoplectic Saint'

Miraculous Deaths and Prodigious Resurrections

Between the seventeenth and eighteenth centuries, rigorism formed the substrate on which the fear of sudden death grew into an unprecedented political, religious and scientific emergency. It represents a further element to take into consideration in deciphering the events in Rome in 1706 and Lancisi's *De subitaneis mortibus*. The heated disputes on divine grace and attrition urged medical and religious élites to take a second look at death. Rigorism, however, did not merely raise the problem, it also pointed towards a solution – that is, it helped foster the naturalisation of the phenomenon.

We must now pull together the threads of the previous chapters. As I have mentioned, experts and laypersons alike agreed that sudden death might occur as divine punishment. The story of Lot's wife (Genesis 19.1–29), of Anania and Sapphira (Acts of the Apostles 5.1–11) and of many others in the Bible exemplified the *mala mors* befalling the heathen and evildoers. Ancient history also abounded in sudden demises that Christian culture had turned into exempla. From Nero and Caligula to Julian the Apostate, killed on the battlefield by the avenging arrow of the True Faith, pagan enemies of God thus met the destiny assigned to vice and cruelty. Similar facts could also be read in the lives of the saints. For instance, in Jacobus de Voragine's *Golden Legend*, the most important hagiographical collection from the Middle Ages, St Pelagius strikes dead and casts into hell the heathen king of the Frisians while St Leodegar smites a sceptic who doubted his miracles. Prodigious tales also saw St Benedict killing his rebel disciple Florentius or, five centuries later, St John of Capestrano punishing a faithless dignitary with sudden death.[1] There was, however, no shortage of counter-examples of righteous men struck dead all of a sudden and yet admitted to heavenly glory, such as St Galdin, who exhaled his last breath at the end of a sermon, or St Homobonus, who expired after reciting his matins. All these sudden demises confirmed the importance of the fateful last moment. It

---

[1]   Jacobus de Voragine, *The Golden Legend: Readings on the Saints*, trans. W.G. Ryan, Princeton, 1993, vol. 2, pp. 373 and 219; G. Klanic Zay, 'Miracoli di punizioni e malefici', in *Miracoli: dai segni alla storia*, ed. S. Boesch Gajano and M. Modica, Rome, 1999, pp. 109–36.

was the befitting seal for the holy life of saints or, conversely, the awful end that struck sinners down unexpectedly, allowing them no time for repentance and reconciliation with God.

In devotional books, stories of sudden deaths inflicted by God or the saints as punishment sometimes featured miracles of momentary resurrection enabling the administration of sacraments. The revival of this theme during the Counter-Reformation was plainly connected with the Tridentine doctrine of justification. Furthermore, the saints' intercession could grant spiritual salvation from sudden death. St Edmund, for instance, resuscitated a man who 'for his crimes was condemned to hell and was thus saved'. In this case, Edmund was additionally aided by virtue of his devotion to the Holy Cross that offered 'special aid to beseech escape from sudden death'.[2] In another legend, St Francis of Assisi brought a woman back to life 'so that she could confess a sin which she had unwittingly omitted'.[3] As mentioned above, stillborn children were brought to special Marian sanctuaries to be reanimated and baptised, since otherwise they were doomed to be buried in unconsecrated ground and to limbo, if not to the flames of hell as many of the strictest rigorist theologians taught.

Thus, in dealing with sudden death early modern clergy wavered between the desire to fight the superstition of those who invariably saw it in the light of divine intervention and the need to exploit it for penitential purposes, in order to govern their flock by instilling the fear of a passing so swift and unexpected as not to permit salvation. For their part, medical writers too believed that sudden death might sometimes have the features of a miracle. In the section *de miraculis* of his *Quaestiones medico-legales*, Paolo Zacchia specifies that one could speak of 'a miraculous death and of disease introduced prodigiously' (*de morte miraculosa et de morbis divinitus immissis*) when, despite 'attentive and diligent inspection' (*exquisita et diligenti inquisitione*), no manifest natural cause could be determined.[4] There also were occurrences of wondrous deaths, like those ensuing from prolonged ecstasy, which was a prodigious fact in itself.[5] As for actual resurrection, it was considered the ultimate miracle, and Zacchia lists it among the highest class of contra-natural miracles – that is, performed by God directly without any recourse to natural forces and, indeed, against the ordinary course of nature. But, warns Zacchia, most of the time a miracle is proclaimed out of ignorance of the real natural causes, and seemingly miraculous deaths

---

[2]   *Devozione al sagro titolo della croce acciò si degni liberare dalla morte subitanea et.varie divozioni per chi desidera di vivere, e morire santamente*, Rome, 1728, p. 99.

[3]   S. Razzi, *Giardino d'essempi, o vero fiori delle vite de' santi, scritte in lingua volgare*, Rome, 1603, p. 71.

[4]   P. Zacchia, *Quaestiones medico-legales*, Lyon, 1661, p. 258; see also P. Grassi, *Mortis repentinae examen*, Modena, 1602, p. 62.

[5]   This was because, in ordinary circumstances, the separation of the soul immediately amounted to death; see Zacchia, *Quaestiones*, p. 267.

and resurrections might be the effect of some occult or metaphysical cause yet to be discovered.

How could natural and supernatural events be distinguished? Where should the dividing line be drawn between natural facts and miracles?

Neo-Tridentine Catholicism, like medicine, also considered the divide between the natural and the miraculous at length. Indeed, rigorists sharply deplored 'superstition' and popular 'corruptions' of faith. The aspiration to reform Baroque piety – if only in reaction against the criticisms of Protestants and freethinkers alike – implied a degree of suspicion of a world view based on wonders. Its proponents denied the unlimited plasticity of Nature, which could be traced back to the Aristotelian heritage, albeit tinged with Platonic elements accumulated over the previous three centuries. Diabolic possessions particularly attracted increasing scepticism,[6] but many other cults and devotions designed to alleviate the fear of death without sacraments came under scrutiny, like the sanctuaries *à répit* for stillborn infants. The Augustinian emphasis on God's omnipotence, once associated with miracles, played a crucial role at this time in what has been termed the mechanisation of the world view or the triumph of natural necessity.[7]

Clement XI's decision to resort to science as a means of explaining what could equally have been regarded as a supernatural phenomenon is particularly significant if set against such a background. In spite of a few attempts to emphasise the miraculous nature of the calamities hitting the Papal States at the beginning of the eighteenth century, there was an evident willingness to curb any prophetic temptations and apocalyptic mood that might be indulged in during those dark days of death and destruction. In truth, the excesses of friars and fanatical worshippers had been repressed with a steady hand for a while, and there was certainly no question of releasing the pressure in such calamitous times.[8]

---

[6]   E. Brambilla, 'La fine dell'esorcismo: possessione, santità, isteria dall'età barocca all'illuminismo', *Quaderni Storici*, 112, 2003, pp. 117–64; A.J. Schutte, *Aspiring Saints: Pretense of Holiness, Inquisition, and Gender in the Republic of Venice, 1618–1750*, Baltimore, 2001; M. Sluhovsky, *Believe not Every Spirit: Possession, Mysticism and Discernment in Early Modern Catholicism*, Chicago, 2007.

[7]   R. Hutchinson, 'Supernaturalism and the Mechanical Philosophy', *History of Science*, 21, 1983, pp. 297–333; D.M. Clarke, *Occult Powers and Hypotheses: Cartesian Natural Philosophy under Louis XIV*, Oxford, 1989; S. Nadler, ed., *Causation in Early Modern Philosophy: Cartesianism, Occasionalism and Preestablished Harmony*, University Park, PA, 1993; M.J. Osler, *Divine Will and the Mechanical Philosophy: Gassendi and Descartes on Contingency and Necessity in the Created World*, Cambridge, 1994. For more general concerns, see L. Daston and K. Park, *Wonders and the Order of Nature, 1150–1750*, New York, 1998.

[8]   E. Brambilla, 'Manuali d'esorcismo, canoni di santità e nuova scienza (fine '600 – primo '700): Indice e Sant'Uffizio tra neoscolastica spagnola e influenze cartesiane', in *Rome et la science moderne: entre Renaissance et Lumières*, ed. A. Romano, Rome, 2008,

As for physicians, they unanimously dismissed supernatural causes, contrary to the interpretation of earlier events like the outbreak of plague in 1656. The causes of death were entirely natural and to be attributed to 'vitriolic, arsenical and nitrous' exhalation, according to da Sylva, or to a 'ferment of an unknown and perverse nature', as suggested by Evangelista, or, as Bernabei believed, to the fashion of wigs. Neither the deeds of evildoers, nor the actions of God were contemplated among the possible explanations, although all medical authors cautioned that everyone's life and death ultimately depended on the supreme divine will. Lancisi's treatise also decidedly favoured the naturalisation of sudden death. Modern mechanical medicine, with its philosophical arguments and anatomo-pathological method, provided a coherent and exhaustive explanation of all strange deadly 'accidents'. Incidentally, mechanical medicine not only extolled the harmony of Nature created by God, but also underscored individual responsibility in leading a healthy life. After all, in the new medical paradigm, wise moderation still coincided with Christian temperance, and so sudden death remained, at least in part, a moral issue.

Rooted in the decline of scholasticism and fostered by the papal political agenda, the naturalisation of sudden deaths thus proceeded hand in hand with the rise of mechanism. Sudden death was actually one further aspect of the demystification of seemingly miraculous phenomena by medicine. For some time already, modern medical and physical doctrines had offered the framework for interpreting instances of religious frenzy in natural terms. Doctors and philosophers of nature, for example, demolished pretences of prodigious fasting by female mystics and devout virgins. In the 1680s, Lancisi himself solved the mystery of a fasting virgin who yet vomited charms and stones. Following Malpighi's teachings, he precluded the possibility that the human body produced anything other than pathological concretions formed out of filaments, and concluded that the supposed charms were in fact concretions similar to polyps.[9] On their side, theologians could draw on modern natural philosophy to purge faith of false beliefs. For instance, in 1670 Boyle's experiments on the

---

pp. 555–93. Repressive measures were also taken in the diocese of Rome to curb exorcists and 'persons possessed or pretending possession'; see ms ASVR, Segreteria, Registro degli editti del Vicario, 7 January 1705; [A. Cuggiò], *Della giurisdittione e prerogative del Vicario e prerogative del Vicario di Roma: opera del canonico Antonio Cuggiò segretario del tribunale di sua Eminenza*, ed. D. Rocciolo, Rome, 2004, p. 81.

9   *Congressus Medico-romanus habitus in aedibus D. Hieronymi Brasavoli die lunae 21. septembris 1682*, Rome, 1682. See also S.A. Mazzuto, *Historia medica coram eruditissimo doctorum coetu in aedibus Brasavolaeis Roma exposita*, Rome, 1685; G. Reali, *Exercitationes binae de convulsione, de motibus convulsivis cum succedaneo hydrope, de lacte, ac de pleuritide*, Rome, 1702. On the naturalisation of bodily concretions, see D. Bertoloni Meli, 'Blood, Monsters, and Necessity in Malpighi's De polypo Cordis', *Medical History*, 45, 2001, pp. 511–22; for similar cases in England, see S. Schaffer, 'Piety, Physic and Prodigious Abstinence', in

composition of water and air were used by the Roman priest Michelangelo Lapi to put forward the idea that drowned people could survive for a while thanks to the air dispersed in water and were eventually brought back to life through natural resuscitation rather than a true (miraculous) resurrection.[10]

Lapi and Lancisi were both referred to years later in the scholarly and comprehensive treatise *De servorum Dei beatificatione et beatorum canonisatione*, published in 1734–38 by Prospero Lambertini – the future pope Benedict XIV. In this work Lambertini reassessed the whole issue of wonders and miracles in Catholic doctrine and practice. In 1706, at the time when sudden death terrorised Rome, Lambertini was a young canon lawyer who stood out for his great learning and for his caustic wit while he was pleading the cause of the Blessed Catherine of Bologna in the Congregation of Rites.[11] In 1708 he was appointed *promotor fidei* of this same congregation, the 'devil's advocate' whose task was to challenge the evidence, particularly miracles, put forward by the supporters of aspiring saints. Since physicians played an essential part in the process of beatification and canonisation and were regularly consulted as expert witnesses, he then worked side by side with the most important representatives of the medical profession, starting with the pope's physician Lancisi. Among other things, acting as a *promotor fidei*, Lambertini flanked Lancisi in disputing the miraculous rescue of a drowned child in the beatification process of the Polish Jesuit Stanislaus Kostka.[12] Lambertini's experience and thorough knowledge of scientific as well as theological and canonical literature were later brought together in *De servorum Dei beatificatione*.[13]

Religio medici: Medicine and Religion in Seventeenth-Century England, ed. O.P. Grell and A. Cunningham, Aldershot, 1996, pp. 171–203.

[10]   M. Lapi, *Discorso sopra il tempo, che si possi star sott'acqua e non morire*, Rome, 1670.

[11]   On Lambertini, see M. Rosa, 'Tra Muratori, il giansenismo e i "lumi": profilo di Benedetto XIV', in his *Riformatori e ribelli nel '700 religioso italiano*, Bari, 1969, pp. 49–85; M.T. Fattori, ed., *Storia medicina e diritto nei trattati di Prospero Lambertini-Benedetto XIV: atti del seminario internazionale Modena-Bologna, 12–13 dicembre 2011*, Rome, 2013; P. Gavit, C.M.S. Johns and R. Messbarger, eds, *Benedict XIV and the Enlightenment: Art, Science and Spirituality*, forthcoming, Toronto, 2015.

[12]   *Benedicti 14 ... doctrina de servorum Dei beatificatione et beatorum canonisatione*, Venice, 1765, pp. 354–8 (originally published in 1734–38). Medical expert opinions and other documents regarding this process are in ms BLR, Lancisi 303, fols 25–33, 47–56, 93–122; ms Lancisi 307, fols 333–61.

[13]   F. Vidal, 'Miracles, Science, and Testimony in Post-Tridentine Saint-Making', *Science in Context*, 20, 2007, pp. 481–508; C. Santing, 'Tiramisù: Pope Benedict XIV and the Beatification of the Flying Saint Giuseppe da Copertino', in *Medicine and Religion in Enlightenment Europe*, ed. O.P. Grell and A. Cunningham, Aldershot, 2007, pp. 79–120. On anatomical artefacts as evidence of miracles, see L. Dacome, 'The Anatomy of the Pope', in *Conflicting Duties: Science, Medicine and Religion in Rome, 1550–1750*, ed. M.P. Donato and J. Kraye, London, 2009, pp. 355–76.

In this bulky work, Lambertini deals with death and the supernatural in two sections. The first concerns last repentance and sacraments: is holiness compatible with sudden death? The author takes a rigorist position, though marking a distance from the strictest Augustinians. Penance and communion on the deathbed are a prerequisite for salvation and even more so for beatification, he states, but those who maintain their heroic virtues intact until the end and whom God singles out through miracles and other signs may be counted among the blessed even if they die in suspicious circumstances and deprived of sacraments.[14]

The second section of *De servorum Dei* on death concerns 'the recall of the dead back to life, or resurrection' (*de revocatione mortuorum ad vitam seu de resuscitatione*). Demonstrating a thorough knowledge of the most recent medical literature, Lambertini takes his cue from the novel conception of death as a process to mark a distinction between authentic resurrections, as rare as they are miraculous and exemplified by Lazarus, mere legends and superstitions, and cases of simple resuscitation from apparent death. The last, especially in the case of apoplexy or drowning, can be explained on the basis of a vast body of medical and philosophical scholarship, including the work of Lancisi, Malpighi, Boyle, Bonet, Hoffmann, Willis and Ettmüller.[15] Finally, in the pages devoted to natural and supernatural healing, Lambertini sums up a thousand-year-old tradition and deems apoplexy the most lethal and difficult to treat of all affections and 'accidents' – truly deserving of the intercession of the saints.[16]

The Apoplectic Saint: the Life, Death and Miracles of Andrew Avellino

Modern medicine and neo-Tridentine 'well-regulated devotion' thus proceeded hand in hand so that a more exact Christian life, a better judgement in religious

---

[14]   *Benedicti 14 ... doctrina de servorum Dei beatificatione*, p. 250.

[15]   In the same epoch, the French theologian and scholar A. Calmet followed along the same lines in his influential *Traité sur les apparitions* of 1746 and expatiated on the distinction between apparent deaths and (rare) true resurrections. It must be noted that Benedict XIV maintained the condemnation of the sanctuaries *à répit* after an inspection carried out by Eusebius Amort, a moderately rigorist theologian and rational philosopher, and author of a critical treatise on mystical visions, *De revelationibus, visionibus et apparitionibus* (1744). For the controversy surrounding vampires and ghosts, see F. Venturi, *Settecento Riformatore*, vol. 1, *Da Muratori a Beccaria*, Turin, 1969; F. Vidal, 'Ghosts, the Economy of Religion, and the Laws of Princes: Dom Calmet's Treatise on the Apparitions of Spirits', in *Gespenster und Politik, 16. bis 21. Jahrhundert*, ed. C. Gantet and F. d'Almeida, Munich, 2007, pp. 103–29. For a more general overview, see R.C. Finucane, *Appearances of the Dead: A Cultural History of Ghosts*, Buffalo, 1984.

[16]   *Benedicti 14 ... doctrina de servorum Dei beatificatione*, p. 346; D. Gorce, *L'oeuvre médicale de Prospero Lambertini (pape Benoît XIV) 1675–1758*, Bordeaux, 1915.

matters and, in the final analysis, a stricter political and religious control could be achieved. It was a matter of disciplining the baroque imaginative, sensual piety, and discriminating the truth from lies, the natural from the supernatural, the divine from the diabolical. Reason illuminated by learning and faith must sift through daemonic possessions, ghostly apparitions and legends of the saints as well as discern the penitent's degree of contrition and the dying patient's state of mind.[17] And it was also a matter of distinguishing holy yet natural deaths from miraculous ones, and the resuscitation of apparently dead persons from authentic resurrection, with the assistance of the most acclaimed experts of natural philosophy and the most learned scholars and theologians.

One figure encompassing all aspects of the Catholic reform of death and dying was the Blessed Andrew Avellino. He had performed genuine miracles of resurrection and lived a truly holy life until he met an even holier death on the altar. Hence, he was ultimately chosen by the Church as the official intercessor and protector from *improvisa et repentina morte*. Following the earthquake of 1703, there had been a revival of the cult of St Emydius. Emydius was a Christian bishop and healer from Late Antiquity who, according to tradition, had freed himself from the hands of pagans through an earthquake. He embodied a primitive, prodigious sainthood that could still serve the 'present necessities' of early eighteenth-century Catholics, such as protection from earthquakes.[18] Against sudden deaths, however, and in order to spur everyone into defending the Roman Catholic Church under attack, Pope Clement XI decided to revive the canonisation process of a Counter-Reformation champion, the Blessed Andrew Avellino of the Theatines, which had been lying for some time with the Congregation of Rites. The solemn

---

[17]   On the 'discernment' of spirits, see G. Zarri, ed., *Storia della direzione spirituale*, vol. 3, *L'età moderna*, Brescia, 2008. On ecclesiastical erudition and the 'purification' of hagiography from ungrounded legends, see, in a vast body of scholarship, B. Kriegel, *Jean Mabillon*, Paris, 1988; J.M. Sawilla, *Antiquarianismus, Hagiographie und Historie im 17. Jahrhundert*, Tubingen, 2009; B. Joassart, *Aspects de l'érudition hagiographique aux XVIIe et XVIIIe siècles*, Geneva, 2011. The expression 'well-regulated devotion' hints at the work of L.A. Muratori, one of the main proponents of early Catholic Enlightenment, on which see the overview by M. Rosa, 'Catholic Enlightenment in Italy', in *A Companion to the Catholic Enlightenment in Europe*, ed. U.L. Lehner and M. Printy, Leiden, 2010, pp. 215–50.

[18]   The adaptation of the traditional hagiography of Emydius to suit recent events is well exemplified in the 'additions' to the *Vita di S. Emidio vescovo d'Ascoli, e martire con un ragguaglio della stessa città* by the Jesuit P.P. Appiani, Rome, 1704 (originally published in 1702, prior to the earthquake). On the cult revival, see A.A. Varrasso, ed., *I terremoti e il culto di sant'Emidio*, Chieti, 1989. On the changing emphasis on medical miracles, which came to be absolutely predominant over other types of miracles in the late seventeenth century and afterwards, see J. Duffin, *Medical Miracles: Doctors, Saints, and Healing in the Modern World*, New York, 2009.

ceremony for the canonisation of this new saint, which took place in 1712, sealed the sudden deaths affair for the papal city while giving it a new universal significance that embraced religion, politics and medicine.

Andrew Avellino was a 'modern' saint in that he had lived in the sixteenth century. His biography perfectly fitted the post-Tridentine ideal of heroic sainthood. Born in Lucania in 1521 and a student of law in Naples, Andrew distinguished himself as an inflexible pastor reforming the lax discipline in the monastery of St Archangel in Baiano at the Archbishop of Naples' behest. In 1556 he joined the congregation of the Clerics Regulars Theatines, founded in 1524 by Gajetan of Thiene and Giovan Pietro Carafa (the future Pope Paul IV), and quickly became one of their leading figures. Master of the novices in 1560, in 1567 he was appointed provost of San Paolo Maggiore, the main Theatine church in Naples, and established himself as a much sought-after spiritual director and confessor. Between 1573 and 1577 Andrew visited the Theatine province of Lombardy and later, in 1590–91, of Campania, imposing a strict Tridentine discipline everywhere he went. His commitment as a zealous reformer made Andrew the victim of no less than three assaults, which he miraculously escaped. Andrew's holy life ended in 1608 with an equally holy death. He was hit by a violent apoplexy while celebrating Mass, but he signalled by a movement of his eyes that he was still capable of receiving communion and extreme unction, before engaging on his deathbed in the fierce yet victorious final battle against the devil and dying peacefully.

Before and after his death, Andrew was venerated as a saint. His cult was sagaciously promoted by the Theatines, who were eager to compete with other Counter-Reformation religious orders like the Jesuits, the Oratorians and the Discalced Carmelites, whose founders were climbing to the status of saints. Thirty-eight miracles credited to Andrew were admitted for the beatification process that began shortly after his demise. These included the prodigious healing of a woman seized by apoplexy who recovered 'speech and cognition', the full recovery of two men struck by apoplectic strokes and the resurrection of a child who had been pronounced dead after smallpox had triggered apoplexy.[19]

Initiated in Naples in 1613, Avellino's process of beatification proceeded swiftly and gained the support of the most notable members of the Neapolitan nobility, among whom the Theatines enjoyed great confidence.[20] By 1616 the Holy Office in Rome had authorised the celebration of a feast in Andrew Avellino's name in the church of San Paolo Maggiore in Naples, where he was

---

[19]   T. Schiara, *Vita di s. Andrea Avellino, chierico regolare*, Rome, 1712, p. 323; the official list of miracles can be read in *Sac. Ritum Congregatione ... canonisationis B. Andreae Avellini ... positio super dubio an et de quibus miraculis constet, superventis post indultam edicto beato venerationem*, Rome, 1695.

[20]   M. Campanelli, 'La Controriforma e i Teatini a Napoli', *Regnum Dei*, 121, 1995, pp. 6–36.

buried. Notwithstanding the fact that he had only been beatified so far, the Blessed Andrew was proclaimed patron of Naples, Palermo and the whole of Sicily, Capua, Cosenza, Nola, Benevento and other minor centres in the Kingdom of Naples. In Rome, the Theatines had a chapel erected in the right transept of the church of San Andrea della Valle, which was under construction. The distinguished painter Giovanni Lanfranco was commissioned to produce a *Morte del Santo* (Saint's Death), which is one of the earliest representations of Avellino's holy death on the altar. Lanfranco also decorated the cupola of the church with a *Gloria del Paradiso* (Heaven's glory) where the Blessed Avellino was portrayed next to St Andrew, to whom the church was dedicated.

The canonical process, however, was abandoned because the cult of Andrew did not conform to the new, stricter rules established by Pope Urban VIII for ascertaining sainthood.[21] It was not until 1671, after the canonisation of their founder Cajetan of Thiene and in a period of rapid expansion of their congregation, that the Theatines devoted themselves to the cause of the Blessed Andrew Avellino with renewed zeal. The devotion was kept alive especially in Naples and in the Southern province of Lucania where he was born. There, several inexplicable events took place that the people immediately considered miracles of his. Hence, the authorisation to resume the procedures for canonisation was obtained by the Congregation of Rites in 1687, whence the Sacra Rota selected eight miracles, on the basis of which Innocent XI finally authorised a new formal apostolic process.

As was customary, in order to facilitate the canonisation process, several new biographies of the Blessed Andrew were produced. The theme of sudden death thus emerged forcefully. Hagiographers etched the portrait of Andrew in the guise of apoplectic saint and protector from sudden death. At one and the same time, they fomented the fear of sudden death and offered a spiritual remedy against it. Accordingly, the illness and death of the Theatine priest, which formed a relatively secondary aspect of his first biography,[22] was fully developed over the years both to strengthen its pastoral significance and to strip it of its terrible, frightening aura. Furthermore, this new account of his death helped channel the fear of *mala mors* into a religiously acceptable experience. The narrative assumed a realistic, almost medical tone, as in the vibrant prose of Anton Giulio Brignole Sale:

---

[21]   P. Burke, 'How to be a Counter Reformation Saint', in *Religion and Society in Early Modern Europe 1500–1800*, ed. K. von Greyerz, London, 1984, pp. 45–55; G. Dalla Torre, 'Santità ed economia processuale: l'esperienza giuridica da Urbano VIII a Benedetto XIV', in *Finzione e santità tra medioevo ed età moderna*, ed. G. Zarri, Turin, 1991, pp. 231–63; S. Ditchfield, 'How not to be a Counter-Reformation Saint: The Attempted Canonisation of Pope Gregory X, 1622–45', *Papers of the British School at Rome*, 60, 1992, p. 379–422; M. Gotor, *I beati del papa: santità, Inquisizione e obbedienza in età moderna*, Florence, 2002.

[22]   G.B. Castaldo, *Vita del padre don Andrea Avellino*, Naples, 1613, pp. 164–6.

> Hence his whole left side struck by a sudden apoplexy, the saint falls into the
> arms of his beloved brothers, devoid of almost all motion, and wholly of language.
> They intend to take him to his cell, but he ... makes sign upon sign in order that
> they must rather take him to the high altar, to feed on the Angelic Bread in that
> extreme hour.[23]

The ultimate battle waged by Andrew against the devil became the emblem
of every Christian's battle in the hour of death and it is described according
to the medical descriptions of apoplexy. Whereas Andrew's first biographer
characterised his agony as the apparition of 'a tempting spirit ... in the form of
an ugly man in tatters, whose sight and temptation horrified the servant of God
so much that his face and body began to turn black',[24] late seventeenth-century
hagiographers concentrated on his physical pain, on the 'frightening blackness'
and the 'horribly inflating visage ... frantic gaze, and increasing breathlessness
in his chest'.[25]

In Andrew's *Life*, written by Giovanni Bonifacio Bagatta at the end of the
seventeenth century, all hagiographic *topoi* regarding the aspiring saint are solidly
established. He is portrayed as the model fisher of souls and reformer, healer and
exorcist, but also as the emblem of Christian attitude in suffering and a powerful
protector against all forms of sudden death, whether by accident or by ailment.[26]
If at the time of his beatification Andrew's powers were not associated with any
particular type of miracle,[27] the focus is now on his death, while his miracles
specialise in neurology, so to speak, and apoplexy, 'lethargies' and epilepsies

---

[23]   A.G. Brignole Sale, *Panegirici sacri ... recitati nella chiesa di Santo Siro di Genova ne'
giorni de' B.B. Gaetano Tiene, et Andrea Avellino*, Venice, 1662, p. 50.

[24]   Castaldo, *Vita del padre don Andrea Avellino*, p. 168. The last fight of saints against
demons was an early Christian topos, see P. Dinzelbacher, 'Der Kampf der Heiligen mit
den Dämonen', in *Santi e demoni nell'alto Medioevo occidentale (secoli V-XI)*, Spoleto, 1988,
pp. 647–95.

[25]   Brignole Sale, *Panegirici sacri*, p. 51.

[26]   G.B. Bagatta, *Vita dell'ammirabile servo di Dio B. Andrea Avellino dell'ordine de
Cherici Regolari*, Naples, 1696.

[27]   The theme of death without sacraments had already been introduced by G.B.
Castaldo, *Vite di tre gloriosi confessori di Christo della religione de padri chierici regulari: il
beato Gaetano Tiene il beato Giovanni Marinoni et il beato Andrea Avellino*, Vicenza, 1627,
pp. 174–5, where Castaldo narrates that Andrew's wondrous apparition stopped a craftsman
from killing a young unmarried woman and her baby 'thus saving the mother from death,
her relatives from guilt, and the baby from death and eternal damnation, as he would have
died without being baptised'. Birth (which was tightly associated with death because of the
dangers of childbirth) was one of St Cajetan of Thiene's 'specialisations', see ibid., pp. 122–3,
and p. 121 for the resurrection of a child '[who was] truly dead, rather than agonising, as he
had no sign of life'.

prevail in the economy of hagiography.[28] Incidentally, this discursive strategy calls numerous physicians to the front of stage, whereas in early biographies they remained in the background.[29] Devotees can now see physicians making their diagnosis and prognosis of Andrew's affliction and standing by powerless while he fights with Satan. Here they come to predict the death of a man who had lost 'in the space of a moment all senses, motion and any apparent sign of life, such that if he were not already dead, he was deemed soon to be dead', on whom they try all 'that their art allowed them to make him return to his senses in any possible way, but all to no avail' and who is finally saved at the contact with the Blessed Avellino's hair. And there they are again, certifying the death of a child 'attacked by multiple diseases at the same time, with an apoplectic accident ... miserably dead' and revived by Andrew's heavenly intercession.[30]

The story of this little apoplectic child, Pietro Paolo Colelli, is a vivid compendium of the themes that increasingly qualified Andrew Avellino for sainthood. As soon as the child died,

> [his] mother burst into a bitter cry at such unexpected event, threw herself over the cradle of the deceased baby ... peering to see whether he exhaled any breath, but in vain; she shook and shook him again, believing that he may be won over by lethargy, but without any profit. Hence, realising he was truly dead, as doctor Domenico Gomesio certified, she raised her cries and lamentations.

---

[28]   Bagatta, *Vita dell'ammirabile servo di Dio B. Andrea*, pp. 230–57, reports recoveries from apoplexies, epileptic fits and from a 'most lethal lethargy' in the name of Avellino. According to G. Sodano, 'Miracolo e canonizzazioni: processi napoletani tra XVI e XVIII secolo', in *Miracoli: dal segno alla storia*, ed. Gajano and Modica, pp. 171–95, Avellino's miracles cannot be seen in relation to any specific pathology, though there are episodes of apoplexy. This situation changed at the end of the seventeenth century at the time of the canonisation, when he 'specialised' in sudden death.

[29]   In early biographies, physicians only appeared to certify the supernatural uncorrupted state of Andrew's corpse and particularly of his blood, a traditional sign of sanctity, on which see G. Sodano, '"Sangue vivo, rubicondo e senza malo odore": i prodigi del sangue nei processi di canonizzazione a Napoli nell'età moderna', *Campania sacra*, 26, 1995, pp. 293–310.

[30]   Bagatta, *Vita dell'ammirabile servo di Dio B. Andrea*, pp. 109–11, 244, 262. A. Burkardt *Les clients des saints: maladie et quête du miracle à travers les procès de canonisation de la première moitié du XVIIe siècle en France*, Rome, 2004, p. 286, highlights that in the process of canonisation, physicians were basically there to testify to their inability to help their patients. However, this did not prevent doctors from acquiring a progressively more significant role as expert witnesses over the centuries. On such evolution, see J. Ziegler, 'Practitioners and Saints: Medical Men in Canonisation Processes in the Thirteenth to Fifteenth Centuries', *Social History of Medicine*, 12, 1999, p. 191–225; D. Gentilcore, 'Contesting Illness in Early Modern Naples: *Miracolati*, Physicians and the Congregation of Rites', *Past and Present*, 148, 1995, pp. 117–48.

The child's distraught father thus goes to San Paolo Maggiore to bury his poor child. In this church, says the biographer, he stops in front of Andrew's tomb 'shedding his tears' to commend him his son's soul. The Theatines at that point put a piece of the Blessed's robe on the crib,

> and behold a wondrous thing: the child already stiff and cold, and dead for many hours, immediately recovered life, began to yawn, stretching out his little hands and body, and looking for the nurse to have the breast, as if he were just awakened from sleep and not raised from the dead.[31]

A similar miracle, the resurrection of a young boy named Scipione Arlei, who had died falling off a cliff, was credited to the Blessed Avellino many years later, in 1678. In this case too, the hagiographical narrative juxtaposes the physician's learning and the saint's power at the threshold of life and death.

> The physician duly pondered the lack of pulse, from the extinguished heat and the privation of senses, and from that large compression in the forehead and dislocation of the vertebrae of the neck, due to which he could not naturally live. He hence deemed ... he was dead, and therefore said he could not do anything but urge [the mother] to go and bury him.

But by virtue of her devotion to Andrew, the boy's mother obtains a miracle, and witnesses her child come back to life with fresh rosy cheeks, as if he had just woken from sleep.[32]

These two resurrections of children already encapsulate crucial issues such as the lethal nature of apoplexy, the distinction between real and apparent death, and the hierarchical order between medical doctors and ecclesiastics. The latter intervene later but more efficaciously than the former because they resort to a supernatural power. Another miracle performed by Andrew Avellino and admitted for his canonisation process works as a parable of the risks that sudden death posed for the salvation of the soul; it also illuminates the respective duties of physicians and priests at the end of life according to the Church. In 1675, Giovan Battista Corizio took part in a celebration in honour of a young priest's first Mass. During the feast, the room full of people dancing collapsed, causing the young man 'a deep wound on the head from which the brain came out, and a fracture of the left arm'. Believed dead, Corizio was carried 'like a corpse' to a nearby house. A local priest, Domenico D'Elefante, tried to wake him to give him the last rites, as he would later testify:

---

[31]   Bagatta, *Vita dell'ammirabile seruo di Dio B. Andrea*, p. 263.
[32]   Ibid., pp. 306–7.

I immediately squeezed his hand to allow him to show any sign of contrition, like bowing his head, or give any other sign. I tried again and again, but no sign ever came, thence I would not give him absolution, and I left him for dead.[33]

The zealous priest consequently left Giovan Battista to assist other injured victims who were still able to receive the sacraments. In other words, he strictly observed the indications of the rigorist sacramental theology, refusing superficial absolution or the administration of sacraments *sub condicione*. Thus, deprived of all sense and motion, the young man was believed to be dead and was abandoned with neither medical nor spiritual assistance. The latter was all the more necessary because the end had caught Giovan Battista unprepared and perhaps in a state of sin, while dancing and celebrating. Only the merciful intercession of the Blessed Avellino, invoked by his mother, brought Corizio back to life and freed him from death and damnation.

Clement XI and the Patron Saints for all 'Present Calamities'

It is unfortunately impossible here to consider in greater detail the probing into Andrew Avellino's miracles during the process for his canonisation that took place at the end of the seventeenth century. It must nevertheless be noted that the arguments of the lawyers and of the expert physicians involved (whose role had increased in the meantime)[34] clearly demonstrate the increasing importance attached to science in vetting – more and more critically – miraculous events. Furthermore, given the nature of Avellino's miracles, the canonisation proceedings aptly attest to the growing interest of science in sudden and apparent death and their religious implications. Particularly with regard to the resurrection of Giovan Battista Corizio, crushed in the collapse of a house, and to the *revocatio ad vitam* of the Scipione Arlei boy, also left for dead, physicians and attorneys debated at length on how to ascertain death, on whether emergency resuscitation

---

[33] 'Informatio super dubio', in *Sac. Ritum Congregatione ... canonisationis B. Andreae Avellini*, p. 42.

[34] *Decreta novissima sacrae rituum congregationis seruanda in causis beatificationum, et canonisationum sanctorum ... D.N. Innocentii 11*, Rome, 1678. On doctors' expert opinion of this period, especially with regard to uncorrupted corpses, see G. Pomata, 'Malpighi and the Holy Body: Medical Experts and Miraculous Evidence in Early Modern Italy', *Renaissance Studies*, 21, 2007, pp. 568–86; B.A. Bouley, 'Contested Cases: Medical Evidence, Popular Opinion, and the Miraculous Body', in *Médecine et religion: collaborations, compétitions, conflits (XIIe–XXe siècles)*, ed. M.P. Donato et al., Rome, 2013, pp. 139–62; for comparison, see G. Fiume, ed., *Il santo patrono e la città. San Benedetto il Moro: culti, devozioni, strategie di età moderna*, Venice, 2000, especially M. Modica, 'I processi settecenteschi di San Benedetto il Moro', pp. 334–53.

procedures could have been applied, and on which diseases and trauma left reasonable hopes for a natural revivescence of the vital motion of blood and air.

Of course, the rise of mechanical natural philosophy and the decline of the Aristotelian metaphysics that for centuries had provided the substratum for the explanation of miracles did not imply the end of miracles altogether. Especially when medical doctors operated in sacred institutions like the Congregation of Rites, they dared not refute the possibility of miraculous events and prodigies. Nevertheless, arguments of medical experts and canonists and their reciprocal expectations underwent changes. They now seemingly traced the dividing line between natural and supernatural events more clearly. The difficulty in defining death was now more acutely perceived than in the past, and spurred a greater need for a precise distinction between mere resuscitation and true resurrection. Since circulatory physiology had made the eventuality of apparent death plausible – that is, a momentary suspension of life motions that was, at least in theory, reversible – medical experts preferably confined themselves to pointing at healing or reanimation, however prodigious they might seem, rather than at miracles.[35]

In the 'age of criticism' of the early Catholic Enlightenment,[36] the prelates of the Congregation of Rites also acted with extreme caution, and therefore admitted only three of the eight miracles put forward for the canonisation of Andrew Avellino. These included the (evangelic) healing of a paralytic boy and the two 'resurrections' mentioned above.[37] On the one hand, despite all philosophical and medical subtleness, the gravity of these cases was obvious to experts and laymen alike; on the other hand, they were endowed of evident exemplarity and were attuned to the religious concerns of the moment. Despite the critical attitude of elites,[38] miracles still represented a symbolic meeting ground where the newest and most sophisticated developments in science and theology could be mediated into popular culture.

---

[35]   *Sac. Ritum Congregatione ... canonisationis B. Andreae Avellini*, in particular on the case of the Arlei boy 'Informatio super dubio', pp. 43–59; medical expert reports form an insert in the volume under the title 'Ponderationes medico physicae' and 'Responsio medica' by B. Santinelli, and 'Iudicium pro veritate' by P. Manfredi.

[36]   See above, note 17.

[37]   The minutes of the voting sessions of the Congregation of Rites have come down to us in *Sac. Ritum Congregatione ... canonisationis B. Andreae Avellini*, in the printed copy held in the VL, Barb LL III 55.

[38]   J. Le Brun, *Bossuet*, Paris, 1970, pp. 61–9. On the socio-cultural fragmentation of Western religious experience between the seventeenth and eighteenth centuries, see M. de Certeau, 'L'inversion du pensable: l'histoire religieuse du XVIIe siècle', in his *L'écriture de l'histoire*, Paris, 1975, pp. 154–77. J. Revel speaks of 'cultural normalization' in late seventeenth-century France in his 'Forms of Expertise: Intellectuals and "Popular" Culture in France (1650–1800)', in *Understanding Popular Culture: Europe from the Middle Ages to the Nineteenth Century*, Berlin and New York, 1984, pp. 255–73.

These three miracles, compounded with the particular circumstances of his death, clearly made Andrew the ideal candidate for the role of protector saint from sudden death without sacraments. Although the formal certification of the miracles of the Blessed Andrew by the Congregation of Rites dated back to 1704, one inevitably gains the impression that the final decree proclaiming the sanctity of Avellino that was issued on 12 May 1707 was in direct connection with the sudden deaths spreading terror in the streets of Rome. In the printed version of this decree, the Cardinal Vicar Carpegna plainly explained that Andrew was canonised so that he might protect Rome 'from the cruel stream of war and mourning'.[39] Of course, Andrew perfectly exemplified the model church reformer and rigorous pastor, and embodied the ideal of heroic sanctity that the neo-Tridentine Church had inherited from the Counter-Reformation. His canonisation was also the just reward for a vital congregation on the rise such as the Theatines were. But Andrew's life, death and miracles made him the natural protector against sudden death too. In his sermons, the Theatine cleric had often insisted on the need for everyone to prepare for death in 'hope and fear'.[40] As a saint, he would perpetually remind the faithful of the importance of preparing for death and of a scrupulous practice of sacraments.

Furthermore, Andrew was one of the patron saints of Naples and other cities and provinces of the Kingdom of Naples that had been conquered by the Habsburgs. His cause had been sponsored by princes and royals of various European states still at war. Therefore, the new saint could very well offer comfort and protection to the whole Catholic flock regardless of national political interests and military conflicts.

It was arguably the dramatic progression of the War of the Spanish Succession, entailing the defeat of the papal army against the Emperor, that convinced Clement XI to celebrate the solemn canonisation of the Theatine in 1712 together with that of Pius V, Felix of Cantalice and Catherine Vigri from Bologna. Each of the new saints, all of whom were Italian, embodied an aspect of the history of the Church that it was keen on exalting for political as well as religious motives: genuine mysticism and righteous government of male and female clergy, pastoral aptitude, prophetic charisma – altogether a thoroughly 'militant sainthood' with martial overtones.[41] On 22 May 1712, a magnificent ceremony was held in the Vatican basilica. The central nave was adorned with panels depicting scenes from the lives of the four new saints. Four episodes from Andrew Avellino's life were represented, including the resurrection of a child

---

[39]   In *Sac. Ritum Congregatione ... canonisationis B. Andreae Avellini*, 18 november 1707.

[40]   A. Avellino, *Trattato della speranza, e del timore, utilissimo a' pusillanimi ... et a' negligenti*, Naples, 1670, on temptations on the point of death esp. pp. 224–6.

[41]   M. Caffiero, *Religione e modernità in Italia: secoli XVII–XIX*, Pisa and Rome, 2000, pp. 27–43.

and an armed assault he had miraculously survived, unmistakably hinting at the Imperial aggression against the Papal States.[42]

The political, as well as the religious and pastoral significance of the solemn canonisations of 1712 were clearly expressed by the pope himself in the homily he recited at the end of the ceremony. Clement XI recalled the 'continuing and repeated calamities besetting the Christian Republic' and the 'misfortunes plaguing our Religion', so great that only divine aid could repair them. The new saints offered 'illustrious examples to imitate' for any Catholic, from bishop to nun. The pontiff fervently begged their protection for Italy, as if he abdicated his wrecked political ambitions:

> Embrace this new Zion, and protect it. ... Protect above all your Italy, Italy that has given you birth, that has brought you up, loved you, given you to Heaven ... Pray the All-Mighty Prince of Peace ... that he may lead the Christian princes, torn in their midst by too long lasting a discord, to the original communion of Christian love, and that he may procure that they join their forces to spread the Kingdom of Jesus Christ.[43]

The celebrations continued throughout the year. Feasts for the new saints were staged everywhere, and St Andrew was celebrated with great pomp in Rome and Naples, and in Spain.[44] A year later, on the anniversary of the solemn canonisation in the Vatican basilica, another grand ceremony was held on the Capitoline Hill in their honour by the artists' academy of San Luca and the literary academy of Arcadia in the presence of 20 cardinals. The halls of the Palazzo dei Conservatori were adorned with canvases depicting Andrew Avellino's holy death and his miracle 'in resurrecting from the dead a young boy fallen off a cliff that his mother beseeched grovelling with her tongue on the floor from the door of the church to the altar of the saint'.[45] The fine folio volume published in 1720 by

---

[42]   *Distinto racconto di quanto si è operato nella canonisatione de quattro santi ... il giorno della SS. Trinità 22 maggio 1712*, Rome, 1712.

[43]   *Homilia ... Clementis XI ... post canonisationem sanctorum Pii Quinti summi pontificis, Andreae Avellini, Felicis a Cantalicio, et Catharinae de Bononia*, Florence, [1712].

[44]   *Raguaglio del ... ottavario fatto ... nella ... Chiesa di S. Andrea della Valle di Roma per la festa del ... Santo ... Andrea Avellino*, Rome, 1712; *Relazione delle feste celebrate in Napoli nel mese di novembre 1712. Per la solenne canonizazione di S. Andrea Avellino della religione de' Chierici regolari*, Naples [1712]; *Oratorio que se ha de cantar en la Real Capilla de Santa Isabel de Clerigos regulares de S. Cayetano, en las ... fiestas, consagradas à ... San Andres Avelino*, [Saragoza, 1712].

[45]   *Il trionfo della fede solennizzato nel Campidoglio dall'Accademia del Disegno il dì 23. di maggio 1713*, Rome, [1713], p. 7; A. Cipriani, ed., *I premiati dell'Accademia 1682–1754*, Rome, 1989, pp. 114–18. On the two academies and Clement XI's cultural policy, see M.P. Donato, 'La capitale au prisme de l'événement: les concours des arts à Rome au XVIIIe siècle',

the Master of Pontifical Ceremonies Giustiniano Chiapponi and containing the official acts of the 1712 canonisation also extolled Andrew in his twofold role of church reformer, suffering armed assault like the Church of Rome under Clement XI, and of well-dying Christian, able to receive the sacraments in spite of his fatal apoplectic stroke.[46] The Church and every Christian could find solace, inspiration and protection in him.

How should the canonisation of Andrew Avellino be interpreted? Was the recourse to the Catholic supreme spiritual weapon of the intercession of saints a repudiation of the previous strategy – that is, tackling sudden death through medicine alone? Should it be considered a reaction, offsetting the pre-eminence of medicine in managing public safety?

Obviously, as mentioned above, in Catholic Europe, and all the more so in papal Rome, the fact that modern medicine could offer a coherent and rational explanation of sudden death, discounting supernatural forces, did not imply a negation of the very existence of the supernatural altogether nor a subversion of the hierarchy between medicine and religion. However, the delicate relationship between the two areas was undergoing appreciable transformation. In the incipient Catholic Enlightenment, a clearer distinction between the two spheres was being drawn, and the choice of having recourse to science to confront a danger which, by virtue of its characteristics and of the peculiar historical circumstances, might have been addressed by faith alone was evidence of the shift in that direction. Precisely for this reason, however, the importance accorded to science had to be matched by facts that were equally significant in religious terms. Andrew Avellino's canonisation was the high point of such symbolical compensation.

After his solemn canonisation, Andrew Avellino was definitively associated with sudden death. In the *Vita di s. Andrea Avellino, chierico regolare*, published in 1712 by Andrew's co-religionist Tommaso Schiara to duly celebrate the new saint, for instance, the unoriginal narrative unfolds much like previous biographies. Yet, much attention is given to his fatal apoplexy on the altar. The book closes with an invocation to the saint that incorporates elements drawn from the medical debate on sudden death and the recent events in Rome, and brings them back within a religious framework:

> Since Rome is subject more than any other city to apoplectic accidents, and since you died of apoplexy ... pray God that He shall mercifully deliver the world,

in *Capitales européennes et rayonnement culturel XVIIIe–XIXe siècles*, ed. C. Charle, Paris, 2004, pp. 97–118. In 1713 Andrew was also celebrated by the Theatines in Milan, Verona, Paris and Naples.

[46] *Acta canonisationis Sanctorum Pii V pont. max, Andreae Avellini, Felicis a Cantalicio, et Catharinae de Bononia*, Rome, 1720, pp. 25–9.

and especially Rome, from such evils, so that sudden death does not destroy our blessed eternal life along with our earthly existence. And because in life you miraculously healed some of your devotees from apoplexy, we shall increase our devotion to you in our spirit in order to obtain from God, by your intercession, the grace to be cured of, or not to fall prey to, apoplectic accidents.[47]

The cultural construction of the patron saint against sudden death continued throughout the eighteenth century. Biography after biography treated the theme of death at length, now extolling Andrew's heroism in facing the last instant, now inviting the faithful to imitate him in their passing, now celebrating Andrew's healing powers over apoplexies and all other deadly 'accidents'.[48] The pastoral and moral arguments that had coalesced around sudden death were built into the cult of the apoplectic saint. The worship of Andrew was meant to nurture the discipline of sacramental life while diluting the terror that had always been associated with unexpected death. A more composed attitude was now encouraged with regard to it, taking the Theatine saint as a model and a guardian. He was the saint 'strong on point of death', 'after death' and 'against death', the

formidable and fully fledged protector that God gave us for that very purpose: and this more than ever in present times, now that sudden apoplectic accidents, and sudden death are becoming so familiar and frequent, and [there is] no hope of any help from other remedies.[49]

Meanwhile, Andrew Avellino's sudden yet holy demise became the standard iconography in the frescos and paintings in the many churches and chapels that were dedicated to him throughout Italy, as well as in the small vignettes and medallions for personal use. Devout Catholics carried such objects on their persons for their protection, or at least to signal their faith and innocence in case they met a lonely unexpected death (an accidental drowning, for example), so that they could at least avert the danger of being left in unconsecrated ground.

---

[47]   Schiara, *Vita di s. Andrea Avellino*, p. 371.

[48]   Ample space is devoted to the Theatine's exemplary death and foreknowledge of his own demise, particularly by the following biographers: G.M. Magenis, *Vita di s. Andrea Avellino, chierico regolare eletto protettore della ecc.ma città di Milano*, Malatesta, Milan, 1740 (first published in Brescia, 1739); T.C. Bem, *Vida de Santo Andre' Avellino Clerigo Regular, especial protector contra accidentes apopleticos, e morte repentina*, Lisbon, 1767; B. Destutt de Tracy, *Vies de S. Gaëtan de Thienne, instituteur de la congrégation des clercs réguliers dits Théatins, du Bienheureux Jean Marinon, de Saint André Avellin et du B. Cardinal Paul Burali d'Arezzo*, Paris, 1774; A.T. Fernandez Moreno, *Vida virtudes y milagros del grande abogado del cielo San Andres Avelino*, Saragoza, [1754].

[49]   The quotes are taken from the chapter titles of G.B. Barzisa, *Le azioni di S. Gaetano Tiene ... e di Sant'Andrea Avellino*, Mantua, 1733, pp. 204–10.

In the eighteenth and nineteenth centuries, the cult of St Andrew Avellino was promoted far and wide and came to be the primary devotion related to death and dying. In the city of Rome, the decisive step was taken in 1751 when Pope Benedict XIV installed the confraternity of Divino amore in the Theatines' main church Sant'Andrea della Valle and changed its name into 'confraternity of saints Cajetan and Andrew Avellino for the protection *a subitanea et improvisa morte*'. In 1763 and in 1767 Clement XIII endowed it with several privileges. Indulgence was granted to those who went to confession on the feast day of St Andrew. As Andrew had died 'struck by apoplexy' but was lucid enough to take the viaticum, the faithful could pray to him to still be able to receive the final sacraments 'if by divine will they were struck by such accidents'. Plenary indulgence was also bestowed upon those who 'in article of death ... utter the most Holy name of Jesus with their lips or, if this were impossible, in their heart, or by other signs ... of repentance', just as the dying Theatine had done.[50]

The foundation of confraternities named after St Andrew and devoted to the preparation for death flourished particularly in the Italian Peninsula but reached far beyond.[51] Indeed, worship of the apoplectic saint would seem to grow in parallel to an increasingly acute perception of sudden death as a real political as well as a public health issue. In some cities, waves of mass panic triggered by 'epidemics' of sudden death similar to that of 1706 in Rome boosted the cult of Andrew Avellino. Giovan Battista Barzisa, a Theatine priest and writer, reported that in Naples, in 1733,

> on account of the occurrence of several sudden deaths, a public novena was held by his sacred sepulchre in the church of San Paolo Maggiore, to implore freedom from such evil from the holy patron saint. Public devotion was equalled by the private piety of many and many faithful who hold him to be the valid defender

---

50   I am quoting from the papal brief of 3 August 1763 included in the booklet *Obblighi de' fratelli e sorelle della Ven: archiconfraternita del divino amore di S. Gaetano e S. Andrea Avellino*, Rome, 1813, p. 11. The office of the saint was approved in 1719, and it was soon followed by a special liturgy, namely *S. Andreae Avellini clerici regularis a Sacra Rituum Congregatione approbatum: pro clericis regularibus sub ritu duplici secundae classis cum octava*, Rome, 1719; *Die 10 Novembris in festo s. Andreae Avellini clerici regularis*, Rome, 1725 (also published in Florence, Rennes, Antwerp and elsewhere); *Missa Sancti Andreae Avellini Confess. Sacerdot. Solemne die X. Novembris*, [Milan, 1730].

51   It would be impossible to list here all the devotions, triduums, novenas and spiritual exercises that were held in honour of St Andrew Avellino as protector from apoplexies and sudden death. Not surprisingly, devotional life followed the dissemination of the congregation of the Theatines in Italy and beyond. Confraternities entitled to St Andrew Avellino were founded in Bologna (1723), Florence (1760), Perugia (1776) and Ferrara (1788).

against apoplectic accidents and a mighty protector during agony, and thus beseech him with daily prayers and devout exercises.[52]

Elements of medical theory were merged into the religious discourse, making the physicians' learning complementary to the power of saints. As a matter of fact, in praying to the saints, writes another Theatine cleric, Gaetano Magenis, in 1740, 'we must resort to the ones who have most distinguished themselves in the type of grace we invoke them for', and this is the reason why a saint who died of apoplexy 'but without losing the use of reason' does protect us 'from sudden death, which *so many apoplectic accidents have by now made so familiar to us*'. Medical and moral arguments converge in making Andrew the saint

> to provide for apoplectic accidents, and assist those among his devotees whom, due to their natural temperament or the disorders of their lives, are prone to apoplexy. In life and after death, he is credited ... with performing so many miracles in this kind of affection: he preserved many lest they be overwhelmed; he cured others who were already affected by it; at least he gave them back the use of reason so to render them capable of receiving the sacraments, and well disposed for a good death.[53]

In the nineteenth century, Andrew Avellino became the object of a further deep and widespread popular devotion, which grew in parallel to the transformation of European cities into modern industrial centres. The related rise in the number of work and road accidents transfigured sudden death, which nonetheless was no less frightening in its industrial version than the sadly familiar apoplexy and syncope. Moreover, Andrew Avellino's worship was fostered by the Catholic Church as part of a new sentimental piety for the humble, in contrast to the increasingly secularised attitude towards death among the upper classes. The latter's impiety was actually often accused by ecclesiastics to be the ultimate cause of 'too frequent the terrible scourge of sudden deaths and apoplectic accidents'.[54] In the nineteenth-century Roman Catholic pastoral strategy, the neo-Tridentine call for a rigorous active penitential preparation for death was in fact abandoned in favour of a more benign attitude.[55] Believers were now invited to keep at bay the fears aroused by sudden death mainly by means of their prayers

---

52   Barzisa, *Le azioni,* p. 209.

53   Magenis, *Vita di s. Andrea Avellino,* pp. 265–6, my italics.

54   *Pagella di aggregazione alla pia opera della devozione al glorioso s. Andrea Avellino,* Rome, 1869, p. 5. See also V. Paglia, 'Le confraternite e i problemi della morte a Roma nel Sei–Settecento', *Ricerche per la storia religiosa di Roma,* 5, 1984, pp. 197–220.

55   M. Vovelle, *La mort et l'Occident de 1300 à nos jours,* Paris, 1983, pp. 548–54, points out that nineteenth-century religion of death witnessed, among other things, the primacy of extreme unction over communion, contrary to the neo-Tridentine pastoral strategy with

to the apoplectic saint Avellino: may he preserve any good Catholic from an evil 'so dangerous and frequent', like unexpected death, gain them 'at least the time to receive the most holy sacraments, and to die in the grace of God', and, whatever the circumstances were, assist them 'at the awful time' of death.[56]

which St Andrew was originally associated; devotion to Andrew Avellino nevertheless remained very popular.

[56] Quotations are taken from the prayer booklet *Divoto esercizio in onore del glorioso sant'Andrea Avellino special protettore contro gli accidenti apoplettici e morte improvvisa*, Rome, 1835.

Epilogue
Was there Ever a Sudden Death 'Epidemic' in Rome?

So far, I have argued that Lancisi and his *De subitaneis mortibus* of 1707 marked a significant step in conceptualising and investigating sudden death. In the eighteenth century, sudden death became a full-fledged topic in medical science, as did death in general. One question remains, though: was there ever a sudden death epidemic in Rome?

Lancisi refuted the claim, and research on the available archival sources seems to support his conclusion. The *libri dei morti* (registers of deceased patients) at the hospital of Consolazione, for instance, report a slight increase in the number of deaths, but no strange occurrence is ever mentioned (Table 1). The commonest registered causes of death are wounds (the hospital specialised in surgery) and fevers, as was usual.[1]

Table 1   Number of deceased patients at the hospital of Consolazione, 1706–1711

Year	Deaths recorded (sample)
1706	35
1707	31
1708	25
1709	26
1710	26
1711	16

The years 1705 and 1706 were relatively quiet for the Confraternity of Orazione e morte, which since 1538 had carried out the charitable task of transferring sick labourers from the countryside to the city's hospitals, and of

---

[1]   Ms ASR, Ospedale della Consolazione, reg. 737, Libro dei morti 1706–15.

burying abandoned corpses. Only 11 and 13 burials respectively are recorded. Charitable burials rose to 17 in 1707, 23 in 1708 and 31 in 1709.[2] No unusual events emerge from the prison surgeon's reports either.[3] The parish registers indicate a regular, if static, population trend too, although they reveal the heavy toll of the 1709 flu epidemic (Table 2).[4]

Table 2   Births and deaths in Rome and Trastevere, 1705–1712

Year	Births (Rome)	Deaths (Rome)	Births (Trastevere)	Deaths (Trastevere)
1705	3979	3065	469	369
1706	4506	4176	381	324
1707	4248	3584	403	407
1708	3530	4812	422	445
1709	4396	6463	379	469
1710	4252	5127	390	504
1711	4252	5127	390	374
1712	4187	4855	359	341

On a closer look, however, these same sources reveal how the tragic events of 1706 induced a more acute perception of sudden death as a public health issue. It came to be of concern not only to physicians, but also to the ecclesiastical and secular governing elites, and to the population at large. Thus, for instance, in the books of the confraternity of Orazione e morte, the record of a first 'dead of sudden death' makes its appearance in April 1707, and is followed by other deadly 'accidents' and 'strokes' noted in subsequent years.[5]

Rome was not the only place where greater attention to the problem of unexpected death was given. In 1724, the health officials in Venice decided to

---

[2]   Data are excerpted from G. Rossi, *L'agro romano tra '500 e '800*, Rome, 1988, pp. 249–50. Charitable burials numbered 21 in 1703, and there were only 9 in 1704.

[3]   Ms ASR, Tribunale del Governatore, Relazioni del medico, reg. 125; Relazioni dei birri, reg. 121.

[4]   M. Cattaneo, *La sponda sbagliata del Tevere: mito e realtà di un'identità popolare tra antico regime e rivoluzione*, Naples, 2004, pp. 163–4, with the addition of further data communicated by Massimo Cattaneo, whom I thank.

[5]   Ms ASVR, Arciconfraternita S. Maria dell'orazione e morte, reg. 726, Libro dei morti 1700–1713, fol. 212. For a similar development in the French colonies, see Y. Landry and R. Lessard, 'Causes of Death in Seventeenth- and Eighteenth-Century Québec as Recorded in the Parish Registers', *Historical Methods*, 29, 1996, pp. 49–57.

collect all the reports of sudden deaths drawn up by physicians in the whole territory of the Venetian Republic. In 1729 they ordered that those who died in suspicious circumstances be subjected to a full autopsy, and archives of the autopsy reports be created for the purpose of study. In the same years, similar measures were taken in Milan, where a medical certificate was now required before allowing burial, and physicians were requested to pay particular attention in dissecting 'the dead from sudden accident'.[6] As the century advanced, while concerns were raised all over Europe about the pernicious influence of cemeteries on public health, an unprecedented emphasis was put on saving lives. Action was urged to prevent hasty burials of apparently dead persons – this extraordinarily powerful collective phobia that surged between the eighteenth and the nineteenth centuries[7] – and to assist endangered citizens. The first society for the rescue of drowned persons saw the light in Amsterdam in 1767, and similar institutions were then founded in Venice, London, Milan and Paris. In Rome, a few months before the invasion of the French Imperial troops in 1808, the Secretary of State, Cardinal Ercole Consalvi, who was the proponent of a moderate reformism, eventually drew the Protomedicate's attention to the abnormal frequency of lethal apoplexies and ordered that 'burial may not be effected unless dissection of the body is done in the presence of two doctors from the College of Physicians, so that they can make their physical observations, and examination'. A 'room for the dead' – that is, a morgue or *Leichenhaus* similar to those created in various European cities to ascertain death and perform autopsy before burial – was arranged in the deconsecrated church of San Lorenzo in Damaso.[8]

---

[6]   N. Filippini, *La nascita straordinaria: tra madre e figlio la rivoluzione del taglio cesareo*, Milan, 1995, p. 151; N. Vanzan Marchini, *I mali e i rimedi della Serenissima*, Vicenza, 1995, p. 111; M. Canella, 'La gestione della morte nel Milanese tra età moderna e contemporanea: l'intervento dello stato dall'indagine conoscitiva all'azione legislativa', in *Specchio della popolazione: la percezione dei fatti e problemi demografici nel passato*, ed. A. Menzione, Udine, 2003, pp. 55–80.

[7]   I. Stoessel, *Scheintod und Todesangst: Äusserungsformen der Angst in ihren geschichtlichen Wandlungen (17.–20. Jahrhundert)*, Cologne, 1983; C. Milanesi, *Morte apparente e morte intermedia: medicina e mentalità nel dibattito sull'incertezza dei segni della morte (1740–1789)*, Rome, 1989; J. Bourke, *Fear: A Cultural History*, London, 2005.

[8]   Ms ASR, Università di Roma, b. 59, fasc. 50. During the short-lived Roman Republic of 1798–99, the church of San Lorenzo in Damaso had been the home of the Legislative organ, the Tribunate, and was not reconsecrated until the papal Restoration in 1815. It should be noted that a new wave of sudden deaths apparently took place in 1772, and was the source of inspiration for Filippo Pirri's *Ragionamento al popolo ... sulle cagioni delle morti improvvise frequentemente accadute nel MDCCLXXII tra gli abitatori di Roma ed istruzioni per potersene garantire a tempo*, Rome, 1773. Notwithstanding the old-fashioned theories on apoplexy and vague aerism, Pirri's book includes instructions for first aid intervention, by then a popular topic in medical writings throughout Europe. On *Leichenhäuser*, see A. Josat, *De la mort et de ses caractères*, Paris, 1854.

In other words, the 'taming of death' by medicine was initiated in the eighteenth century both in theory and in practice, in terms of medical surveillance of the population from birth to death. Control over death was a substantial part of the new discourse on the authority of medical doctors and one foundation of the expanding social role of medicine in Enlightenment Europe, and eventually of nineteenth-century hygienism. My claim is that this development first began in the Rome of Clement XI, where the political circumstances and the social and intellectual context enhanced a new stance on death and on the corpse as an object of science, as well as a new medical interventionism vis-à-vis the dying. Modern natural philosophy and religious rigorism created the pre-conditions for medicine to take a fundamental step into the territory of death.

The 'taming of death', however, soon moved away from Rome to countries where Enlightenment reforms were being implemented. In the papal city, the alliance between doctors and the ecclesiastical monarchy shattered rather quickly, ostensibly because of the intrinsic impossibility of truly secularising the management of life and death. After Clement XI's initial openings, subsequent pontificates witnessed the waning of physicians' authority over the end of life, despite rather brief instances of collaboration. A clear signal was given as early as 1725, under Benedict XIII Orsini, when the Roman synod renewed the apostolic excommunication for physicians who visited patients who had not fulfilled their religious obligations, 'which in our time is often overlooked by doctors, whence many sick people die without receiving sacraments and even without the sacramental confession'.[9] Rather tellingly, in 1729 the confraternity of the Sacro Cuore di Gesù (Sacred Heart of Jesus) for protection from sudden death was instituted at the hospital of San Gallicano. This new hospital for skin diseases had just been built in the popular area of Trastevere with the bequest that Lancisi had made for a new female ward at the hospital of Santo Spirito. The brothers of the confraternity had the charitable task to serve the sick at the hospital and to

> wear a sack of raw canvas cloth tied with a rope around the waist, with a white wooden rosary of the Lord hanging by their left side; the head always covered and the feet bare in sandals, observing perpetual silence, [they have] the duty to pray for [protection against] apoplectic accidents and sudden deaths.[10]

Along with the apoplectic saint Andrew Avellino, the cult of the Sacred Heart was in fact to serve as a further antidote for the fear of sudden death. The

---

9   G. Catalani, *Rituale romanum Benedicti papae XIV jussu editum et auctum, perpetuis commentariis exornatum*, Padua, 1760, vol. 1, p. 347; L. Fiorani, *Il Concilio romano del 1725*, Rome, 1977, p. 251.

10   Ms ASVR, Confraternita del S. Cuore di Gesù in s. Teodoro, Atti 1729–1732, vol. 1, fols 2–3.

first associate of the new confraternity was unsurprisingly the French Jesuit Joseph Gallifet, who was the most tireless proponent of devotion to the Sacred Heart.[11] Benedict XIV Lambertini followed similar policies. He promoted improvements in health care and burial practices, but it would be wrong to view these as enlightened innovations, since they followed the Church's agenda only, and merely updated and strengthened the political and religious trends which had emerged at the turn of the seventeenth and eighteenth centuries.[12] In this context, sudden death was prevalently dealt with as a religious issue, reviving the pastoral and charitable impetus with regard to the end of life.[13]

According to several historians, the second half of the eighteenth century witnessed a gradual easing of the ancient collective fear surrounding sudden death. This was no longer perceived as the ultimate bad death, but on the contrary as a rather convenient way to leave earthly existence, avoiding the pain and discomfort of agony. What was once considered in Christian ethics as the supreme moment of any person of faith to fight against evil was now seen as an inconvenience to escape.[14]

In truth, the religious attitude towards sudden death was evolving too. Indeed, in the course of the eighteenth century the fears that had surrounded swift and unexpected passing for century past seemingly subsided. For Catholics there was now some hope that physicians and priests would do their best to

---

[11]   V. Paglia, 'Le confraternite e i problemi della morte a Roma nel Sei-Settecento', *Ricerche per la storia religiosa di Roma*, 5, 1984, pp. 197–220, esp. pp. 214–18. On Gallifet, see D. Menozzi, *Sacro cuore: un culto tra devozione interiore e restaurazione cristiana della società*, Rome, 2001, pp. 28–44.

[12]   Benedict XIV had, for instance, a new cemetery and an anatomical theatre built at Santo Spirito hospital, where medical assistance was also improved. However, he dissolved the perpetual magistrate of the College of Physicians, which had made an essential contribution to the affirmation of a greater public role of physicians in Rome.

[13]   With the bull *Pia mater Catholica ecclesia* of 5 April 1747 (now in *Sanctissimi Domini nostri Benedicti Papae XIV Bullarium*, vol. 5, Mechelen, 1827, pp. 204–21), Benedict XIV put order into the bishops' prerogatives regarding blessing and indulgences for the dying, allowing a more benevolent approach. In the same period and at the pope's behest, parish priests were invited to specify the circumstances of their parishioners' deaths in the parish books, noting whether they had been 'natural, violent, unexpected or sudden'; see Catalani, *Rituale Romanum Benedicti papae XIV*, vol. 2, p. 356.

[14]   R. Favre, *La mort dans la littérature et la pensée française au siècle des Lumières*, Lyon, 1978, pp. 99–103; L.M. Beier, 'The Good Death in Seventeenth-Century England', in *Death, Ritual and Bereavement*, ed. R. Houlbrooke, London, 1989, pp. 43–61; P. Vecchi, *Salute, morte e compensazione nel Settecento francese*, Pisa 1990; R. Houlbrooke, 'The Age of Decency: 1660–1760', in *Death in England*, ed. P. Jupp and C. Gittings, Manchester, 2000, pp. 174–201; M. Sozzi, 'Il medico contro la morte: l'Encyclopédie e la concezione illuministica del morire nella seconda metà del XVIII secolo', in *Il medico di fronte alla morte (secoli XVI–XXI)*, ed. G. Cosmacini and G. Vigarello, Turin, 2008, pp. 79–109.

intervene quickly and save their souls in case of accidents. There was, above all, the consolation of spiritual clemency on the deathbed. A reaction emerged against the traditional pastoral care of the dying focused on terror, in which sudden death had played a prominent role.[15] A more benign attitude towards the dying came to the fore, which softened the severity of contritionist theology and rigorist morals in the end-of-life sacramental practice and piety. In a way, the canonisation of Andrew Avellino had already pointed in this direction, and late eighteenth-century Catholicism followed it.

By then, the Enlightenment had done the rest in changing collective attitudes. The general secularisation of the attitude towards life and death transformed the perception of sudden death as well. This new sensibility, reminiscent of Epicurean ideas, was encapsulated in the article *Mort – histoire naturelle de l'homme* that the Chevalier de Jaucourt wrote for Diderot and d'Alembert's *Encyclopédie*. The fear of death is presented as a cultural and religious artefact, since death is nothing but an imperceptible step:

> We stop living by imperceptible degrees. The exhaustion of our forces annihilates all senses and excites in us only vague sensation, like we feel when we give ourselves up to dreaming ... and the decisive moment comes without our suspecting it and without our thinking about it.

Death, he continues, whether natural or caused by disease, is painless, except for some acute affections triggering convulsions. The lack of awareness of the approaching end thus takes on a positive connotation. Furthermore, as physicians were now expected to assist their patients until the very end, de Jaucourt also criticises practitioners who 'after having pronounced a death sentence, relinquish the victims to their pain, to priests and to the wails of their family'.[16]

Hence, the wise man ought not to think about death, nor should he take special dispositions for the eventuality of a swift and unexpected demise, which might, in fact, be the best way to end one's days. According to Menuret de Chambaut, who wrote the medical section of the entry *Mort*:

> Sudden death is an abrupt cessation of the vital motions, without any considerable external change; it is a swift transition, often without any apparent cause, from the most florid exercise of all functions to utter inaction. We stop living at the

---

15   D. Roche, 'La mémoire de la mort', *Annales ESC*, 31, 1976, pp. 76–119; J. McManners, *Death and the Enlightenment: Changing Attitudes to Death Among Christians and Unbelievers in Eighteenth-Century France*, Oxford, 1981, p. 201. A new sensibility also emerged among English Puritans, as attested by the beautiful sermon by B. Grosvenor, *Observations on Sudden Death, Occasioned by the Late Frequent Instances of it, Both in City and Country*, London, 1720.

16   *Encyclopédie*, Neuchâtel edn, vol. 10, 1765, pp. 716–18.

moment in which health seems best assured and danger most remote, in the midst of games, at banquets, at revelries, or in the arms of a gentle, quiet sleep. This is what made ancient philosophers wish to die in this way ... It is the least unpleasant death, averting suffering ... that does not allow time to fall into that terrible sense of annihilation, that despondency which is often unseemly for a philosopher ... One has no time to regret life.

Moreover, Menuret de Chambaut continues, given the distinction between imperfect and absolute death, sudden death allows some hope for resuscitation. True, 'the time that elapses from imperfect death to absolute death is undetermined', but for those who die a sudden or violent death, the interval is commonly longer, as demonstrated by cases of people who 'by means of appropriate rescue measures, or by themselves, have returned to life'.[17] The prospect of a return to life of those unfortunate ones struck by sudden diseases or accidents was at that time trivialised in medical discourse and philanthropic literature, and indeed constituted a powerful argument for supporting the dissemination of rescue societies in major European cities.[18]

Are we to conclude that by the end of the eighteenth century sudden death had turned from a terrifying eventuality into the ideal good death, unburdened of its most terrible physical and spiritual implications and mitigated by the hope of a return to life thanks to the doctor's intervention? Not really. The Enlightenment ideal of the good death was in fact a peaceful end, awaited in full consciousness until the moment when the dying slipped into eternal sleep, without pain, assisted by the physician and loved ones.[19] It was an ideal that did not in fact differ much from the Christian narrative of a serene passing, trusting in God's mercy and comforted by the sacraments and the prayers of priest and family. For Enlightenment unbelievers and the Catholic devout alike, albeit for different reasons, sudden death was now rather an event to be actively fought. In any case, doctors were now trusted to prevent it, to try and reverse it and, ultimately, to explain and make it acceptable.

---

[17] Ibid., pp. 718–19.

[18] W. Whiter, *A Dissertation on the Disorder of Death; or That State of the Frame Under the Signs of Death Called Suspended Animation, to Which Remedies Have Been Sometimes Successfully Applied*, Norwich and London, 1819.

[19] D. Porter and R. Porter, *Patient's Progress: Doctors and Doctoring in Eighteenth-Century England*, Cambridge, 1998; A. Carol, *Les médecins et la mort: XIXe–XXe siècles*, Paris, 2004; S. Lauter, *Geschichten vom Tod: Tod und Sterben in Deutschschweizer und oberdeutschen Selbstzeugnissen des 16. und 17. Jahrhunderts*, Basel, 2007, pp. 91–8.

Index